Hot Topics in
Urology

This h

Commissioning Editor: Rebecca Schmidt
Project Development Manager: Joanne Scott
Project Manager: Rory MacDonald
Illustration Manager: Bruce Hogarth
Designer: Andy Chapman
Illustrator: Robert Britton

Hot Topics in Urology

Edited by

Roger S Kirby MA MD FRCS(UROL) FEBU
Professor of Urology
St George's Hospital
London, UK

Michael P O'Leary MD MPH
Associate Professor of Surgery
Harvard Medical School
Senior Surgeon, Division of Urology
Brigham and Women's Hospital
Boston, MA, USA

SAUNDERS

Edinburgh • London • New York • Oxford • Philadelphia • St Louis • Sydney • Toronto • 2004

SAUNDERS
An imprint of Elsevier Limited

First published 2004

ISBN 0-7020-2674-3

British Library Cataloguing in Publication Data
A catalogue record for this book is available from the British Library

Library of Congress Cataloging in Publication Data
A catalog record for this book is available from the Library of Congress

Notice
Medical knowledge is constantly changing. Standard safety precautions must be followed, but as new research and clinical experience broaden our knowledge, changes in treatment and drug therapy may become necessary or appropriate. Readers are advised to check the most current product information provided by the manufacturer of each drug to be administered to verify the recommended dose, the method and duration of administration, and contraindications. It is the responsibility of the practitioner, relying on experience and knowledge of the patient, to determine dosages and the best treatment for each individual patient. Neither the publisher nor the editors assume any liability for any injury and/or damage to persons or property arising from this publication.

Printed in China

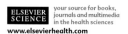
your source for books, journals and multimedia in the health sciences
www.elsevierhealth.com

The Publisher's policy is to use paper manufactured from sustainable forests

Contents

Contributors

Gregory S Adey MD
Clinical Fellow in Surgery, Harvard
Medical School
Brigham and Women's Hospital
Harvard Medical School
Boston, MA, USA

Christopher Anderson MBChB FCS(Urol) SA
Consultant Urologist
Department of Urology
St George's Hospital
London, UK

Daniela E Andrich MD MSc MRCS
Professor of Urology
Institute of Urology and Nephrology
University College London Medical
School
London, UK

Kenneth Anson MS FRCS(Urol)
Consultant Urological Surgeon
Department of Urology
St George's Hospital
London, UK

Simon RJ Bott FRCS
Urology and Nephrology Research
Fellow
The Institute of Urology
London, UK

Culley C Carson MD
Professor and Chief in Urology
Division of Urology
University of North Carolina
Chapel Hill, NC, USA

Xavier Cathelineau MD
Professor of Urology and Head of
Department
Department of Urology
Institut Mutualiste Montsouris
Paris, France

Jonathan P Coxon MA MRCS
Research Fellow in Urology
Department of Urology
St George's Hospital
London, UK

Jeremy Crew MA MD FRCS(Urol)
Consultant Urological Surgeon
Urology Department
The Churchill Hospital
Oxford, UK

Ara Darzi MD FRCS FRCSI FRC PSG
Professor of Surgery
Academic Surgical Unit
Imperial College School of Medicine
London, UK

John M Fitzpatrick MCh FRCSI FCUrol(SA) FRCS(Glas) FRCS
Professor of Surgery
Department of Surgery
Mater Hospital
University College Dublin
Dublin, Ireland

Charlotte L Foley MRCS
Urology and Nephrology Research
Fellow
The Institute of Urology
London, UK

Michael Froehner MD
Fellow in Urology
Department of Urology
University Hospital Carl Gustav Carus
Dresden, Germany

Martin E Gleave MD FRCSC FACS
Professor of Surgery, University of
British Columbia,
Director of Clinical Research, The
Prostate Center at VGH
Division of Urology
Vancouver General Hospital
Vancouver, Canada

Irwin Goldstein MD
Professor
Department of Urology
Boston University School of Medicine
Boston, MA, USA

Rebecca Greenhalgh MBBS AFRCSI
Urology Research Fellow
Department of Urology Research
St George's Hospital
London, UK

Oliver W Hakenberg MD PhD FEBU
Senior Staff Urologist, Urology
Surgeon
Department of Urology
University Hospital Carl Gustav Carus
Dresden, Germany

Erik Havranek BSc MBBS MCRS(Eng)
Research Fellow in Urology
Department of Urology Research
St George's Hospital
London, UK

Graham Jackson FRCP FESC FACC FAHA
Consultant Cardiologist
Cardiothoracic Department
St Thomas' Hospital
London, UK

Burkhard Jansen MD
Vice President, Clinical Development
OncoGenex Technologies
Adjunct Professor
Department of Surgery
University of British Columbia
Vancouver, Canada

Noel N Kim PhD
Research Assistant Professor in
Urology
Department of Urology
Boston University School of Medicine
Boston, MA, USA

Michael G Kirby MBBS LRCP MRCS FRCP
Director of the Hertfordshire Primary
Care Research Network
Letchworth, UK

Roger S Kirby MA MD FRCS(Urol) FEBU
Professor of Urology
St George's Hospital
London, UK

Chryssanthos Kouriefs MBChB(hon) MRCS Eng
Specialist Registrar in Urology
St George's Hospital
London, UK

Shirley Mak MBChB MRCS
Urology Research Registrar
Urology Research Centre
St George's Hospital Medical School
London, UK

Hideaki Miyaki MD PhD
Head, Department of Urology
Hyogo Medical Centre for Adults
Akashi, Japan

Colm Morrissey PhD
Postdoctoral Fellow
Department of Surgery, Mater
Misericordiae University Hospital
Conway Institute of Biomolecular and
Biomedical Research
University College Dublin
Dublin, Ireland

Ricardo M Munarriz MD
Assistant Professor of Urology
Department of Urology
Boston University School of Medicine
Boston, MA, USA

**Anthony R Mundy MS FRCP
FRCS**
Professor of Urology
Institute of Urology and Nephrology
University College London Medical
School
London, UK

Michael P O'Leary MD MPH
Associate Professor of Surgery
Harvard Medical School
Senior Surgeon, Division of Urology
Brigham and Women's Hospital
Boston, MA, USA

**Grenville M Oades BSc(Hons)
MRCS**
Research Fellow in Urology
Department of Urology
St George's Hospital
London, UK

Uday Patel MRCP FRCR
Consultant Radiologist
Department of Radiology
St George's Hospital
London, UK

Sophie H Pattison BSc, MBChB
Patient Safety Training Facilitator
Postgraduate Medical Centre
St George's Hospital
London, UK

Rachel N Pauls MD
Fellow in Urogynecology
Good Samaritan Hospital
Cincinnati, OH, USA

Matthew Perry MD BSc FRCS
Specialist Registrar in Urology
Department of Urology Research
St George's Hospital
London, UK

Wade J Sexton MD Maj USAF MC
Staff Urologist
Division of Urology
Willford Hall Medical Center
Lackland, TX, USA

**Jyoti Shah BSc MD MRCS
DHMSA**
Specialist Registrar in Urology
Department of Surgery, Academic
Surgical Unit
Imperial College of Medicine
St Mary's Hospital
London, UK

Graeme S Steele MD FCS
Assistant Professor
Brigham and Women's Hospital
Boston, MA, USA

Peter K Stevenson BA(Hons)
Chief Instructor in Human Factors
Training
MyTravel Airways
Manchester, UK

**Edward Streeter MA BM BCh
MRCS**
Research Fellow
Department of Urology
Churchill Hospital
Oxford, UK

Ian M Thompson MD
Professor and Chief - Division of
Urology
Division of Urology, Department of
Surgery
Health Sciences Center at San
Antonio
San Antonio, TX, USA

Abdul M Traish BSc MBA PhD
Professor of Biochemistry and
Urology
Center for Advanced Biomedical
Research
Boston University School of Medicine
Boston, MA, USA

Guy Vallancien MD
Professor of Urology
Department of Urology and
Nephrology
Institut Mutualiste Montsouris
Paris, France

**Nicholas A Watkin MA MChir
FRCS(Urol)**
Consultant Urological Surgeon
Department of Urology
St George's Hospital
London, UK

R William G Watson BSc PhD
College Lecturer – Director of the
Surgical Research Laboratory
Department of Surgery, Mater
Misericordiae University Hospital
Conway Institute of Biomolecular and
Biomedical Research
University College Dublin
Dublin, Ireland

Manfred P Wirth MD
Professor of Urology
Department of Urology
University Hospital Carl Gustar Carus
Dresden, Germany

Foreword

What a unique idea – devoting a monograph to new and innovative developments in the field of urology, for urology has always been a specialty that prided itself in pioneering advances in medical therapy, surgical procedures and technology. Many of these developments have not only expanded and refined the practice of urology but have also impacted on the advances in other specialties as well. For example, urologists were the initial endoscopists and as the practice expanded from the bladder to the ureter and kidney, these basic techniques were also utilized in many other medical and surgical specialties including gastroenterology, gynecology and general surgery. Innovative surgical procedures such as urinary diversion have led to expanded utilization of bowel or other non-urinary tissue in such diverse areas as bladder augmentation and replacement and urethral reconstruction.

Roger Kirby and Michael O'Leary, the editors of *Hot Topics in Urology*, have brought together experts on both sides of the Atlantic and called upon them to detail their thoughts and experiences in varied but important areas including sexual dysfunction, oncology, voiding dysfunction, genitourinary reconstruction and imaging. The topics are not only new but practical and pertinent to clinical practice. New and evolving surgical procedures are reviewed as are the use of additional or adjuvant treatments to help improve operative approaches. When appropriate, many chapters draw upon basic research advances that have led to the development and implementation of improvements in clinical care. Very appropriately, an important chapter is directed at reducing medical errors in urology.

There is no doubt that this text will be used by many urologists and the material in it will benefit many of the patients under their care. One can only look forward to Hot Topics 2 which will most certainly be needed in the ever evolving and innovative field of urology.

Martin I Resnick MD
Lester Persky Professor of Urology
Chairman, Department of Urology
Case Western Reserve University
Cleveland, Ohio

Preface

Urologists are busy people, but the nature of our work makes it imperative that we stay absolutely up to date. Patients increasingly arrive armed with a sheaf of internet printouts relating to their particular problem. If their doctor is not up to speed on the latest "hot topic" their confidence quickly disappears and they soon look elsewhere for advice. But which of us has time to plough through all the urological journals or to read all four volumes of Campbell's Urology, worthy though they undoubtedly are?

With these thoughts in mind we asked some of the key movers and shakers in urology in both Europe and the US to write an up-to-the-minute overview of their own favourite hot topic. The result is a compilation of 21 excellent chapters covering some of the most controversial areas in contemporary urology. Male and female sexual dysfunction, benign and malignant prostate disease, the overactive bladder, renal and penile cancer, upper tract imaging and the state of the art for urethral stricture surgery are all elegantly reviewed here. The ensemble is rounded off with a highly topical chapter on error reduction in urology.

We hope that this book not only captures the flavour of excitement that characterises modern urology but also predicts some key future advances. It can be read during one trans-Atlantic flight, so sit back, relax and read on.

Roger Kirby and Michael O'Leary
June 2003

1

Premature ejaculation
Michael P O'Leary

Introduction

Since the introduction of pharmacotherapy for the treatment of erectile dysfunction, men with sexual disorders have become less reluctant to discuss their problems with health care providers. Nevertheless, ejaculatory disturbances, and early ejaculation (PE) in particular are still likely under-reported. The uncertainty regarding the prevalence of the condition along with an unclear definition and confusing data about etiology and efficacy of therapy, much of which is published in other than the urologic literature, combine to make this a difficult topic even for the expert in sexual dysfunction, let alone the practicing urologist. This chapter attempts to summarize what is currently known about this very common condition and focuses on a practical approach to management.

Physiology of ejaculation

Efferent sympathetic nerves arise from spinal segments at T10–L2 to form the lumbar sympathetic ganglia which encircle the aorta and coalesce in the midline as the hypogastric plexus just below the aortic bifurcation. This gives rise to hypogastric nerves which course through the pelvis and terminate as postganglionic fibers at the bladder neck, seminal vesicles, vasa and prostate. With acetylcholine as the neurotransmitter, sympathetic flow stimulates contraction in these structures, while somatic stimulation of the bulbo and ischio-cavernous muscles in this area is under the influence of the pudendal nerve. Supraspinal control of this process is less well understood although the medial preoptic area as well as the locus ceruleus appear to be important cortical centers.

Prevalence

It is unclear how many men have PE. In fact, there is no clear consensus on the definition, although the American Psychiatric Association's *Diagnostic and Statistical Manual IV*[1] (DSM-IV) categories have become widely accepted:

1. Persistent or recurrent ejaculation with minimal stimulation before, on, or shortly after penetration and before the person wishes it. The clinician must take into account the factors that affect duration of the excitement phase, such as age, novelty of the sexual partner or situation and recent frequency of sexual activity.
2. The disturbance causes marked distress or interpersonal difficulty.
3. The PE is not due exclusively to the direct effects of a substance (e.g. withdrawal from opioids).

The DSM-IV definition is purposefully broad, but recent studies give some indication of what should be considered normal versus early ejaculation. Rowland and colleagues evaluated 26 men with PE and compared them with 13 age-matched, sexually functional men on ejaculatory response during coitus and masturbation.[2] Mean ejaculatory latency during vaginal penetrative sex was 1.5 min in the PE group and 5.6 min in controls. Interestingly ejaculation during masturbation yielded different results. PE men had similar latency times to normals (n = 4.5 min). Further-more, the frequency of reported sexual activity (intercourse or masturbation) was similar in both groups, questioning a long-held theory to explain PE, namely that it results from long intervals between attempts to ejaculate or fewer opportunities to learn control.

Another important definitional distinction may be subtypes of PE. Is it a lifelong or acquired problem ('global' vs 'situational')? These distinctions may not be important to a urologist but can have implications for psychological counseling, or during experimental investigation. Time to ejaculation (measured from beginning of stimulation – usually vaginal intromission) is generally the metric reported in most PE studies.[3] Other continuous variables have also been reported (e.g. number of intravaginal thrusts). All are at best subjective, and reproducibility for investigational purposes is problematic. We have recently developed a mechanical device in an effort to achieve more reproducible stimulation, especially for use in trials of pharmacologic agents. Most studies rely on the male study subject using a stopwatch and recording the time from intromission to ejaculation. The reproducibility of this form of measurement is questionable. Our device applies continuous vibratory stimulation to the penis and ejaculatory latency times have been reproducible in both normal subjects as well as men with PE.[4]

More recently, we added a portable recorder to the device.[5] Within the device, an indium–gallium-filled stretch transducer is placed around the shaft of the penis, measuring sustained changes in penile tone (i.e. tumescence) and pulsatile responses (i.e. ejaculation) (Fig. 1.1). The device is connected to a laptop computer.

The small loop in the center foreground is placed around the base of the penis. Recording is via an indium–gallium-filled stretch transducer. The data are downloaded into the laptop. The stimulation parameter, time to erection, and ejaculatory latency are all recorded automatically and can be subsequently downloaded for data analysis. This device should facilitate studies of PE in men and be particularly useful in clinical trials of interventions.

Epidemiology

Community-based studies of the prevalence of PE range from 4%[6] to as high as 29%.[7] Studies from primary care settings suggest that PE is more

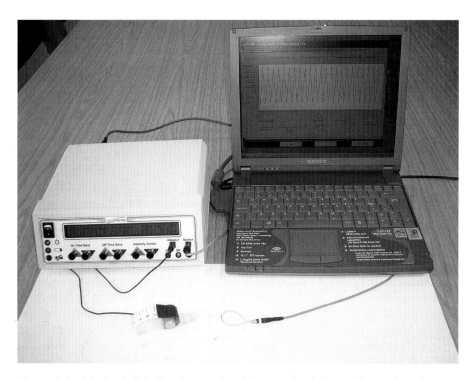

Figure 1.1 Mechanical device that applies vibratory stimulation to the penis and measures ejaculatory latency times via an indium–gallium-filled stretch transducer.

prevalent with estimates from 31% in the US[8] to as high as 66% in Germany.[9] Curiously, somewhat lower estimates are reported from sexual dysfunction clinics, with ranges around 20–25%.[10] Nevertheless, PE is a common condition, and likely more prevalent than has been reported.

Etiology

What causes men to ejaculate before they or their partner desire? Until recently, the answer to this question was thought to be largely behavioral. Recently however, investigators have questioned whether local penile response may be altered in men with PE. Xin and colleagues investigated penile sensory levels using biothesiometry in men with PE and compared them to normals. In normal men, biothesiometric measurements of vibratory threshold increased with age, but were significantly decreased ($p < 0.001$) without age dependency in men with PE.[11]

In follow-up studies, this group further examined penile hypersensitivity by evaluating somatosensory-evoked potentials in men with PE and normals.[12] Mean latency of dorsal nerve and glans penis somatosensory-evoked potentials was 1.51 and 6.80 msec shorter, respectively, in PE men than in controls. Xin et al thus concluded that PE men have greater cortical representation of sensory stimuli from the glans penis, which facilitates rapid ejaculation. Other investigators, however, have not been able to show penile hypersensitivity in men with PE and suggest that other somatic or cognitive factors may be responsible.[13] For example, certain behavioral characteristics may predispose to PE such as early sexual experiences that promote rapid ejaculation (e.g. fear of being 'caught' or sex with a prostitute).

Therapy

In the past, most treatments for PE were behavioral. In 1956, Semans[14] described the pause technique. Masters and Johnson[15] modified this to the 'pause/squeeze' technique in 1970. Subjects are counseled to stop penile stimulation at the 'moment of inevitability',[16] defined as a period immediately prior to ejaculation when cessation of stimulation can postpone orgasm. Subjects are instructed to squeeze the penis forcibly momentarily then resume stimulation. This process, when repeated, is thought to train the individual to recognize the premonitory sensation immediately preceding ejaculation and learn better control. As late as the early 1990s this was still felt to be the 'current treatment of choice for this disorder',[17] at least in the psychiatric literature. However, as early as 1980 pharmacologic therapy was proposed as possibly efficacious.

Pharmacologic therapy (see Table 1.1)

Clomipramine was one of the first pharmacologic agents evaluated in the treatment of PE. Goodman found it to be superior to placebo.[18] In 1984 the beta-blocker propranolol was evaluated in 12 men by Cooper and Magnus.[19] No improvement in time to ejaculation was noted. Beretta et al[20] evaluated phenoxybenzamine, a non-specific alpha-adrenergic antagonist in 15 men, 8 of whom reported improvement. 'Dry ejaculation' was noted as a side effect of treatment. This most probably describes retrograde ejaculation as a consequence of bladder neck relaxation, although phenoxybenzamine and other alpha-blockers may also affect seminal emission and/or vasal smooth muscle contraction. No subsequent reports have advocated the use of alpha-blockers for PE.

Table 1.1 Pharmacologic treatment for premature ejaculation

Agent	Reported benefit	Reference
Clomipramine	Superior to placebo	Goodman[18]; Abdel-Hamid et al[23]
Propranolol	No efficacy	Cooper & Magnus[19]
Phenoxybenzamine	Minor benefit	Beretta et al[20]
Paroxetine	Superior to placebo	McMahon & Touma[21]; Abdel-Hamid et al[23]
Sertraline	Superior to placebo	Kim & Paick[22]; Abdel-Hamid et al[23]
Sildenafil	Superior to placebo	Abdel-Hamid et al[23]

McMahon and Touma reported two single-blind, placebo-controlled, crossover studies of 26 and 42 men with PE.[21] Using paroxetine, mean pretreatment ejaculatory latency time was less than 30 sec for both studies. In the first study either paroxetine, 20 mg or placebo was taken 3–4 hours prior to intercourse. Crossover was performed after 4 weeks of treatment plus an additional 3 weeks drug-free washout period. At 4 weeks, mean ejaculatory latency was 3.2 min in the paroxetine group and 0.45 min in the placebo group (p < 0.001). There were no adverse events reported. In the second study, 10 mg of paroxetine or placebo was given daily for 2 weeks followed by 20 mg or placebo as needed 3–4 hours prior to intercourse. Mean ejaculatory latency time was 4.3 min in the paroxetine daily and 5.8 min in the as-needed phases versus 0.9 min and 0.6 min in the placebo arm (p < 0.001). Adverse events were reported in 17% (anejaculation in 3/42, anorexia 1/42, gastric upset 3/42, reduced libido 2/42). These authors conclude that paroxetine is effective in treating PE. The study further suggests that better ejaculatory control is achieved by treating daily for a short period (2 weeks) followed by 'as-needed' (prn) use.

Another selective serotonin reuptake inhibitor (SSRI), sertraline, has also been studied with both daily and prn use. Kim and Paick[22] reported increased ejaculatory latency times from 23 ± 19 sec prior to treatment to 5.9 ± 4.2 min using 50 mg sertraline daily. Similar results were achieved when 50 or 100 mg sertraline was used on a prn basis. Peak plasma levels are achieved at 4–8 hours so these authors recommend taking the drug at 5 p.m. in the evening of expected intercourse.

Abdel-Hamid et al[23] compared an SSRI (clomipramine, sertraline and paroxetine), sildenafil, and the pause/squeeze technique in a prospective randomized, double-blind, crossover study that was not placebo controlled. A total of 31 men with PE were randomized into a 4-week treatment arm of one of these five treatment modalities. At the end of the study period all subjects noted a significant improvement over baseline. Clomipramine, sertraline and paroxetine were all superior to the pause/squeeze technique. Interestingly, sildenafil was superior to all other treatments in prolonging ejaculatory latency time. The mechanism for this is unclear, although reduced performance anxiety, more prolonged erection, or some central effects involving increased c-GMP activity are possible explanations.

Topical and herbal agents

Large varieties of over-the-counter prescriptions are available for the treatment of PE which range from oral herbal remedies to creams and other topical applications. One Internet search revealed products such as 'Indian God Lotion', 'Kwang's Solution', 'Stud 100' and 'Ironwood', the precise contents of which are unknown. There are of course few studies on such remedies. However, Choi et al[24] investigated a topical agent comprised of Ginseng Redix Alba, Angelicae Gigantic Radix, Cistancis Herba, Zanthoxylli Fructs, Torlidis Semen, Asiasari Radix, Caryophylli Flos, Cinnamon Cortex, and Bufonis Veneum which had been previously shown to increase penile vibratory threshold, prolong ejaculatory latency and reduce the amplitude of penile somatosensory-evoked potentials.[25] A randomized, double-blind, placebo-controlled trial was conducted on 106 men who were instructed to apply the cream to the glans penis 1 hour prior to intercourse. Mean ejaculatory latency time was prolonged from 1.37 ± 0.12 min to 10.92 ± 0.95 min in the treatment group vs 2.45 ± 0.29 min in the placebo group. Mild local burning was reported in 18%, while no partner effects were observed. SS cream was developed in Korea and is not commercially available in the US.

Conclusion

Of all male sexual dysfunctions, premature ejaculation is perhaps the most prevalent as it occurs to most men at some point in their sexual lives. A precise definition is still problematic, although most studies seem to agree that an ejaculatory latency time of less than 1–2 min is bothersome enough to most men to consider seeking treatment. Such treatment now consists principally of oral medication – namely SSRIs, although phosphodiesterase inhibitors such as sildenafil show promise. None of these drugs has label approval for the treatment of PE at this time, but as our understanding of the prevalence of this very common condition improves, we can expect the market basket of potentially effective products to increase dramatically.

References

1. American Psychiatric Association. Diagnostic and statistical manual of mental disorders, 4th edn. Washington DC: ASA; 1987.
2. Rowland DL, Strassberg DS, de Gouveia Brazao CA, Slob KA. Ejaculatory latency and control in men with premature ejaculation: an analysis across sexual activities using multiple sources of information. J Psychosom Reg 2000; 48:69–77.
3. Rowland DL, Cooper SE, Schneider M. Defining premature ejaculation for experimental and clinical investigators. Arch Sex Behav 2001; 30(3):235–253.
4. O'Leary M, Wylie M. Assessing ejaculatory latency in normals and in men with early ejaculation. Use of a new automated device. J Urol 2001; 165:1105A.
5. Dinsmore W, O'Leary M, Ralph D, Wyllie M. Automated recording of ejaculatory latency in an office or 'at home' setting. J Urol 2002; 167:Abstract 640.
6. Fugl-Meyer AR, Sjogren Fugl-Meyer K. Sexual disabilities, problems, and satisfaction in 18–74 years old Swedes. Scand J Sexol 1999; 3:79–105.
7. Laumann EO, Paik A, Rosen RC. Sexual dysfunction in the United States. JAMA 1999; 281:537–544.
8. Read S, King M, Watson J. Sexual dysfunction in primary medical care: prevalence, characteristics and detection by the general practitioner. J Pub Health Med 1997; 19:387–391.
9. Aschka C, Himmel W, Ittner E, Kochen M. Sexual problems of male patients in family practice. J Fam Pract 2001; 50:773–778.
10. Goldmeier D, Keane FE, Carter P, et al. Prevalence of sexual dysfunction in heterosexual patients attending a Central London genitourinary medicine clinic. Int J STD AIDS 1997; 8:303–306.
11. Xin ZC, Chung WS, Choi YD, et al. Penile sensitivity in patients with primary premature ejaculation. J Urol 1996; 156:979–981.
12. Xin ZC, Choi YD, Alra KH, Choi HK. Somatosensory evoked potentials in patients with primary premature ejaculation. J Urol 1997; 158:451–455.
13. Rowland DL, Haensel SM, Blom JHM, Slob AK. Penile sensitivity in men with premature ejaculation and erectile dysfunction. J Sex Marital Ther 1993; 19:189–197.
14. Semans JH. Premature ejaculation: a new approach. South Med J 1956; 49:353–357.
15. Masters WH, Johnson VE. Human sexual response. Boston: Little Brown; 1970.
16. Westheimer RK. Encyclopedia of sex. New York: Continuum; 2002.
17. St Lawrence JS, Madakasira S. Evaluation and treatment of premature ejaculation: a critical review. Int J Psychiatry Med 1992; 22(1):77–97.
18. Goodman RE. An assessment of clomipramine in the treatment of premature ejaculation. J Int Med Res 1980; 8(suppl 3):53–59.
19. Cooper AJ, Magnus RV. A clinical trial of the beta blocker propranolol in premature ejaculation. J Psychosom Res 1984; 28(4):331–336.
20. Beretta G, Chelo E, Fanciullacci F, Zanollo A. Effect of an alpha-blocker agent (phenoxybenzamine) in the management of premature ejaculation. Acta Eur Fertil 1986; 17(1):43–45.
21. McMahon CG, Touma K. Treatment of premature ejaculation with paroxetine hydrochloride as needed: two, single blind placebo controlled crossover studies. J Urol 1990; 161:1826–1830.
22. Kim SW, Paick JS. Short-term analysis of the effects of as needed use of sertraline at 5pm for the treatment of premature ejaculation. Urology 1999; 54: 544–547.
23. Abdel-Hamid IA, El Naggar EA, El Gilany AH. Assessment of as needed use of pharmacotherapy and the pause/squeeze technique in premature ejaculation. Int J Impot Res 2001; 13:41–45.
24. Choi HK, Jung GW, Moon KH et al Clinical study of SS-cream in patients with lifelong premature ejaculation. Urology 2000; 55:257–261.
25. Xin ZC, Seong DH, Choi HK. A double blind clinical trial of SS cream on premature ejaculation. Int J Impot Res 1994; 6(suppl):D73.

2

New developments for the treatment of erectile dysfunction: present and future

Culley C Carson

Introduction

Over the last two decades, the physiology and molecular biology of erection and erectile dysfunction has been carefully studied and translational research has led not only to an elucidation of the physiology of erection, but also significant progress in the diagnosis and treatment of men with erectile dysfunction (ED). Basic science laboratory investigation has elucidated the anatomy, physiology and pharmacology of the corpus cavernosum as well as the neurophysiology and vascular physiology of erectile function. Similarly, the mechanism of erection and its dependence upon the neurogenic, arterial and venous systems to produce erectile rigidity continues to be studied. Further, the importance of androgen support of erectile function, both in the corpus cavernosum level and in the central nervous system is being studied both clinically and in the basic science laboratories. Investigations into smooth muscle physiology, endothelial cell function, central nervous system control with the identification of neurotransmitters such as nitric oxide (NO) and vasoactive intestinal polypeptide (VIP) in the corpus cavernosum have led to the design, development and use of specific pharmacologic agents to recreate the normal physiology of the corpus cavernosum and restore erectile function in men previously termed 'impotent'.

Prevalence of ED

ED is highly prevalent. The Massachusetts Male Aging Study (MMAS) has documented the high prevalence, which reaches 52% in men over age 40. This prevalence increases with age and exceeds 70% in men over age 65. Laumann et al[1] also examined sexual dysfunction prevalence in US men and women in a younger cohort of patients. Their results also support the high prevalence and suggest that the major complaint in younger men is ejaculatory disorders with > 30% complaining of premature ejaculation. Worldwide epidemiologic studies have confirmed the high prevalence rates in men of all ages (Table 2.1). Despite this high prevalence, less than 10% of men have received therapy for ED.

Molecular physiology of erection

Initial stimulation for erection is in the central nervous system via excitatory visual, tactile, psychologic or other stimuli. These cortical stimuli descend from the cerebral cortex to lower centers in the midbrain. Recent studies have documented the role of the nucleus paragigantocellularis (nPGi) in moderating excitatory and inhibitory stimuli from the midbrain to the descending tracts of the spinal cord. Dopaminergic centers in the midbrain – mainly the medial preoptic area (MPOA) and the paraventricular nucleus – are primarily responsible for these functions and their impulses are relayed through the locus ceruleus before entering the nPGi. Descending impulses are either

Table 2.1 Worldwide prevalence of erectile dysfunction

Population	Age (years)	Percentage
Cologne, Germany	30–80	19.2
Spain	25–70	18.9
Perth, Australia	40–69	33.9
Krimpen, Netherlands	50–78	11.0
London, UK	16–78	19.0

excitatory or inhibitory and stimulate the penile vascular structures through the non-adrenergic, non-cholinergic (NANC) nerves in the penis. These nerves are responsible for the production of nitric oxide (NO), which is the principal neurotransmitter controlling erectile function. This neurophysiology is increasingly important as newer agents are designed to stimulate central nervous system control of erectile and indeed sexual activity.

For an erection to occur from a vascular standpoint, the central cavernosal arteries of the corpora cavernosa must dilate to increase blood flow to the penis. This increased blood flow and the production of NO from nerve endings in the smooth muscles forming the lacunar spaces of the corpora cavernosa produces lacunar smooth muscle relaxation.[2] Once smooth muscle relaxation has occurred, blood flows rapidly into the lacunar spaces increasing the volume in the corpora. Subsequent compression and elongation of the subtunical veins draining the corpora cavernosa produce decreased venous outflow and increased intracorporeal pressure. Pressure in the corpora cavernosa is supplemented by contraction of the perineal muscles resulting in a high-pressure rigid erection satisfactory for sexual activity. On a subcellular level, control of smooth muscle activity is dependent upon intracellular calcium flux. Neurotransmitters and endothelium-derived factors influence the flow of intracellular calcium balancing penile flaccidity and rigidity.

The principal substance responsible for smooth muscle relaxation is the neurotransmitter nitric oxide (NO).[3] Nitric oxide is produced from the precursor L-arginine through the enzyme nitric oxide synthase (NOS). Nitric oxide subsequently diffuses into smooth muscle cells, activates the secondary neurotransmitter system guanylate cyclase, which converts guanosine triphosphate (GTP) into cyclic guanosine monophosphate (cGMP). This secondary neurotransmitter activates the intracellular sodium pump system, opening potassium channels and producing a decrease in intracellular potassium and calcium with resultant smooth muscle relaxation. cGMP is metabolized through enzymatic breakdown by phosphodiesterase type 5 (PDE-5), which results in closing of potassium channels, increased intracellular calcium and smooth muscle contraction[4] (Fig. 2.1).

Signal transduction pathways (Fig. 2.1a)

Nitric oxide (NO) is the first messenger in the cGMP pathway and probably the principal neurotransmitter mediating tumescence.[5] NO is a gas and diffuses directly into the smooth muscle cell. Here it attaches to the heme moiety of guanylate cyclase, stimulating it to generate cGMP, which in turn activates protein kinase G (PKG). The catalysis of cAMP formation by adenylate cyclase is stimulated by vasoactive intestinal peptide (VIP), prostaglandin E-1 (PGE-1) and beta-adrenoreceptor agonists. Adenylate cyclase is coupled to the various membrane-bound receptors for these first messengers by G proteins. Once formed, cAMP activates protein kinase A (PKA). Activated PKA and PKG both phosphorylate certain proteins to cause the closure of calcium channels and sequestration of intracellular free calcium, resulting in decreased calcium concentration and relaxation of the muscle cell. It is probable that the coordinated activation of both the cAMP and cGMP pathways participates in the physiology of erection.

Agonists: effect on mechanisms of the smooth muscle pathway (Fig. 2.1b)

As well as depending upon the level of intracellular signal transduction via the second messengers cAMP and cGMP, relaxation of penile smooth muscle also depends on adequate levels of both agonists and the expression of their receptors. Cholinergic nerves seem to have an agonistic modulatory role on the other neuroeffector mechanisms by inhibiting adrenergic-mediated constriction and promoting relaxation mediated by non-adrenergic, non-cholinergic (NANC) nerves. NO is agonistic for the cGMP pathway. NO is released by NANC nerves in response to sexual stimulation and by the corpus cavernosum endothelium in response to blood flow sheer stress. The catalysis of cAMP formation is stimulated by VIP, prostaglandins and beta-adrenoreceptor agonists. VIP is released by NANC nerves innervating cavernous tissue. PGEs are the most abundant prostanoids synthesized by the cavernous muscle. PGE-1 and -2 relax trabecular smooth muscle and also have a role in inhibiting smooth muscle contraction via alpha-adrenergic receptors. Stimulation of beta-adrenergic receptors by catecholamines such as adrenaline mediates penile smooth muscle relaxation and in part counteracts the

(a)

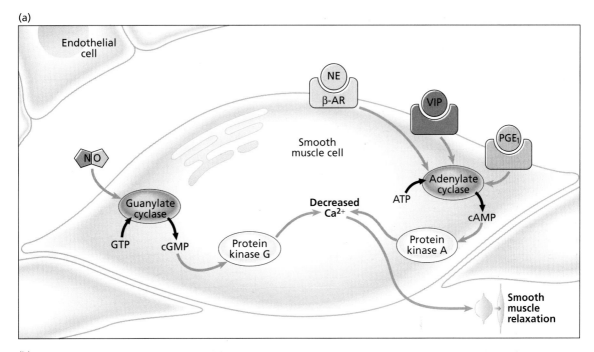

(b)

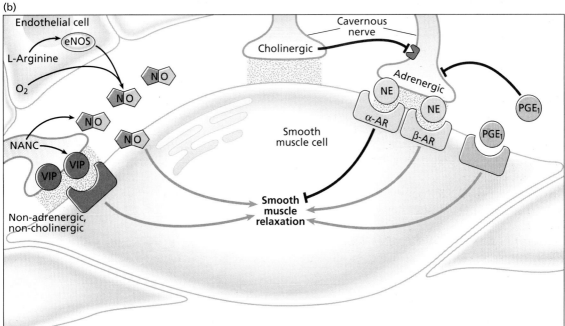

Figure 2.1 (a) Signal transduction pathways. (b) Agonists: effect on mechanisms of the smooth muscle pathway. *Continued*

(c)

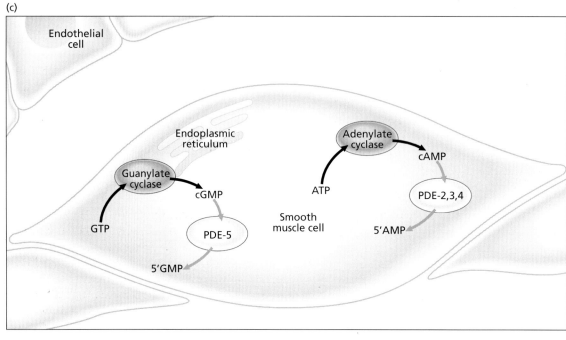

(d)

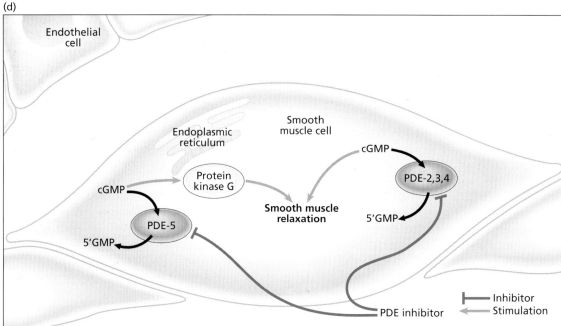

Figure 2.1, cont'd (c) Phosphodiesterases. (d) PDE-5 inhibition: general principles. (See text for full explanation.)

constrictor effects mediated by alpha-adrenergic receptors.[6]

Phosphodiesterases (PDEs) (Fig. 2.1c)
PDEs are enzymes that regulate the intracellular concentration of cyclic nucleotides. cAMP and cGMP in penile smooth muscle cells are hydrolyzed by PDEs, so reducing their concentration, ultimately leading to detumescence. PDE-5 is specific to the NO–cGMP pathway in human cavernous tissue; PDEs 2, 3 and 4 are involved in deactivating cAMP.

PDE-5 inhibition: general principles (Fig. 2.1d)
PDE inhibitors are agents that inhibit the activity of PDEs by competing with cyclic nucleotides for PDE active sites. Cyclic nucleotides can then no longer be deactivated by PDE and thus accumulate within the cell. The efficacy of any PDE inhibitor depends on its selectivity for PDE isoenzymes and its potency in blocking their enzymatic action.

Other neurotransmitters involved as co-transmitters include vasoactive intestinal polypeptide (VIP) and prostaglandins, which act through the adenylate cyclase pathway and its secondary neurotransmitter cyclic adenosine monophosphate (cAMP).[7,8]

Smooth muscle relaxation is counter-balanced by neurotransmitters and substances which produce smooth muscle contraction.[9] These agents, present in the normal corpus cavernosum, may be increased by high sympathetic tone caused by physical and psychologic stressors. The vasoconstrictor norepinephrine is the principal agent responsible for smooth muscle contraction. Norepinephrine is released from the sympathetic nerve endings in the corpora cavernosa and activates the alpha-1 adrenoceptors raising intracellular calcium and producing smooth muscle contraction.[10] Other similar molecules may also be involved in smooth muscle contraction. These include endothelin-1, prostaglandin F2 and epinephrine.[2]

Levels of these local neurotransmitters as well as central nervous system substances that can be manipulated pharmacologically have led to the revolution in the pharmacologic treatment of erectile dysfunction.

Pharmacologic treatment of ED

Pharmacologic treatment of ED using intracavernosally injected phenoxybenzamine and subsequently papaverine and phentolamine began in 1983.[11] Other injectable, oral and topical agents have been designed, used and marketed for the treatment of erectile dysfunction with enhanced activity and decreased morbidity. Development continues in laboratory and clinical trials of agents used to achieve and maintain an erection by newer, more focused medications.

Androgen treatment

Among the first agents used for the restoration of potency was the male hormone testosterone. Recent research has demonstrated that testosterone is necessary for the function of the enzyme nitric oxide synthase (NOS) in the corpus cavernosum. Deficient testosterone in laboratory animals results in decreased corpus cavernosum smooth muscle relaxation. Delivery systems for patients deficient in testosterone, however, have been suboptimal. Oral agents available in the US have resulted in rapid hepatic metabolism, hepatotoxicity, no specific serum testosterone response and frequently inadequate serum androgen levels. Oral agents such as testosterone undecanoate, not available in the US, enhances serum testosterone without significant hepatotoxicity.[12] The development of long-acting testosterone esters administered by injection results in initial supranormal blood levels of testosterone for up to 3 days following injection. With this treatment, an immediate peak is followed by a nadir approximately 21 days after injection.

The introduction of transdermal patches to provide testosterone using polymeric membrane patches currently permits a sustained release of testosterone for at least 22 hours. The maximum testosterone level with these devices occurs early in the morning, declining late in the evening in a fashion similar to the physiologic production of testosterone under the control of pituitary hormones. These testosterone patches require application on a daily basis and can be applied to scrotal or non-scrotal skin. While they are clearly more expensive than oral or injectable testosterone, their more physiologic pattern of administration may provide advantages over oral or injectable testosterone treatment.[12]

More recent developments in the treatment of hypogonadism and androgen deficiency in the aging male (ADAM) has included the introduction of an effective testosterone gel (Androgel®). This has improved upon the transdermal route of administration by enhancing ease of use and decreasing dermatologic adverse events while maintaining effectiveness. Testosterone gel is applied each morning after a shower with expected peak levels between 8.00 and 10.00 a.m., declining until the next application the following morning. This pattern replicates the normal diurnal curve of physiologic testosterone production. Caveats include maintaining a dry surface for 2 hours to allow absorption, and avoiding contact of the applied gel with the female partner for 2 hours. Serum testosterone levels should be monitored in 4 weeks and then at 6-monthly intervals with a prostate specific antigen. Annual evaluation of lipid profile, liver enzymes and blood count are also suggested to avoid some of the side effects of testosterone replacement. The effectiveness of testosterone gel appears to be equivalent to that of the transdermal patches. Androgel® is available as a 1% solution in 2.5 and 5 g packets. Patients may need more than one packet each day to maintain a normal testosterone level.

Oral agents

Oral medications for the treatment of erectile dysfunction have been unreliable prior to the development of the currently available oral agents. Trazodone, an antidepressant agent that produces selective inhibition of central nervous system serotonin uptake to increase dopamine turnover with some peripheral alpha-adrenergic blocking activity has been used in an effort to restore erectile function.[13] Intracavernosal injection of trazodone in the laboratory produces some tumescence, but not full erection. Several investigators, however, have demonstrated no clear advantage of trazodone administration over placebo in the treatment of men with even mild erectile dysfunction.[14]

Yohimbine, long considered an aphrodisiac in men, produces its effect through blockade of alpha-2 adrenergic receptors.[15] Yohimbine, in vitro, produces significant corpus cavernosum smooth muscle relaxation; however, the majority of adrenergic receptors in penile erectile tissue are alpha-1 type and the effectiveness of alpha-2

blockade in vitro is most likely a presynaptic effect which is less efficient in producing erection than alpha-1 blockade. In animal models, alpha-2 blockade increases sexual arousal and activity, but direct intravenous infusion of yohimbine in normal volunteers did not produce significant penile tumescence.[16] Clinical trials with yohimbine have not produced significant erectile improvement compared with placebo.[15-17] Adverse effects of yohimbine may include significant blood pressure elevation and even hypertensive crisis.[18] Delequamine is a newer alpha-2 adrenoreceptor antagonist one hundred times more selective than yohimbine.[19] It has good bioavailability in a 5–8 hour half-life. Clinical studies, however, have failed to reveal significant improvement in restoration of erections compared with placebo and its continued clinical development is unlikely.

L-Arginine, the precursor of nitric oxide, has been suggested as an oral supplement for patients with erectile dysfunction.[20] Placebo-controlled trials using two 800 mg doses daily for 2 weeks demonstrated an improvement in erectile function compared with placebo in a small group of patients. Most patients in this study had minimal erectile dysfunction.[21]

Newer oral agents are now available for clinical use and many newer agents are in various stages of clinical trials. The twenty-first century will see many new pharmacologic approaches to the treatment of ED. Sildenafil, the first of these agents to be approved in 1998 for clinical use has revolutionized the evaluation and treatment of erectile dysfunction.[22] Sildenafil was originally conceived as an anginal agent for its vasodilatory effects. Sildenafil is a selective inhibitor of phosphodiesterase type 5, the enzyme that breaks down cGMP in the corpus cavernosum.[23,24] This novel agent has few side effects, and significantly enhances the smooth muscle relaxation of the corpora cavernosa by increasing cGMP concentrations in the smooth muscle cell and facilitating erection. Placebo-controlled clinical trials involving more than 3000 patients followed for as long as 4 years has demonstrated a statistically significant improvement in erectile function compared with placebo.[22] More than 70% of men taking sildenafil reported improved erections compared with 10–30% of men receiving placebo. Sildenafil, available in 25, 50 and 100 mg doses, is taken

1 hour before sexual activity with optimal tissue levels occurring approximately 60 min after oral administration. Data from clinical trials have demonstrated improved erectile function in patients with a cross-section of etiologies of erectile dysfunction. This includes patients with diabetes (57%), spinal cord injury (60%), hypertension (70%), post radical prostatectomy (60%) and mild depression (80%).[25–27] Sildenafil is safe and effective in patients taking a variety of other medications. The results in men after radical prostatectomy are best achieved in those who have undergone a nerve-sparing procedure. Zippe et al[28] reported an 80% response in men undergoing bilateral nerve-sparing procedures versus non-responders with a non-nerve-sparing medical prostatectomy. After brachytherapy for prostate cancer, sildenafil is likewise effective with 80.6% excellent responses reported by Merrick et al.[29] After external beam radiation therapy for prostate cancer, Weber and colleagues[30] reported 85% responses without androgen deprivation therapy and 50% in radiation plus androgen deprivation. Kedia et al[31] reported a 71% response in 21 patients with 12/15 (80%) of responders requiring a 100 mg dose.

Adverse affects of sildenafil include mild headache, facial flushing, dyspepsia and nasal congestion. A temporary but reproducible blue tint to vision has also been demonstrated due to its inhibitory effect of PDE-6 in the photosensory cells of the retina. In clinical studies, however, discontinuation caused by adverse events was no different between active drug and placebo.[22]

The most important contraindication to sildenafil is in those patients taking nitrates for cardiac disease. These include drugs such as nitroglycerin, isosorbide, sodium nitroprusside or any other nitrate-associated medications.[32] Because sildenafil is metabolized in the liver through the cytochrome p450 isoenzyme pathway, agents which inhibit cytochrome p450 may reduce metabolism and clearance of sildenafil. These agents include cimetidine, erythromycin and ketoconazole. These caveats also apply to the newer PDE-5 inhibitors as metabolism and nitrate effects are 'class effects' and are common to all similar agents.

Newer PDE-5 inhibitors

Several other PDE-5 inhibitors are in various stages of development. Two agents which have completed advanced clinical trials and have significant clinical data available are vardenafil and tadalafil. These two agents vary in some significant areas including chemical structure, PDE selectivity, biochemical potency and duration of action (Table 2.2). While head-to-head trials of these newer agents with sildenafil and each other have not yet been performed, it is important to understand some of the basic differences in these compounds, review the available clinical experience and prepare for the use of these agents in clinical practice.

Vardenafil

Vardenafil is a PDE-5 inhibiting agent being developed by Bayer. It is similar to sildenafil in its chemical structure but may be more specific for the PDE-5 enzyme. Its half-life ($t_{1/2}$) is similar to sildenafil (see Table 2.3). Early studies have documented its efficacy in pivotal, as well as special populations of men with ED.

Table 2.2 PDE-5 inhibitor relative selectivity to non-PDE-5 Isoforms

PDE Isoenzyme	Sildenafil	Tadalafil	Vardenafil
PDE 1	> 80	> 10 000	> 200
PDE 2	> 1000	> 10 000	> 14 000
PDE 3	4000	> 10 000	> 3000
PDE 4	> 1000	> 10 000	> 5000
PDE 6	9	780	200
PDE 7-10*	–	> 10 000	–

*Tadalafil is known to inhibit PDE-11

Table 2.3 Comparison of sildenafil and newer PDE-5 inhibitors

Indicator	Sildenafil	Tadalafil	Vardenafil
Company	Pfizer	Lilly	Bayer
Tmax (h)	1	2	< 1
$T_{1/2}$ (h)	3–5	17.5	3–5
Metabolism	Hepatic	Hepatic	Hepatic
Onset of action (min)*	30–60	30–45	20–45
Duration (h)*	4	> 24	4

*Methodology of studies to determine these parameters is not equivalent.

Tadalafil (Cialis®)

Tadalafil is a unique PDE-5 inhibitor, chemically unrelated to sildenafil or vardenafil. It has been shown to be effective in mild, moderate and severe ED of a variety of etiologies. Its major difference is its half-life and duration of action (see Table 2.3). With its 17.5-hour half-life, it can be taken daily or less often with expected continued activity. Side effects and adverse events appear to be similar to the other agents.

Apomorphine

Apomorphine has also been long known as an erectogenic agent in both animals and man.[2] Its use as a subcutaneous agent was demonstrated more than a decade ago. Unfortunately, when used in the laboratory to stimulate erection, adverse events from this direct injection included severe nausea and vomiting. Heaton et al, however, were able to formulate a sublingual administration, which has preserved the erectogenic activity while decreasing the noxious side effects.[33] Apomorphine stimulates postsynaptic dopamine receptors in the hypothalamus and is effective as a precoitus oral agent. Phase III studies have demonstrated more than 60% durable erections 20–40 min following sublingual administration of apomorphine.[34] Adverse events continue to include nausea, hypotension, persistent yawning and occasional vomiting. At high doses, as many as 20% of men require regular antiemetic therapy. Lower doses, which will be used clinically, however, are less associated with this troublesome adverse event. Apomorphine is currently the only central nervous system acting agent available for treatment of erectile dysfunction. This and other newer central nervous system agents may be combined with peripherally active agents to enhance response rates. Andersson et al[35] have demonstrated an additive effect of apomorphine and sildenafil in rats.

The first centrally acting agent to be approved for use for ED is sublingual apomorphine. Currently available only in Europe, apomorphine is currently under review in the US by the Food and Drug Administration. Apomorphine has long been known as erectogenic and now is thought to stimulate the D1 and D2 receptors in the midbrain. While it is likely that the D2 receptors are inhibitory, the D1 receptors appear to be associated with the erectogenic activity.

Phentolamine

The use of phentolamine as an intracavernosal injection agent has long been known to produce tumescence. This non-selective alpha-adrenergic antagonist also possesses some antiserotonin activity and has a direct dilatory effect on corpus cavernosum smooth muscle and blood vessels. Early studies demonstrated the effect of phentolamine on patients with mild erectile dysfunction with 42% of patients developing functional erections satisfactory for sexual activity.[36] Trials of oral phentolamine (Vasomax) demonstrated a 60% satisfactory erection rate compared with placebo responses of approximately 40%.[37] Patients chosen for these studies had mild to moderate erectile dysfunction. The effect of oral phentolamine in patients with severe erectile dysfunction was somewhat less satisfactory. Side effects and adverse events from oral phentolamine are similar to those of other alpha-blockers and include headache, hypotension, tachycardia and nasal congestion. Recent results in laboratory animals have demonstrated benign neuroendocrine tumors in certain species of rodents. As a result, oral phentolamine trials are currently on hold until more data are available in other animal species to confirm the safety of this agent.

Injectable agents

The use of injectable vasoactive agents for the stimulation of erectile function began in 1983 with the dramatic presentation by Brindley at the American Urologic Association Meeting in Las Vegas, Nevada.[11] Following his stimulating discussion and graphic demonstration of the effectiveness of intracavernosal injected pharmacoactive agents, the international urologic community began the widespread use of these agents in patients of all ages. Subsequently, physiologic investigation of the corpus cavernosum smooth muscle demonstrated that the phenoxybenzamine used by Brindley caused corpus cavernosum smooth muscle relaxation with increased intracavernosal blood flow and decreased venous outflow. Studies using animal as well as human corpus cavernosal tissue strips demonstrated the effectiveness of papaverine, phentolamine and prostaglandin E-1 (PGE-1) in the relaxation of corpus cavernosum smooth muscle.[9,38] It is apparent from dose–response curves that papaverine and phentolamine completely relax the corporal tissue with a very rapid precipitous response. This completeness of relaxation with steep response may explain the increased incidence of prolonged erection with papaverine and phentolamine compared with PGE-1. Relaxation with PGE-1 is less complete and the response is more gradual with a decreased slope, indicating a wider concentration range of relaxant response.

While papaverine and PGE-1 have been used alone, various combinations of papaverine, phentolamine and PGE-1 have been widely prescribed. While PGE-1 alone appears to be the agent most commonly used, its expense, shorter half-life and discomfort at the injection site have assured the continued use of the papaverine–phentolamine combination in some patients. In patients where this two-drug combination fails to produce satisfactory erectile function, a three-drug therapy known as Trimix may salvage non-responders. This combination of papaverine, phentolamine and PGE-1 permits a reduced dosage of each agent with increased safety and decreased morbidity:

- Papaverine's pharmacologic function occurs as a result of increasing intracellular cAMP concentrations with subsequent decrease in calcium concentration and smooth muscle relaxation of all vascular structures in the penis.
- Phentolamine functions through its activity as a non-selective alpha-adrenoceptor blocker inhibiting smooth muscle contraction.
- Prostaglandin E-1, a prostanoid, produces smooth muscle relaxation in both the corpus cavernosum and arteriolar structures in the corpus cavernosum through the cAMP pathway, decreasing intracellular calcium concentrations.[39] Satisfactory erections from injection of prostaglandin E-1 at dose range (from 5 to 40 μg) are in excess of 70%, with prolonged erections occurring in 1% and corpus cavernosum fibrosis in only 2.7%.[40,41]

Other combinations of injectable agents are available internationally. A combination of phentolamine and vasoactive intestinal polypeptide (VIP) has been approved in several European countries.[42–44] This combination product (Invicorp, Senetec) has responses equivalent to PGE-1 without penile pain and aching. Moxisylyte, a selective alpha-1 receptor blocking substance, has also been approved for use in several European countries.[45] This agent, which relaxes smooth muscle in a fashion similar to phentolamine has a reported success rate of 70% at doses of 10–30 mg. Adverse events include prolonged erection (1%) and corpus cavernosum fibrosis (1.5%). Comparisons between moxisylyte and PGE-1 demonstrate stronger penile rigidity and higher success for PGE-1 but decreased penile pain and discomfort with moxisylyte.[46]

The improved understanding of smooth muscle physiology and agents producing relaxation has resulted in the development of K_{ATP} channel openers for the treatment of ED. These novel substances, which require intracavernosal injection, are being studied in early clinical trials with excellent, predictable erections without penile pain.[47,48]

Topical and intraurethral therapy

Alternative methods for the introduction of pharmacoactive agents into the corpus cavernosum have been investigated widely. Topical intraurethral and other methods of medication delivery may produce adequate erectile function in patients without the morbidity of self-injection. Topical application has included transcutaneous and urethral absorption of a variety of pharmacologic agents. Minoxidil, an antihypertensive agent that produces significant arterial dilation as a potassium channel opener has been applied topically as a 2% solution.[49] While the results of minoxidil application were superior to placebo, satisfactory rigidity was not obtained for clinical use. Nitroglycerin, an older established vasodilator, can be applied transcutaneously using an ointment formulation.[50,51] A randomized, placebo-controlled, double-blind trial demonstrated a significant response in patients treated with nitroglycerin patches with satisfactory erectile function in 21 of 26 patients with mild erectile dysfunction. Side effects included headache and penile erythema.[52] Because topical nitroglycerin is rapidly absorbed through vaginal mucosa, patients using transcutaneous or ointment-based nitroglycerin for erectile dysfunction must be advised to wear a condom during sexual activity. A newer preparation of prostaglandin E-1 in SEPA gel has undergone early trials. McVary et al[53] report 67–75% satisfactory erections within 60 min using visual sexual stimulation. More than 75% of all men (both placebo and PGE-1) reported glans discomfort.[53]

The intraurethral application of alprostadil (PGE-1) has been demonstrated in multiple studies and through clinical practice.[54,55] A pellet containing PGE-1 is delivered to the urethra through the medicated urethral system for erection (MUSE) delivering prostaglandin E-1 to the corpus cavernosum providing smooth muscle relaxation through activation of the adenylate cyclase system reducing intracellular calcium and producing smooth muscle relaxation. Phase III trial results have documented erectile function in as many as 66% of men with erectile dysfunction of a variety of etiologies.[54] Doses available range from 125 to 1000 µg and side effects of treatment include urethral pain and urethral trauma. Porst[55] compared intraurethral and intracavernosal injected prostaglandin E-1 with a significantly higher success rate and decreased side effects with injection of prostaglandin E-1 at lower doses compared with intraurethral application of prostaglandin E-1. The use of the MUSE system for oral medication failures and in selected patients with unsatisfactory erections with penile prostheses establish a niche for this method of treatment of erectile dysfunction. Recent studies using a combination of the selective alpha-1 blocker prazosin resulted in minimal but significant increase in efficacy over single drug therapy.

Newer injectable agents currently in clinical trials include direct ATP-sensitive potassium channel openers administered by injection. These agents – which are stable, do not require refrigeration and produce no penile pain after injection – appear to have substantial advantages over currently available injectable agents.

Gene therapy

Gene therapy for the treatment of ED may be one of the ideal locations for the use of this novel and ground-breaking technology. Already many investigators have used nitric oxide synthase or potassium channel opening agents transfected by gene therapy to treat in vivo ED with good success.[56] These experiments have been used in diabetes, vasculogenic and trauma models of ED with high success rates. These treatments in vivo, however, require redosing every 1–3 months by direct injection. In the future, therefore, a diabetic man with ED might have to see his physician three

to four times a year for an injection that would result in a restoration of his normal ability to obtain and maintain an erection. Other types of gene therapy may also be useful in restoring androgen production, sensitivity and reduce ADAM.

Penile prostheses

Prosthetic implants to restore erectile function have been used successfully for many years. Indeed, the introduction of the inflatable penile prosthesis by Scott et al in 1973 initiated the modern era of evaluation and treatment of erectile dysfunction.[57] This sentinel work began the active use of prosthetic devices and the active treatment of erectile dysfunction by urologists. Other prosthetic devices have also been used; however, the inflatable penile prosthesis is the most often implanted prosthesis today in the US.[58,59] Rehabilitation of men with erectile dysfunction with these devices was never successful.[60] Development of newer synthetic materials in the 1950s and 1960s allowed improved prosthetic design and acceptance. The silicone-based materials used for the construction of penile implants based on the development of silicone elastomer revolutionized the durability, acceptance and decreased complications of these prosthetic devices. Although an increase of local tissue silicone levels have been documented, systemic effects of these silicone elastomers without silicone gel appear to be safe and without significant side effects.[60] Even local levels of silicone identified are far less for silicone elastomer than gel-containing devices.[60] Modern penile prostheses, both inflatable and non-inflatable, have excellent patient–partner satisfaction results and a mechanical failure rate that continues to decline. A multicenter study published in 2000 reports a greater than 90% 5-year and greater than 70% 10-year survival with more than 90% of patients satisfied with the function of their prosthesis and willing to undergo implantation of a penile prosthesis subsequently.[61] This study is mirrored by other single and multi-institutional studies of various penile implants.[60] Despite long-term use and laudable successes, challenges and complications, as well as morbidity may be associated with some penile prosthesis implantation.

Recent developments in penile prosthesis design have included efforts to decrease the incidence of infection-associated failures. Both American Medical Systems (AMS) and Mentor Corporation have introduced concepts that will decrease these tragic complications. While the Mentor device coating Resist™ has yet to be introduced to the market, this hydrophilic coating is similar to that used on stents and catheters. The Resist™ coating has been used in vitro and in clinical trials with commonly used topical antibiotic solutions to decrease the early adherence of bacteria to the implanted device. This coating results in a longer lasting adherence of antibiotic agents and has been reported to last 24–36 hours and result in fewer Staphylococcus-related colonizations and infections. As a result of the hydrophilic properties, bacteria are less likely to adhere to the surface early in the postoperative period. Its true effectiveness awaits formal clinical trials and clinical experience.

The AMS three-piece inflatable prostheses are now available with a coating called InhibiZone®. This coating consists of a combination of minocycline and rifampin, which remains on the implant fabric for up to 3 days. This combination antibiotic coating is targeted at the most common infection-related pathogens – the Gram-positive staphylococci such as *S. epidermidis*. Early postoperative results have demonstrated an advantage in both first and repeat implants compared with historical and contemporary implant infection rates for prostheses implanted without InhibiZone®.

Summary

With newer novel methods for the treatment of erectile dysfunction, urologists and other health care providers can offer men with erectile dysfunction a variety of solutions suited to their pathophysiology, etiology and personal needs. Because many patients fail to maintain treatment with injectable and more invasive therapeutic alternatives, oral treatment and combinations of agents appear to be the best method for treatment of men who do not respond to simple oral therapy.[62] Heaton et al[63] have suggested a method of pharmacologic treatment of erectile dysfunction including central and peripheral medications which produce stimulation or facilitation of erectile function. By applying this grid to a decision tree once multiple oral and injectable medications are available, urologists with a knowledge and expertise in erectile dysfunction may design therapeutic programs for individual patients refractory to simple single oral therapy.[63]

References

1. Laumann EO, Paik A, Rosen RC. Sexual dysfunction in the United States: prevalence and predictors. JAMA 1999; 281:537–544.
2. Andersson KE, Wagener G. Physiology of penile erection. Physiol Rev 1995; 75:191–236.
3. Raijfer J, Aronson WJ, Bush PA, et al. Nitric oxide as a mediator of the corpus cavernosum in response to non-cholinergic non-adrenergic neurotransmission. N Engl J Med 1992; 326:90–94.
4. Holmquist F, Andersson KE, Fovaeus MN, Hedlund H. Potassium channel openers for relaxation of isolated erectile tissue from rabbit. J Urol 1990; 144:146–151.
5. Lue TF. Erectile dysfunction. N Engl J Med 2000; 342:1802–1813.
6. Saenz de Tejada I, et al. Anatomy, physiology and pathophysiology of erectile function. In: Jardin A, ed. Erectile dysfunction. Plymouth: Health Publications; 2000:65–102.
7. Kim YC, Kim JA, Hagan PO, Carson CC. Modulation of vasoactive intestinal polypeptide (VIP) mediated relaxation by nitric oxide and prostanoids in the rabbit corpus cavernosum. J Urol 1995; 153:807–810.
8. Iwanaga T, Hanyu S, Tamaki M. VIP and other bioactive substances involved in penile erection. Bio Med Res 1992; 2:71–73.
9. Kerfoot WW, Schwartz LB, Hagen PO, Carson CC. Characterization of contracting and relaxing agents in human and rabbit corpus cavernosum. Surg Forum 1991; 42:688–689.
10. Kim SC, Ooh MM. Norepinephrine involvement in response to intracorporeal injection of papaverine in psychogenic impotence. J Urol 1992; 147:1530–1532.
11. Brindley GS. Pilot experiments on the action of drugs injected into the human corpus cavernosum penis. Br J Pharmacol 1986; 87:405–500.
12. Morales A, Heaton JPW, Carson CC. Andropause: misnomer for true clinical entity. J Urol 2000; 163:705–712.
13. Carson CC, Mino RD. Priapism associated with trazodone therapy. J Urol 1988; 139:369–370.
14. Costibile RA, Spevak M. Oral trazodone is not effective therapy for erectile dysfunction: a double blind placebo controlled study. J Urol 1999; 161:1819–1822.
15. Montorsi F, Strambi LF, Guazzoni G, et al. Effect of yohimbine in psychogenic impotence: a randomized double-blind placebo controlled study. Urology 1994; 44:732–736.
16. Susset JG, Tessier CD, Wincaze J, et al. Effect of yohimbine hydrochloride on erectile impotence: a double-blind study. J Urol 1989; 141:1360–1363.
17. Vogt HJ, Brandall P, Kockott G, et al. Double-blind placebo controlled safety and efficacy trial with yohimbine hydrochloride in the treatment of non-organic erectile dysfunction. Int J Impot Res 1997; 9:155–161.

18. Ruck B, Shih RD, Marcus SM. Hypertensive crisis from herbal treatment of impotence. Am J Emerg Med 1999; 17:317–318.

19. Tallentire D, McRae G, Spedding M, et al. Modulation of sexual behavior in the rat by a potent alpha 2 antagonist delequamine (RS-15385-197). Br J Pharmacol 1996; 118:63–72.

20. Melman A. L-Arginine and penile erection. J Urol 1997; 158:686.

21. Zorgniotti AW, Lizza AF. Effective large doses of nitric oxide precursor L-arginine on erectile failure. Int J Impot Res 1994; 6:33–34.

22. Goldstein I, Lue TF, Padma-Nathan H, et al. Oral sildenafil and the treatment of erectile dysfunction. N Engl J Med 1998; 338:1397–1404.

23. Moreland RB, Goldstein I, Traish A. Sildenafil: a novel inhibitor of phosphodiesterase type 5 in human corpus cavernosum smooth muscle cells. Life Sci 1998; 62:309–318.

24. Ballard SA, Gingell CJ, Tang K, et al. Effects of sildenafil on the relaxation of human corpus cavernosum tissue in vitro and on the activities of cyclic nucleotide phosphodiesterase isoenzymes. J Urol 1998; 159:2164–2167.

25. Virag R. Indications and early results of sildenafil (Viagra) in erectile dysfunction. Urology 1999; 54:1073–1077.

26. Guiliano F, Hultling C, El Masry WS, et al. Randomized trial of sildenafil for the treatment of erectile dysfunction in spinal cord injury. Ann Neurol 1999; 46:15–21.

27. Rendell MS, Rajfer J, Wilson P, et al. Sildenafil for the treatment of erectile dysfunction in men with diabetes: a randomized controlled trial. JAMA 1999; 281:421–426.

28. Zippe CD, Kedia S, Kedia AW, Pesquealotto F. Sildenafil citrate (Viagra) after radical retropubic prostatectomy. Urology 1999; 54:583–586.

29. Merrick GS, Butler WM, Lief JH, et al. Efficacy of sildenafil in prostate brachytherapy patients with erectile dysfunction. Urology 1999; 53:1112–1116.

30. Weber DC, Bieri S, Kuntz JM, Miralbell R. Prospective pilot study of sildenafil for treatment of post radiotherapy erectile dysfunction in patients with prostate cancer. J Clin Oncol 1979; 17:3444–3449.

31. Kedia S, Zippe CD, Agarwal A, et al. Treatment of erectile dysfunction with sildenafil citrate after radiation therapy for prostate cancer. Urology 1999; 54:308–312.

32. Kloner RA, Zusman RM. Cardiovascular effects of sildenafil citrate and recommendations for its use. Am J Cardiol 1999; 84:11–17(N).

33. Heaton JPW, Morales A, Adams MA, et al. Recovery of erectile function after oral administration of apomorphine. Urology 1995; 45:200–206.

34. Padman Nathan H, Fromm S, Ruff D, et al. Efficacy and safety of apomorphine SL vs placebo for male erectile dysfunction. J Urol 1998; 159:241–243.

35. Andersson KE, Gamalmaz H, Waldeck K, et al. The effect of sildenafil on apomorphine evoked increases in intracavernous pressure in the awake rat. J Urol 1999; 161:1707–1712.

36. Gwinup G. Oral phentolamine in nonspecific erectile insufficiency. Ann Intern Med 1988; 109:162–163.

37. Wagner G, Lacy S, Lewis R. Buccal phentolamine: a pilot trial for male erectile dysfunction at three separate clinics. Int J Impot Res 1994; 6:D78.

38. Virag R. Intracavernous injection of papaverine for erectile failure. Lancet 1982; 2:938.

39. Lee LM, Stevenson RW, Szasz G. Prostaglandin E-1 versus phentolamine–papaverine for the treatment of erectile impotence: a double-blind comparison. J Urol 1989; 141:549–550.

40. Linet OI, Ogring FG. Efficacy in safety of intracavernosal alprostadil in men with erectile dysfunction. N Engl J Med 1996; 334:873–877.

41. Stakl W, Hasun R, Marberger N. Prostaglandin E-1 in the treatment of erectile dysfunction. World J Urol 1990; 8:84–86.

42. McMahon CG. A pilot study for the role of intracavernosal injection of vasoactive intestinal polypeptide (VIP) and phentolamine mesylate in the treatment of erectile dysfunction. Int J Impot Res 1996; 8:233–236.

43. Kiely EA, Bloom SR, Williams G. Penile response to intracavernosal vasoactive intestinal polypeptide alone and in combination with other vasoactive agents. Br J Urol 1989; 64:191–194.

44. Gerstenberg TC, Metz T, Ottesen B, Fahrenkrug J. Intracavernous self-injection with vasoactive intestinal polypeptide and phentolamine in the management of erectile failure. J Urol 1992; 147:1277–1279.

45. Hermabessiere J, Costa CFP. Efficacy in safety assessment of intracavernous injection of moxisylyte in patients with erectile dysfunction: a double-blind placebo controlled study. Int J Impot Res 1994; 6:D147.

46. Buvat J, Costa P, Moralier D, et al. Double-blind multicenter study comparing alprostadil alpha cyclodextrin with moxisylyte chlorohydrate in patients with chronic erectile dysfunction. J Urol 1998; 159:116–119.

47. Benevides MD, Parivar K, Vick RN, et al. Intracavernosal injection of a potassium channel opener to treat erectile dysfunction. J Urol 1999; 161(suppl):212.

48. Moon DG, Byum HS, Kim JJ. A KATP-channel opener as a potential treatment modality for erectile dysfunction. Br J Urol 1999; 83:837–841.

49. Cavalini G. Minoxidil and capsaicin: an association of transcutaneous active drugs for erection facilitation. Int J Impot Res 1994; 6:D71.

50. Heaton JPW, Morales A, Owen J, et al. Topical glyceryl trinitrate causes measurable penile arterial dilation in impotent men. J Urol 1990; 143:729–731.

51. Nunez BD, Andersson DC. Nitroglycerine ointment in the treatment of impotence. J Urol 1993; 150:1241–1243.

52. Cavallini G. Minoxidil versus nitroglycerin: prospective double-blind control trial in transcutaneous erection facilitation for organic impotence. J Urol 1991; 146:50–53.

53. McVary KT, Polepalle S, Riggi S. Topical prostaglandin E1 SEPA gel for the treatment of erectile dysfunction. J Urol 1999; 162:726–731.

55. Padma-Nathan H, Hellstrom WJG, Kaiser FE, et al. Treatment of men with erectile dysfunction with transurethral alprostadil. N Engl J Med 1997; 336:1–7.

55. Porst H. Transurethral alprostadil with MUSE versus intracavernous alprostadil: a comparative study in 103 patients with erectile dysfunction. Int J Impot Res 1997; 9:187–192.

56. Schenk G, Melman A, Christ G. Gene therapy: future therapy for erectile dysfunction. Curr Urol Rep 2001; 2(6):480–487.
57. Scott FB, Bradley W, Timm G. Management of erectile impotence: use of implantable inflatable prosthesis. Urology 1973; 2:80–84.
58. Small MP, Carrion HM, Gordon JA. A small Carrion penile prosthesis: a new implant for the management of impotence. Urology 1975; 5:479–485.
59. Jhaveri FM, Rutledge R, Carson CC. Penile prosthesis implantation surgery: a statewide population based analysis of 2354 patients. Int J Impot Res 1998; 10(4):251–254.
60. Kim JH, Carson CC. History of urologic prostheses for impotence. Prob Urol 1993; 7:283–288.
61. Carson CC, Mulcahy JJ, Govier FE. Efficacy, safety and patient satisfaction outcomes of the AMS 700CX inflatable penile prosthesis: results of a long-term multicenter study. AMS 700CX Study Group. J Urol 2000; 164(2):376–380.
62. Fundaram CP, Thomas W, Pryor LE, et al. Long term follow-up of patients receiving injection therapy for erectile dysfunction. Urology 1997; 49:932–935.
63. Heaton JPW, Adams MA, Morales A. Therapeutic taxonomy of treatments for erectile dysfunction: an evolutionary imperative. Int J Impot Res 1997; 9:115–121.

3

Erectile dysfunction and cardiovascular disease

Graham Jackson and Michael G Kirby

Sex is an intrinsic part of society and culture and influences all aspects of modern day life. In a recent global survey, more than 80% of men and 60% of women aged 40–80 who took part, said sex was an important part of their overall lives.[1]

It is not surprising that the survey found that sex is especially important for men, who at adolescence compete to lose their virginity, seeing it as a sign of success, and in adulthood still judge themselves on the size, firmness and staying power of their erections. As adults, men continue to place huge significance on how many sexual partners they have had, and the frequency at which sexual intercourse takes place.

Throughout history, perceptions in society have been such that men are expected to be the stronger gender. Macho stereotyping has led to men having a very functional view of their bodies. They expect their body to continue working, regardless of the task they set for it. If sexual intercourse is prevented because the man cannot get a sufficient erection, the consequences can be distressing, and can impact negatively not only on his sense of well-being, but also on his relationship with his partner.[2] Being able to attain and maintain an erection is not simply about being able to have sex. The actual act of sexual intercourse is just a small part of a much bigger picture. An inability to perform this basic function actually poses a direct threat to a man's core belief in himself, and can be an extremely traumatic event.

The term impotence (traditionally applied to erection difficulties, before erectile dysfunction became the name more widely used today) derives from the Latin phrase for 'loss of power'. Although 'impotence' is now less commonly used, men still associate erectile dysfunction with lack of strength and vitality, and automatically connect the condition with the opposite of all that they consider masculine. The embarrassment men feel about the condition means that on average less than a third of men with erection problems have summoned the courage to ask for medical help.

Erectile dysfunction (ED) is defined as the inability to achieve and/or maintain an erection sufficient for satisfactory sexual activity[3] for a period of longer than 3 months. At present, it is estimated that over three million men suffer from erection problems in the UK and over 140 million men worldwide.[4] The projections for 2025 show a prevalence of approximately 322 million men worldwide with ED.[4] ED is one of the most common male sexual problems and becomes progressively more prevalent as men get older.

Cardiovascular disease and ED

Normal erectile function requires the coordination of psychologic, neurologic, hormonal and vascular factors. ED is associated with organic and psychogenic conditions that disturb the interplay of these components.

The physiology of erection (discussed in more detail in Chapter 2) involves a complex chain of events resulting in the dilation of penile blood vessels, increased blood flow and subsequent erection.[5] As an erection requires the successful flow of blood into the penis, factors that affect the arterial vasculature will obviously impact upon erectile function. The vascular endothelium provides the link between ED and cardiovascular disease, as it plays a vital role in the regulation of the circulation (Fig. 3.1).

Hypertension, ischemic heart disease, hypercholesterolemia and diabetes can all lead to abnormalities of the vascular smooth muscle and extracellular matrix. Endothelial cell dysfunction can precede the formation of atherosclerotic

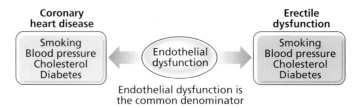

Figure 3.1 Endothelial link between cardiovascular disease and erectile dysfunction.

plaques and is common in cardiovascular disease and diabetic patients.[6] Although vasculogenic problems such as cardiovascular disease are the most common cause of organic ED, regardless of the primary etiology, it should be highlighted that often a psychologic element coexists with the organic cause.

Psychogenic factors may well contribute to ED in cardiovascular patients, and in the majority of men with ED a psychologic component will also contribute to their problem. An erection relies partly upon messages based on visual, auditory, olfactory or imaginative stimuli being sent from the brain to the spinal cord. Therefore, psychologic dysfunction might inhibit stimuli from the brain and block normal erection. Some men with primarily psychogenic ED may suffer from a cardiovascular condition, which could be contributing to their ED. In short, psychologic and cardiovascular causes commonly coexist and should not be thought of as being mutually exclusive.

Prevalence of ED in the cardiovascular patient

Risk factors
The Massachusetts Male Aging Study (MMAS) conducted between 1987 and 1989 in men aged 40–70 years is probably the most widely cited study of the incidence of ED. Although this study identified age to be the strongest risk factor for ED, it also found, after age adjustment, that men with heart disease, diabetes or hypertension are up to four times more likely to develop complete ED compared with men who do not suffer from these chronic conditions.[7]

A report from an 8-year follow-up sample of the MMAS population confirmed the prevalence of moderate or complete ED, in patients with cardiovascular risk factors, to be 31% compared with 19.6% in the age-matched, disease-free control group.[8] The study also showed that two associated risk factors in particular (i.e. low levels of high-density lipoprotein and hypertension) were significantly correlated with ED.

Key risk factors for cardiovascular disease are summarized in Table 3.1. The greater the number of risk factors present, the greater the overall risk of worsening cardiovascular status.

It is estimated that between 39 and 64% of male patients with cardiovascular disease suffer from ED.[9] Cardiovascular disease is generally subdivided into four conditions: atherosclerosis, coronary artery disease, hypertension and peripheral vascular disease. Any of these four conditions can predispose the patient to developing ED.

Another study has confirmed a significant prevalence of ED in patients who have experienced a previous myocardial infarction (44%), in those with untreated hypertension (17%) and treated hypertension (25%).[10,11]

Table 3.1 Key risk factors for cardiovascular disease

Cardiovascular disease	Associated clinical conditions
Hypertension	Ischemic heart disease
Hyperlipidemia	Angina
Diabetes	Post-myocardial infarction
Smoking	Left ventricular failure
Chronic renal disease	Congestive heart failure
Obesity	Arrhythmias
Ethnic background, e.g. Asian	
Increasing age	
Excess alcohol	
Male gender	

Lifestyle, e.g. sedentary, depression

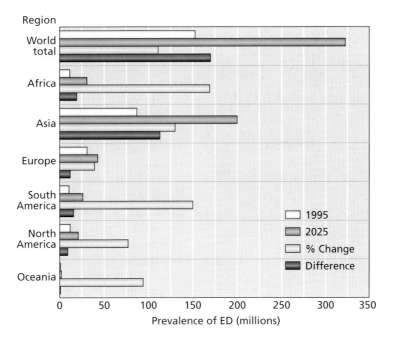

Figure 3.2 The probable worldwide increase in the (age-adjusted) prevalence of erectile dysfunction between 1995 and 2025.[4] (From United Nations data,[12] the most conservative (lowest) projection was used. Prevalence estimates of ED used were from the MMAS 1987–89 for ages 40–69 and from MMAS 1995–97 for ages 70–79.)

A worldwide problem

Figure 3.2 shows the probable worldwide increase in the (age-adjusted) prevalence of erectile dysfunction between 1995 and 2025. The number of men suffering from ED is set to double in the majority of countries, illustrating the importance of raising awareness of the condition and treatment options available.

Impact of ED on patients with cardiovascular disease

ED has a profound effect on all aspects of a patient's psychologic and social functioning, including his capacity to work, maintain social and family roles and sustain self-esteem.[13] It has been shown that quality of life can be substantially diminished by ED.[14–16] Approximately 65% of men with ED say that their ED makes them feel worried or anxious and makes them lack confidence, and nearly a quarter (24%) say that their ED makes them feel unattractive. As human beings our sexuality is inextricably linked to our overall health, happiness and sense of wellness. Global data show that nearly 70% of people describing their health as 'excellent' also reported that their physical relationship with their partner was very/extremely pleasurable in the past year. A similar trend could also be seen between emotional and sexual health.[1]

ED also has a huge impact on the patient's relationship with his partner. Nearly three-quarters of women whose partner has ED, say that the man usually initiated sexual activity,[17] but when the man suffers from ED, he often fears that he may not be able to 'finish what he starts' and consequently withdraws from sexual activity completely. This lack of physical affection can put a huge strain on a relationship, and the lack of kissing and cuddling can be particularly upsetting to the woman who may start to believe her partner no longer finds her attractive. In some cases the woman may fear that her partner is having an affair, as the man will often choose to work long hours and come home 'tired'.

Evidence for the effect on relationships comes from a survey of 3693 men seen by RELATE counselors who found that one in four men who

Table 3.2 Impotence Association survey results, 2000 and 2001[21]

Effect on quality of life and relationships	Percentage of men
Depressed or made to feel depressed by ED	32
Worried and anxious	65
Lacking confidence	62
Negative feelings caused by ED	46
Relationship difficulties	35
Worsened relationship	28
Breakdown in relationship	7
Stopped forming relationships	12

required these services had some degree of ED.[18] An Impotence Association survey in 1997 found that 20% of men with ED had broken relationships as a result of their condition.[19] Just over 8% of patients had actually considered ending their relationship because of ED, and 27% of couples in which the man had a sexual problem had significant marital problems.[20] Results of Impotence Association surveys in 2000 and 2001 are presented in Table 3.2.

Despite the huge impact ED clearly has on the patient, men are still reluctant to come forward and seek help for their condition. Just under half of men with ED failed to tell their urologist and, of these, 71% said embarrassment was the main reason for not broaching the subject.[22]

> **Key to remember:**
> 'If doctors don't ask, patients won't tell.'

ED as a marker for cardiovascular disease

It is important for health care professionals to be proactive in discussing ED with their patients not only for the reasons cited above, but also because ED can be the first detectable sign of other serious medical conditions, such as heart disease. Curkendall et al[23] showed that among 980 men who did seek help because of their ED, 18% were suffering unknowingly from hypertension and 5% from ischemic heart disease. Managing ED can play a large role in helping health care professionals to reduce this huge number of deaths. Although the

symptoms of early cardiovascular disease are not always immediately obvious, ED is an obvious symptom and proactive identification would enable earlier diagnosis of cardiovascular disease as well as early identification of those patients who are likely to have heart problems in the future.

Early identification of men who suffer from ED would also be beneficial on a global scale. The World Health Organization has the ambition to reduce the death rate from heart disease and related illnesses such as stroke throughout the world. According to the World Health Organization's 1997 health report, diseases of the heart and circulatory system accounted for more than 15 million deaths per year. Even though methods of prevention are now well known, the number of deaths due to heart attack and stroke are expected to continue to rise around the world. The epidemic of coronary heart disease is expected to emerge first in those who are financially better off and to spread to those who are less well off.[24] Perhaps this spread could be slowed if awareness of ED and its causes were raised amongst patients and health care professionals.

ED can be also be used as a marker for cardiovascular disease progression and severity. This is illustrated by patients with single-vessel ischemic heart disease having firmer erections and less difficulty in obtaining an erection than those with two- or three-vessel disease.[25] The penis can therefore be seen to act as an indicator of cardiovascular status

Management of ED in patients with cardiovascular disease

Good medical practice means taking a holistic approach towards diagnosis before initiating treatment. The underlying cause of ED in patients should be established and, where possible, treated before, or at the same time, as initiating therapy specifically for the ED – determining not only the physical causes in the individual, but also any accompanying psychologic factors contributing to the condition. Regardless of the precipitating factors, there is usually a psychogenic component involved, especially if the patient has delayed in coming forward to seek help. Even if it is suspected that the ED has an organic cause such as cardiovascular disease or diabetes, psychosexual therapy should be considered, and can often complement other treatments.

Today, there is a wide range of licensed therapies available for managing ED in the general population. These include:

- oral medication (i.e. sildenafil citrate, apomorphine sublingual)
- intracavernosal injection or transurethral alprostadil
- vacuum constriction devices and penile implants.

These are all suitable for managing ED in patients with cardiovascular disease as long as the manufacturer's instructions and guidelines are followed. The advantages and disadvantages of each treatment option are the same for the cardiovascular patient as for any other, and do not increase the overall cardiovascular risk in patients with diagnosed cardiovascular disease, provided they are used correctly. The exceptions to this are patients on warfarin who may experience increased risk of bruising with injections, urethral bleeding with intraurethral alprostadil and hematoma with a vacuum device. Caution is also advised in men taking the combination of clopidogrel and aspirin. In addition, sildenafil, tadalafil and vardenafil are contraindicated in patients taking nitrate and nicorandil therapy, and use of apomorphine is cautioned.

Hypotensive episodes have been reported if sildenafil is taken in the 4 hours after doxazosin and until this is clarified (dose, formulation of doxazosin), sildenafil is not advised in this time period.

Involving the partner

Partners are not always involved in the process of establishing the cause of the man's ED, and appropriate treatment options. This is a concern, because over half of the time clinicians may decide to alter their diagnosis and treatment options if they take the partner's views into account.[26]

Some partners have either, subconsciously or unconsciously, affected a potentially successful outcome of management of their partner's condition. Partners should be given the opportunity to discuss any concerns or problems they may have, and which treatment option they would be most happy with their partner using. Female partners should also be asked about significant life changes, such as the menopause or a hysterectomy, and whether these have affected self-perception. It is common for women to feel less feminine or attractive to their partner after these events. Nearly two-thirds of men with ED say that their partners have negative emotions towards their condition. Therefore, it should be explained that irritability, depression and emotional and social withdrawal are all normal reactions to ED for both partners.

The hypertensive patient

The relatively small difference in ED prevalence between patients with untreated and treated hypertension can be explained because there are a number of drugs that may cause ED in the cardiovascular patient (Table 3.3), the most frequent being antihypertensive agents. Reports have indicated an incidence range of 20–80% with

Table 3.3 Drugs linked to ED

Cardiovascular drugs	*Psychotropic drugs*
Thiazide diuretics	Major tranquilizers
Beta-blockers	Anxiolytics and hypnotics
Calcium antagonists	Tricyclic antidepressants
Centrally acting agents:	Selective serotonin reuptake inhibitors
— methyldopa	
— clonidine, reserpine	*Endocrine drugs*
— ganglion blockers	Antiandrogens
Digoxin	Estrogens
Lipid-lowering agents	Luteinizing hormone-releasing hormone analogs
Angiotensin converting enzyme inhibitors	Testosterone
Recreational drugs	*Others*
Alcohol	Cimetidine, ranitidine
Marijuana	Metoclopramide
Amfetamines	Carbamazepine
Cocaine	
Anabolic steroids	
Heroin	

methyldopa, 5–43% with propranolol and 4–32% with thiazide diuretics.

There is little evidence to show that changing cardiovascular drug therapy will have a positive influence on erectile function. However, if the erection problems started at the same time as the patient began taking a specific medication, it seems logical to assume a change to an alternative medication would be beneficial, but only if this can be achieved safely. Any improvements in ED are likely to occur within 2–4 weeks and should be evaluated in the context of their impact on the underlying disease they are being used to treat.

For example, where a link is suspected between the initiation of a beta-blocker for the treatment of hypertension and the onset of ED, alpha-blockers or angiotensin II receptor antagonists could be alternative options to consider. However, beta-blockers are likely to have beneficial effects upon post-myocardial infarction (MI) patients and in those with heart failure. They should not be stopped abruptly or without consideration of overall risk.[27] It is important to consider that the development of ED may be due to the condition being treated, such as hypertension, ischemic heart disease or atherosclerosis, rather than the drugs used.

Risk assessment of patients diagnosed with cardiovascular disease

The cardiac risk of sexual activity in men with diagnosed cardiovascular disease is minimal in properly assessed patients.[28]

In the case of strokes, these occur most commonly at night and in the early morning, regardless of sexual activity. Many patients who have suffered strokes may incorrectly believe there is a strong relationship between the two, as these are the times when the majority of people have sex. Sex does not significantly increase the risk of stroke and could even offer protection against fatal coronary events.[29]

The incidence of ED ranges from 44 to 64% in patients who have previously had an MI.[9,10] Here, ED could occur as a result of the general risk factors for cardiovascular disease that may have led to the MI (the ED may well have been present before the MI took place). It may also result from psychogenic causes, because patients often believe that sexual intercourse is likely to trigger another

attack and this fear negatively impacts on the ED and future management. The partner often feeds into these fears, which highlights the importance of providing counseling to both patient and partner together as a couple. If ED is mainly psychogenic in cause, it is possible that following advice and reassurance and initial treatment, the patient may have a spontaneous return of his erections. Table 3.4 outlines a management algorithm for patients diagnosed with cardiovascular disease according to graded risk.[30]

Patients who fall into the low risk category can usually be assessed and treated for their ED without the need for further investigations into their cardiac status and/or referral to a specialist. Patients who are classified as being at intermediate risk should not resume sexual activity or undergo treatment for ED until their cardiac status has been re-evaluated and they have been restratified into either the high risk or low risk category. High risk patients should not be managed in primary care, but instead be referred to a specialist for cardiac assessment before commencing ED treatment. Management of ED in patients with cardiovascular disease will always take second place to stabilizing their cardiovascular status and optimizing drug therapy for cardiovascular symptoms.

Assessing a patient's normal physical abilities can also be a useful guide in determining their ability to undertake sexual activity without triggering further cardiovascular events. An exercise tolerance test will provide a useful guide based on the METs system: in scientific terms, the level of cardiac exertion for an activity can be expressed as the metabolic equivalent of the task (MET).[31] One MET refers to the relative energy demand of oxygen usage in the resting state, approximately 3.5 ml oxygen/kg body weight/min.

If a patient can achieve 5–6 METs without significant ischemia (> 2 mm ST segment depression), arrhythmias or a fall in systolic blood pressure, the patient is not at risk during their normal sexual activity. By asking the patient to walk 1 mile on the flat in 20 minutes, 5–6 METs can be achieved. If the patient experiences chest pain, irregular heartbeat or extreme shortness of breath during any of these tests, the patient's cardiovascular condition and its management should be further investigated before sexual activity should be

Table 3.4 Management algorithm according to graded risk

Grading of risk	Cardiovascular status upon presentation	ED management recommendations for the primary care health professional
Low risk	Controlled hypertension Asymptomatic ≤ 3 risk factors for CAD, excluding age and gender Mild valvular disease Minimal/mild stable angina Post successful revascularization CHF (I)	Manage within the primary care setting Review treatment options with patient and his partner (where possible)
Intermediate risk	Recent MI or CVA (i.e. within last 2–6 weeks) LVD/CHF (II) Murmur of unknown cause Moderate stable angina Heart transplant Recurrent TIAs Asymptomatic but >3 risk factors for CAD excluding age and gender	Specialized evaluation recommended (e.g. exercise test for angina, echocardiography for murmur) Patient to be placed in high or low risk category, depending upon outcome of testing ED treatment can be initiated but exercise testing recommended to stratify risk
High risk	Severe or unstable or refractory angina Uncontrolled hypertension (SBP>180 mmHg) CHF (III, IV) Recent MI or CVA (i.e. within last 14 days) High risk arrhythmias Hypertrophic cardiomyopathy Moderate/severe valve disease	Refer for specialized cardiac evaluation and management Treatment for ED to be deferred until cardiac condition established and/or specialist evaluation completed

CAD, coronary artery disease; CHF, congestive heart failure, CVA, cerebral vascular accident; ED, erectile dysfunction; LVD, left ventricular dysfunction; MI, myocardial infarction; SBP, systolic blood pressure; TIA, transient ischemic attack

resumed. If the patient is deemed 'unfit' for sexual activity, once the cardiovascular condition has been effectively controlled, a graduated exercise program should be started and, using the same criteria, the patient's exercise tolerance re-assessed at a later date. Figure 3.3 quantifies the level of exertion (MET) associated with a range of daily activities and can be used to compare the current level of physical activity against that required during sexual intercourse.

Risk assessment summary

- Intercourse with an established partner equates to 2–3 METs with an upper range of 5–6 METs depending on how vigorous the activity is and the sexual positions adopted.
- 3–4 METs is equivalent to walking 1.5 km (1 mile) in 20 minutes on the level.
- The baseline risk from suffering an MI during normal daily life is extremely low and estimated to be in the region of one chance in a million for a healthy adult and 10 chances in a million per hour for a patient with pre-existing cardiovascular disease.[32]
- It has been estimated that the relative risk of triggering an MI occurring in the 2 hours

following sexual activity increases 2.5-fold above baseline in the non-cardiovascular patient and increases to approximately 30 chances in a million per hour for the 2 hours after sex in the cardiac patient.

- Overall in the general population, research suggests that sexual activity is a likely contributor to the onset of an MI in just less than 1% of cases and is 50% less in the physically fit.
- Antianginal therapy, such as beta-blockers may reduce the number of METs for a given degree of exercise by reducing the heart rate and blood pressure response to exertion.

Many patients with cardiovascular disease and ED (when it has been established they are suitable for treatment) may just want a 'quick fix' for their erection problems. However, a full assessment is necessary and crucial to identify the diseases, psychosocial factors and other risk factors that may cause or maintain ED. It is recommended a medical history should therefore be taken, focusing on risk factors such as cigarette smoking, hypertension, alcoholism, drug abuse, trauma and, where clinically initiated, endocrine problems including hypothyroidism, low testosterone levels and hyperprolactinaemia.

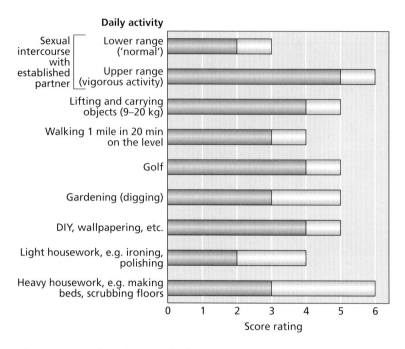

Figure 3.3 Daily activities with their corresponding MET score rating.

Oral therapy in men with ED and cardiovascular disease

Sildenafil citrate (Viagra™)

The most widely recognized and first-line treatment is sildenafil, a phosphodiesterase type 5 (PDE-5) inhibitor. This is based on extensive published literature demonstrating an efficacy and safety profile. Sildenafil shows improvements in erections in 70% of patients with ischemic heart disease, versus 20% on placebo.[33] The same efficacy is seen with hypertension.[34,35] Pelliccia et al[36] reported that sildenafil is well tolerated in patients with chronic stable angina whose symptoms and exercise test response are well controlled by beta-blocker therapy. In men with exercise-limiting angina, sildenafil can actually increase the duration of exercise before anginal pain is experienced.[37]

Efficacy

The clinical efficacy of sildenafil has been evaluated in more than 4400 men worldwide, aged 19–87 years. Twenty-one randomized placebo controlled trials all showed a statistically significant effect of sildenafil compared with placebo; the mean duration of ED in these patients (with mixed etiologies) was 5 years. The results of these trials showed that sildenafil is effective, in the presence of sexual stimulation, at restoring erectile function and improving intercourse rates in a wide spectrum of patients, including those with cardiovascular disease and in patients taking a wide variety of concomitant medications. Treatment-related improvements in erections were reported by 70–90% of patients receiving sildenafil compared with only 10–30% of patients receiving placebo.[38]

Goldstein et al[39] evaluated the efficacy of sildenafil in men with ED of organic, psychogenic or mixed causes. A 24-week double-blind, dose–response study was conducted in which 532 men were treated with sildenafil or placebo. Efficacy was assessed by changes in mean international index of erectile function (IIEF) scores for frequency of penetration and frequency of maintained erections. Each dose of sildenafil was significantly better than placebo (p < 0.001) and increasing doses of sildenafil were associated with improved erectile function.

Safety

Any side effects of sildenafil are usually mild and transient, dose-related and completely reversible when the drug is withdrawn. However, it is advisable to show caution with sildenafil, which is contraindicated in the presence of nitrate therapy, as some patients may not be aware they are taking nitrates and only recognize their drugs by trade names. Organic nitrates and nitric oxide donors promote vascular smooth muscle relaxation by the same cyclic guanosine monophosphate (cGMP) mechanism of vasodilation as endogenous nitric oxide (NO). Although sildenafil and nitrates act on different points in the NO–cGMP pathway, the hemodynamic effects of both agents result from increases in cGMP levels. Since sildenafil and nitrates both cause cGMP-induced vasodilation, taken together, a significant reduction in blood pressure can result.

There are two options for cardiovascular patients taking nitrates, in whom it is considered safe to resume sexual activity:

- As nitrates have no prognostic value, the patient could consider being transferred to an alternative anti-ischemic therapy. In most angina patients this is possible. If the patient is in any way a complex case, then the change in medication should be based on advice from a cardiologist.
- Suggest an alternative form of therapy for the ED, ensuring the patient/partner are counseled as to the medical reasoning behind this. Apomorphine may offer the best option when sildenafil is contraindicated (although caution is still advised), as the central mode of action is by stimulating postsynaptic dopamine receptors (D1 and D2) and not on the nitric pathway as with sildenafil. Apomorphine is given sublingually and is a powerful emetic, which explains some of the side effects.[40] It is effective only in mild cases of ED and success rates vary, but average 45% compared to placebo (35%). Because apomorphine addresses the central component, it will only be effective when the endothelial dysfunction is not severe.[41]

At present there are no official studies published on when sildenafil can be prescribed after a nitrate has been used, or when a nitrate can be given after sildenafil has been used. An official guide can be found in the American College of Cardiology (ACC)/American Heart Association (AHA) Expert Consensus Document which states that the administration of a nitrate may be considered 24 hours after a sildenafil dose, with the patient's

hemodynamic response carefully monitored.[42] A reasonable estimate would be that sildenafil could be prescribed 1 week after permanent discontinuation of a long-acting oral nitrate. However, this would not be appropriate if the patient's cardiovascular status had deteriorated.

Health care professionals should advise patients who are prescribed sildenafil that they should not keep nitrates in the house, to avoid any risks of taking these accidentally. As with all patients who experience activity-related angina, patients taking sildenafil who experience chest pain during sexual intercourse should be advised that they should stop the sexual activity and either sit or stand, as this reduces preload and can ease the symptoms in a similar way to nitrates. If their anginal symptoms do not quickly improve with rest, it should be seen as an emergency and medical advice should be sought immediately. Patients must be instructed to notify medical staff on presentation to the Emergency Room if sildenafil has been taken. Otherwise patients should consult their family doctor regarding their angina before attempting to have sex again.

Follow up
Regular review of cardiovascular status and ED response is recommended. This can improve patient/couple therapy compliance, confidence and technique and any emergent sexual or relationship issues. Regular follow up of cardiovascular patients being treated for ED provides an ideal and effective opportunity to address other cardiovascular risk factors and improve treatment outcomes.[43] Patients should be encouraged not to give up if their erections do not return with the initial treatment dose. Efficacy rates can be improved by nearly a third with effective patient follow up[44] focusing on advice and discussing concerns on how to best take treatments.

Alternative PDE-5s
Licenses for vardenafil and tadalafil have recently been approved in the United Kingdom and Europe. There are broad similarities in clinical efficacy between these and sildenafil. Also as with sildenafil, the side effects at this early stage appear to be mild and transient and include headaches and dyspepsia. Tadalafil and vardenafil exhibit a higher PDE-5:PDE-6 selectivity ratio than

sildenafil, which may reduce color vision changes. There is a low risk of facial flushing associated with use of tadalafil, but back pain and myalgia have been reported.[45]

The time to onset of effect differentiates tadalafil and vardenafil from sildenafil. In particular, vardenafil has a shorter mean time to maximum plasma concentration than both tadalafil and sildenafil. Dedicated onset-of-effect studies for all substances will establish whether this translates into a real advantage.[45]

Tadalafil has a longer plasma clearance half-life ($t_{1/2}$) than vardenafil and sildenafil after oral dosing. Although the half-life required for an optimal 'window of opportunity' remains a matter of discussion, a very long half-life may offer both advantages and disadvantages. The longer duration of action may enhance spontaneity of sexual activity, but the slower clearance may have safety implications,[45] especially in cardiovascular patients who are taking nitrate therapy, where the risk of concomitant use of the drug and nitrates is increased.

In the future, it will be important to investigate with clinical trials and real world experience, the differing profiles of treatments for ED, with particular regard to the onset and duration of action, and the role of foreplay in sexual activity. Important, however, is the potential to expand the use of PDE-5 inhibitors to increasing numbers of men with ED.

PDE-5s in the future

Studies currently being undertaken are investigating other benefits of PDE inhibitors for use in the future. However, although the following information outlines potential added benefits of ED treatment, there is currently no license for sildenafil to be used in these indications and the author cannot recommend the use of sildenafil for these indications.

Severe pulmonary hypertension

Severe pulmonary hypertension is a debilitating disease, which often affects young people. One of the current treatments is continuous intravenous administration of epoprostenol. This can be limited because side effects and infections are common, and the costs involved are high because of the long-term administration of the drug. Although sample sizes are currently quite small and long-term

observations lacking, initial studies have shown that sildenafil is a potent pulmonary vasodilator, which acts with inhaled iloprost to cause strong pulmonary vasodilation in both severe pulmonary arterial hypertension and chronic thromboembolic pulmonary hypertension.[46]

Effect on endothelial function

Another study found that acute and chronic low dose sildenafil treatment in type 2 diabetic patients had a favorable effect on endothelial function. This benefit of PDE-5 inhibition not only has implications for the treatment of ED, but also for the potential prevention of cardiovascular events in people with type 2 diabetes.[47]

ED prevention

PDEs may help to prevent ED developing in the first place. Preliminary studies have found that sildenafil taken at bedtime produces significantly improved nocturnal erectile activity. Night-time erections contribute to the maintenance of the morphodynamic integrity of smooth muscle cells within the corpora cavernosa, and so there may be the potential for medications to offer prevention of deterioration of the cavernosal smooth muscle and hence maintain erectile function. Further studies are needed to verify whether this initial finding may constitute the basis for the use of sildenafil as a means of preventing ED.[48]

Conclusions

- Risk factors associated with ED increase with age and overlap extensively with risk factors for cardiovascular disease.
- ED may be the first presenting symptom of a patient with previously undiagnosed cardiovascular disease. Health care professionals should proactively question patients about sexual function, affording the opportunity to identify and diagnose coexisting conditions, which can then be treated early. Furthermore ED can act as a marker for cardiovascular disease progression.
- The cardiac risk associated with sexual activity for stable cardiovascular patients is minimal following proper assessment. The majority of cardiovascular patients with ED can be effectively treated in primary care according to published guidelines.

Key considerations	New York Heart Association classification of congestive heart failure	
• A myocardial infarction or stroke can be triggered by exertion, anger, emotion or, more rarely, sexual activity but in many cases the trigger is unknown. No guarantees can be given that a person with pre-existing cardiovascular disease is 100% risk-free from suffering further cardiovascular adverse events in the short or long term, even with a normal exercise test or ECG. However, the objective is to minimize this risk, through appropriate risk assessment.	Class I	Patients with cardiac disease but with no limitation during ordinary physical activity
	Class II	Slight limitations caused by cardiac disease. Activity such as walking causes dyspnea
• It is recognized that an exercise ECG is likely to have been conducted as part of the standard management process for many post-MI or angina patients, while under specialist care. If the MI is recent (< 6 weeks) or if the health care professional is uncertain about symptom limitations, consideration should be given to further exercise testing.	Class III	Marked limitation; symptoms are provoked easily, e.g. by walking on the flat
	Class IV	Breathlessness at rest

• Many treatments are currently available and suitable for use in the cardiovascular patient; however sildenafil is the recommended first-line therapy in the majority of ED patients.

• Successful treatment is highly beneficial, as surveys have shown that nearly 90% of those men with ED who were treated successfully said it improved their life.

• In patients with a history of cardiovascular disease, sildenafil is effective in achieving and maintaining an erection. Sildenafil can be used in patients taking concurrent cardiovascular medications, with the exception of nitrate and nicorandil therapy, which are absolutely contraindicated with sildenafil.

The importance of sexual health to overall health is often overlooked by individuals, health care professionals and by society in general to the detriment of all. The impact sexual health has on a person's overall well-being, especially the cardiovascular patient, can no longer be dismissed – it is as important as diet and exercise.[1]

References

1. Pfizer. The Pfizer global study of sexual attitudes and behaviours. New York: Pfizer Inc.; 2002.
2. Market and Opinion Research International (MORI). Attitudes towards erectile dysfunction: a survey of men aged 40+. London: MORI; 1998.
3. Wagner G, Saenz de Tejada I. Update on male erectile dysfunction. BMJ 1998; 316:678–682.
4. Ayta IA, McKinlay JB, Krane RJ. The likely worldwide increase in erectile dysfunction between 1995 and 2025 and some possible policy consequences. BJU Int 1999; 84:50–56.
5. Sullivan ME, Thompson CS, Dashwood MR, et al. Nitric oxide and penile erection: is erectile dysfunction another manifestation of vascular disease? Cardiovasc Res 1999; 43:658–665.
6. Kirby M. Lipid management can reduce CHD in diabetes. Best Practice 2001; 31–32.
7. Feldman HA, Goldstein I, Hatzichristou DG, et al. Impotence and its medical and psychosocial correlates: results of the Massachusetts Male Aging Study. J Urol 1994; 151:54–61.
8. Feldman HA, Elias MF, Durante R, et al. Antihypertensives, heart medications, and erectile dysfunction: cross-sectional associations in a large random sample of Massachusetts men. Br J Urol 1997; 80:99.
9. Bortolotti A, Parazzini F, Colli E, Landoni M. The epidemiology of erectile dysfunction and its risk factors. Int J Androl 1997; 20:323–334.
10. Wabrek AJ, Burchell RC. Male sexual dysfunction associated with coronary heart disease. Arch Sex Behav 1980; 9:69–75.
11. Bulpitt CJ, Dollery CT, Carne S. Change in symptoms of hypertensive patients after referral to hospital clinic. Br Heart J 1976; 38:121–128.
12. United Nations. World population prospects: the 1996 revision. New York: United Nations; 1997.
13. Zurowski K, Kayne H, Goldstein I. The social and behavioral costs of organic impotence. Baltimore: American Urological Association; 1994.
14. Fugl-Meyer AR, Lodnert G, Branholm IB, Fugl-Meyer KS. On life satisfaction in male erectile dysfunction. Int J Impot Res 1997; 9:141–148.
15. Litwin MS, Nied RJ, Dhanani N. Health-related quality of life in men with erectile dysfunction. J Gen Intern Med 1998; 13:159–166.
16. Jonler M, Moon T, Brannan W, et al. The effect of age, ethnicity and geographical location on impotence and quality of life. Br J Urol 1995; 75:651–655.
17. Carroll JL, Bagley DH. Evaluation of sexual satisfaction in partners of men experiencing erectile failure. J Sex Marital Ther 1990; 16:70–78.
18. McCarthy P, Thoburn M. Psychosexual therapy at RELATE: a report on cases processed between 1992 and 1994. Rugby, Warwickshire: RELATE Center for Family Studies and RELATE Marriage Guidance; 1996.
19. Impotence Association Survey. London: Conducted by Taylor Nelson AGB Healthcare; 1997.
20. Catalan J, Hawton K, Day A. Couples referred to a sexual

dysfunction clinic: psychological and physical morbidity. Br J Psychiatry 1990; 156:61–67.

21. Impotence Association Survey. London: 2000 and 2001.

22. Baldwin KC, Ginsberg PC, Harkaway RC. Underreporting of erectile dysfunction among men with unrelated urologic conditions. Abstract presented at Annual Meeting of the American Urological Association, Atlanta, 2000.

23. Curkendall SM, Jones JK, Glassier D, Goehring E. Incidence of medically detected erectile dysfunction and related diseases before and after Viagra (sildenafil citrate) [Abstract 324]. Eur Urol 2000; 37(suppl 2):81.

24. Heart disease – a global perspective. http://www.healthpromotion.ie/hearts/ change_of_heart/global.html.

25. Greenstein A, Chen J, Miller H, et al. Does severity of ischemic coronary disease correlate with erectile function? Int J Impot Res 1997; 9:123–126.

26. Tiefer L, Meleman A. Interviews of wives: a necessary adjunct in the evaluation of impotence. Sex Disabil 1983; 6:167–175.

27. Management of stable angina pectoris. Recommendations of the Task Force of the European Society of Cardiology. Eur Heart J 1997; 18:394–413.

28. Feldman HA, McKinlay JB, Durante R, et al. Erectile dysfunction, cardiovascular disease, and cardiovascular risk factors. Br J Urol 1997; 80:90.

29. Ebrahim S, May M, Schlomo BY, et al. Sexual intercourse and risk of ischemic stoke and coronary heart disease: the Caerphilly study. J Epidemiol Community Health 2002; 56:99–102.

30. Jackson G, Betteridge J, Dean J, et al. A systematic approach to erectile dysfunction in the cardiovascular patient: a consensus statement – update 2002. Int J Clin Pract 2002; 56:663–671.

31. Wilson PK, Farday PS, Froelicher V, eds. Cardiac rehabilitation: adult fitness and exercise testing. Philadelphia: Lea & Febiger; 1981.

32. Müller JE, Mittleman A, Maclure M, et al and the Determinants of Myocardial Infarction Onset Study Investigators. Triggering myocardial infarction by sexual activity. Low absolute risk and prevention by regular physical exertion. JAMA 1996; 275:1405–1409.

33. Conti CR, Pepine CJ, Sweeney M. Efficacy and safety of sildenafil citrate in the treatment of erectile dysfunction in patients with ischemic heart disease. Am J Cardiol 1999; 83:29C–34C.

34. Price D and the Sildenafil Study Group. Sildenafil citrate (Viagra) efficacy in the treatment of erectile dysfunction in patients with common concomitant conditions. Int J Clin Pract 1999; 102(suppl):21–23.

35. Kloner RA, Brown M, Prisant LM, Collins M and the Sildenafil Study Group. Effect of sildenafil in patients with erectile dysfunction taking antihypertensive therapy. Am J Hypertens 2001; 14:70–73.

36. Pelliccia F, et al. Effects of phosphodiesterase-5 inhibition on myocardial ischemia in patients with chronic stable angina in therapy with beta-blockers. J Am Coll Cardiol 2000; 35:339.

37. Fox KM, Thadani U, Ma PTS, et al. Time to onset of limiting angina during treadmill exercise in men with erectile dysfunction and stable chronic angina: effect of sildenafil citrate. Circulation 2001; 104:II601–II602.

38. Osterloh I. Update on the efficacy and safety of Viagra. VII International Symposium of Andrology, Palma, Mallorca, 2000.

39. Goldstein I, Lue TF, Padma-Nathan H, et al. Oral sildenafil in the treatment of erectile dysfunction. N Engl J Med 1998; 338:1397–1404.

40. Lue TF. Erectile dysfunction. N Engl J Med 2000; 342:1622–1626.

41. Jackson G. Cardiovascular safety in erectile dysfunction treatment. Br J Diabetes Vascular Dis 2002; 2:301–304.

42. Cheitlin MD, Hutter AM Jr, Brindis RG, et al. ACC/AHA expert consensus document. Use of sildenafil (Viagra) in patients with cardiovascular disease. J Am Coll Cardiol 1999; 33:273–282.

43. Guay AT, Perez JB, Jacobson J, Newton RA. Efficacy and safety of sildenafil citrate for treatment of erectile dysfunction in a population with associated organic risk factors. J Androl 2002; 23:113.

44. Hatzichristou DG, Apostolidis A, Bekos A, et al. Sildenafil failures may be due to inadequate instructions and follow-up: a study on 100 non-responders. 4th Congress of the European Society for Sexual and Impotence Research (ESSIR), Rome, 2001.

45. Snow KJ. Erectile dysfunction in patients with diabetes mellitus – advances in treatment with phosphodiesterase type 5 inhibitors. Br J Diabetes Vascular Dis 2002; 2:282–287.

46. Ghofrani HA, Wiedemann R, Rose F, et al. Combination therapy with oral sildenafil and inhaled iloprost for severe pulmonary hypertension. Ann Intern Med 2002; 136:515–522.

47. DeSouza C, Parulkar A, Lumpkin D, et al. Acute and chronic effects of low dose sildenafil on endothelial function in type 2 diabetes. 61st Scientific Sessions of the American Diabetes Association; 2001:50.

48. Montorsi F, Maga T, Strambi LF, et al. Sildenafil taken at bedtime significantly increases nocturnal erections: results of a placebo-controlled study. Urology 2000; 56:906–911.

4

Management of female sexual dysfunction

Ricardo Munarriz, Noel N Kim, Rachel Pauls, Abdul Traish and Irwin Goldstein

Introduction

Well-designed, random-sample, community-based epidemiologic investigations of women with sexual dysfunction are limited. Current data reveal that up to 76% of women have some type of sexual dysfunction.[1,2] US population census data suggest that approximately 10 million American women aged 50–74 self-report complaints of diminished vaginal lubrication, pain and discomfort with intercourse, decreased arousal and difficulty achieving orgasm. Recently, Laumann et al[3] found that sexual dysfunction is more prevalent in women (43%) than in men (31%) and is associated with various psychodemographic characteristics such as age, education, and poor physical and emotional health. More importantly, female sexual dysfunction is associated with negative sexual relationship experiences. Despite the high prevalence of sexual dysfunction in women, there are very few centers worldwide that practice a comprehensive and multidisciplinary investigation and management of sexual dysfunction in women.

Management of patients with female sexual dysfunction begins with the identification and diagnosis of the problem relationships and is based on the patient self-report in conjunction with a clinical evaluation. Sexual dysfunction in women is defined as disorders of sexual desire, arousal, orgasm and/or sexual pain, which results in significant personal distress and may have an impact on the quality of life. Although each specific condition can be separately defined in medical terms, clinically there is significant overlap in afflicted patients. The Report of the International Consensus Development Conference on Female Sexual Dysfunction classified female sexual dysfunction into:

I. Sexual desire disorders:

IA. *Hypoactive sexual desire disorder*, which is the persistent or recurrent deficiency (or absence) of sexual fantasies/thoughts, and/or desire for, or receptivity to, sexual activity, which causes personal distress.

IB. *Sexual aversion disorder*, which is the persistent or recurrent phobic aversion to and avoidance of sexual contact with a sexual partner, which causes personal distress.

II. Sexual arousal disorder:

Sexual arousal disorder is the persistent or recurrent inability to attain or maintain sufficient sexual excitement, causing personal distress. It may be expressed as a lack of subjective excitement or a lack of genital (lubrication/swelling) or other somatic responses.

III. Orgasmic disorder:

Orgasmic disorder is the persistent or recurrent difficulty, delay in, or absence of attaining orgasm following sufficient sexual stimulation and arousal, which causes personal distress.

IV. Sexual pain disorders:

IVA. *Dyspareunia* is recurrent or persistent genital pain associated with sexual intercourse.

IVB. *Vaginismus* is recurrent or persistent involuntary spasm of the musculature of the outer third of the vagina that interferes with vaginal penetration, which causes personal distress.

IVC. *Non-coital sexual pain disorder* is recurrent or persistent genital pain induced by non-coital sexual stimulation.

Each of these diagnoses may be subtyped as: A. lifelong vs acquired type; B. generalized vs situational type; C. etiologic origin (organic, psychogenic, mixed, unknown).[4]

In some cases, it may be necessary for physicians to carefully enquire about sexual functioning, paying special attention to the sensitivity of the topic and to the patient's comfort levels. Validated sexual questionnaires, such as the Female Sexual

Function Index and the Sexual Distress Scale may be helpful tools in the evaluation of sexual function. The cornerstone of the patient evaluation is a comprehensive and detailed sexual, medical and psychosocial history, physical examination and focused laboratory testing. Specialized diagnostic tests such as biothesiometry or genital vascular studies (duplex Doppler ultrasound, although not always indicated, may corroborate the impressions discovered on the initial evaluation). It should be stressed that the secondary psychologic reaction to these organic factors must not be ignored.

Anatomy and physiology of genital sexual arousal

There is a paucity of data concerning the anatomy, physiology and pathophysiology of sexual function in women. The female external genitalia consist of various structures. The vagina is a midline cylindrical organ that connects the uterus with the external genitalia. The vaginal wall consists of three layers:

- an inner *mucous* type stratified squamous cell epithelium supported by a thick lamina propria, that undergoes hormone-related cyclical changes
- the *muscularis* composed of outer longitudinal smooth muscle fibers and inner circular fibers
- an *outer fibrous layer*, rich in collagen and elastin, which provides structural support to the vagina.

The vulva, bounded by the symphysis pubis, the anal sphincter and the ischial tuberosities, consists of labial formations, the interlabial space, and erectile tissue. The *labial formations* are two paired cutaneous structures:

- the *labia majora* are fatty folds covered by hair-bearing skin that fuse anteriorly with the mons veneris, or anterior prominence of the symphysis pubis, and posteriorly with the perineal body or posterior commissure
- the *labia minora* are smaller folds covered by non-hairy skin laterally and by vaginal mucosa medially, that fuse anteriorly to form the prepuce of the clitoris, and posteriorly in the fossa navicularis.

The *interlabial space* is composed of the vestibule, the urinary meatus and vaginal opening and is bounded by the space medial to the labia minora, the fossa navicularis and the clitoris. The clitoris is a 7–13 mm Y-shaped organ comprised of glans, body and crura.[5] The body of the clitoris is surrounded by tunica albuginea and consists of two paired corpora cavernosa composed of trabecular smooth muscle and lacunar sinusoids. finally, the vestibular bulb consists of paired structures located beneath the skin of the labia minora and represents the homolog of the corpus spongiosum in the male.

There is limited understanding of the precise location of autonomic neurovascular structures related to the uterus, cervix and vagina. Uterine nerves arise from the inferior hypogastric plexus formed by the union of hypogastric nerves (sympathetic T10–L1) and the splanchnic fibers (parasympathetic S2–S4). This plexus has three portions: vesical plexus, the rectal plexus and the uterovaginal plexus (Frankenhauser's ganglion), which lies at the base of the broad ligament, dorsal to the uterine vessels, and lateral to the uterosacral and cardinal ligaments. This plexus provides innervation via the cardinal and uterosacral ligaments to the cervix, upper vagina, urethra, vestibular bulbs and clitoris. At the cervix, sympathetic and parasympathetic nerves form the paracervical ganglia. The larger one is called the uterine cervical ganglion. It is at this level that injury to the autonomic fibers of the vagina, labia and cervix may occur during hysterectomy. The pudendal nerve (S2–S4) reaches the perineum through Alcock's canal and provides sensory and motor innervation to the external genitalia.

Large gaps exist in our knowledge of how the central nervous system controls female sexual function. Limited data suggest that descending supraspinal modulation of female genital reflexes emanates from:

- brainstem structures such as the nucleus paragigantocellularis (inhibitory via serotonin), locus ceruleus (norepinephrine, nocturnal engorgement during rapid eye movement (REM) sleep) and midbrain periaqueductal gray
- hypothalamic structures such as the medial preoptic area, ventromedial nucleus and paraventricular nucleus
- forebrain structures such as the amygdala.

Multiple factors interact at the supraspinal levels to influence the excitability of spinal sexual reflexes such as: gonadal hormones; genital sensory information via the mylenated spinothalamic pathway and the unmyelinated spinoreticular pathway; and input from higher cortical centers of cognition.

The sexual arousal responses of the multiple genital and non-genital peripheral anatomic structures are largely the product of spinal cord reflex mechanisms. The spinal segments are under descending excitatory and inhibitory control from multiple supraspinal sites. The afferent reflex arm is primarily via the pudendal nerve. The efferent reflex arm consists of coordinated somatic and autonomic activity. One spinal sexual reflex is the bulbo-cavernosus reflex involving sacral cord segments S2, 3 and 4 in which pudendal nerve stimulation results in pelvic floor muscle contraction. Another spinal sexual reflex involves vaginal and clitoral cavernosal autonomic nerve stimulation resulting in clitoral, labial and vaginal engorgement.

In the basal state, clitoral corporal and vaginal smooth muscles are under contractile tone. Following sexual stimulation, neurogenic and endothelial release of nitric oxide (NO) plays an important role in clitoral cavernosal artery and helicine arteriolar smooth muscle relaxation.[5] This leads to a rise in clitoral cavernosal artery inflow, an increase in clitoral intracavernosal pressure, and clitoral engorgement. The result is extrusion of the glans clitoris and enhanced sensitivity.

In the basal state, the vaginal epithelium reabsorbs sodium from the submucosal capillary plasma transudate. Following sexual stimulation, a number of neurotransmitters including NO and vasoactive intestinal peptide (VIP) are released modulating vaginal vascular and non-vascular smooth muscle relaxation. Dramatic increase in capillary inflow in the submucosa overwhelms Na-reabsorption leading to 3–5 ml of vaginal transudate, enhancing lubrication essential for pleasurable coitus. Vaginal smooth muscle relaxation results in increased vaginal length and luminal diameter, especially in the distal two-thirds of the vagina. Vasoactive intestinal polypeptide is a non-adrenergic, non-cholinergic neurotransmitter that plays a role in enhancing vaginal blood flow, lubrication and secretions.[6]

In vivo animal studies

Data derived from in vivo animal models indicate that estrogen but not androgens modulate genital blood flow, vaginal lubrication and vaginal tissue structural integrity. It should be noted that estradiol levels used in these studies were supraphysiologic with potential pharmacologic effects different from those achieved physiologically.[7–12] Although estrogen replacement increases vaginal lubrication and restores vaginal epithelial integrity, this therapy may not be appropriate for all patients, due to associated risk of breast and endometrial cancer.

Limited data are available on the effects of vasoactive substances on genital hemodynamics. Park et al[10] demonstrated that injection of papaverine hydrochloride and phentolamine mesylate into the vaginal spongy muscularis layer increased vaginal wall pressure and vaginal blood flow. We have shown that sildenafil administration caused significant increase in genital blood flow and vaginal lubrication in intact and ovariectomized animals.[13] However, this response was more pronounced in animals treated with estradiol. These data suggested that the nitric oxide–cyclic guanosine monophosphate (NO–cGMP) pathway is involved, at least in part, in the physiologic mechanism of female genital arousal and that sildenafil facilitates this response in an in vivo animal model.[14] The effects of apomorphine, a non-selective dopamine receptor agonist, on genital blood flow were investigated by Tarcan et al[15] who suggested that systemic administration of apomorphine improved clitoral and vaginal engorgement by increasing clitoral intracavernosal and vaginal wall arterial inflow.

In summary, data derived from in vivo animal models indicate that vasoactive agents play a role in genital arousal. Although sildenafil and apomorphine enhanced genital blood flow in the animal model, clinical use of vasoactive agents remains controversial.

Organ bath studies

Data reported from several laboratories suggest that NO is a key pathway in mediating clitoral smooth muscle relaxation.[16,17] However, in the vagina, NO appears to play only a partial role in mediating smooth muscle relaxation.[18] VIP also induces vaginal smooth muscle relaxation yet its exact functional role remains to be determined.[19–23] Functional alpha-adrenergic receptors are expressed in the vagina and mediate norepinephrine-induced contraction.[24–26] We have observed that androgens but not estrogens at pharmacologic doses enhance smooth muscle relaxation.[27] Further studies with hormonal manipulations at physiologic doses are necessary to establish the role of hormones on vaginal smooth muscle relaxation.

Cell culture studies

Park et al[28] and Traish et al[29] recently subcultured and characterized human and rabbit vaginal and clitoral smooth muscle cells and investigated the synthesis of second messenger cyclic nucleotides in response to vasodilators and determined the activity and kinetics of phosphodiesterase (PDE) type 5. These studies suggest that cultured human and rabbit vaginal smooth muscle cells retained their metabolic functional integrity and this experimental system should prove useful in investigating the signaling pathways that modulate vaginal smooth muscle tone. Investigation of the distribution of nitric oxide synthase (NOS) in the rat vagina in response to ovariectomy and estrogen replacement was recently performed using immunohistochemical analyses with n-NOS and e-NOS antibodies.[30] Estrogen replacement resulted in significant increase in e-NOS and n-NOS expression, when compared with NOS in intact animals. It was suggested that estrogen plays a critical role in regulating vaginal NOS expression of the rat vagina and that NO may modulate both vaginal blood supply and vaginal smooth musculature.

More recent studies have shown the opposite observation. They found that rabbit vaginal NOS activity was considerably reduced by treatment with estradiol or estradiol and progesterone.[31,32] This discrepancy in NOS regulation by estrogen in these studies may be due to species differences or to methods for assessment of NOS expression and activity. We have used both immunochemical (Western blots) and enzymatic activity assays to determine regulation of vaginal NOS in the rabbit model. In this study we demonstrated that nitric oxide synthase was predominantly expressed in the proximal vagina.[33] The reason for this tissue distribution is yet to be determined. We further observed that ovariectomy enhanced NOS activity in the proximal vagina, suggesting specific regulation of NOS by sex steroid hormones. Treatment of ovariectomized animals with estrogens resulted in decreased expression and activity of NOS in vaginal tissue, consistent with the research by Al-

Hijji et al.[31] In contrast, treatment of ovariectomized animals with androgens resulted in increased NOS expression and activity. These observations suggest that NOS in vaginal tissue is regulated by androgens and estrogens in an opposite manner.

Sexual, medical and psychosocial history

A detailed and comprehensive sexual history should include past and present assessment of sexual desire (libido), arousal and orgasmic capabilities. In addition to physiologic sexual responses, overall sexual satisfaction should also be assessed.

The medical history should include focused questions on the patient's chronic/medical illness (e.g. diabetes, anemia, renal failure), neurologic illness (e.g. spinal cord injury, multiple sclerosis, lumbosacral disc disease), endocrinologic illness (e.g. hypogonadism, hyperprolactinemia, thyroid disorders), atherosclerotic vascular risk factors (e.g. hypercholesterolemia, hypertension, diabetes, smoking, family history), medications/recreational drug use (e.g. antihypertensives, antidepressants, alcohol, cocaine), pelvic/perineal/genital trauma (e.g. bicycling injury), genital pain (Table 4.1), surgical (e.g. hysterectomy, laminectomy, vascular bypass surgery) and psychiatric history (e.g. depression, anxiety).

Given the personal, interpersonal, social and occupational implications of sexual problems, a brief psychosocial history is mandatory in every patient. Current psychologic state, self-esteem,

Table 4.1 Etiology of genital/sexual pain

Superficial or external	Deep or internal

Infectious/inflammatory:
  Genital herpes
  Sexually transmitted diseases
  Recurrent vaginal infections
  Vestibular adenitis
	Endometriosis
	Uterine fibromas
	Ovarian cyst and tumors
	Adhesions
	Pelvic inflammatory disease

Tumors:
  Neuroma
  Fibroepithelial polyp
  Inclusion cysts
  Papillomas
  Melanoma
  Squamous cell carcinoma	

Genital myofascial pain syndrome	
Vaginismus	

history of sexual trauma/abuse as well as past and present relationships and social and occupational performance should be addressed.

Physical examination

In addition to a detail vascular and neurologic examination, a careful and systematic examination of the external genitalia using magnifying surgical loops and Q-tip evaluation of the external genitalia may confirm aspects of the medical history (e.g. vestibular adenitis (Fig. 4.1a) and neuropathies), and occasionally reveal unsuspected physical findings such as paraclitoral neuromas (Fig. 4.1b).

Laboratory testing

Laboratory testing is strongly recommended. Standard serum chemistries, complete blood count and lipid profiles may elucidate vascular risk factors such as hypercholesterolemia, diabetes, and renal failure. Serum thyroid-stimulating hormone (TSH) determination may be indicated in select cases.

The integrity of the hypothalamic–pituitary–gonadal axis should be examined in every patient with sexual dysfunction. Adrenal and ovarian androgens, estrogens and follicle-stimulating hormone (FSH) and luteinizing hormone (LH) testing are strongly recommended. It is unclear which testosterone assay (total, free, bioavailable) is the best; however there is a consensus that at least one of these assays should be performed. Total androgen production is best reflected by the total testosterone, but the available testosterone is best measured by free testosterone value, as determined by equilibrium dialysis. Whenever total or free testosterone is measured, the value of circulating sex hormone binding globulin (SHBG) has to be taken into consideration. To evaluate adrenal androgen status, it is recommended that dehydroepiandrosterone sulphate (DHEA-S) levels be obtained. Androgen values should be ideally determined in the morning and in the mid-third of the menstrual cycle, but this recommendation makes clinical practice extremely difficult.

Although pituitary adenomas are a rare cause of sexual dysfunction, this potentially life-threatening disease and reversible cause of sexual dysfunction should not be forgotten.

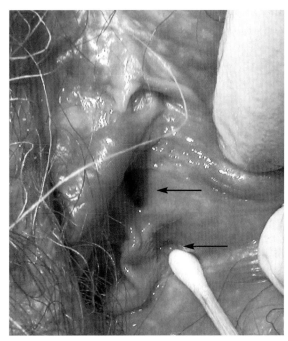

(a)

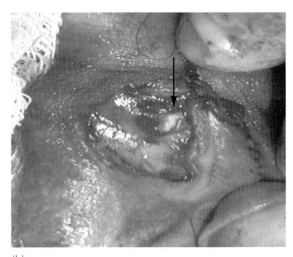

(b)

Figure 4.1 (a) Vestibular adenitis. (b) Paraclitoral neuroma.

Patient/partner education

Patient and partner education is a critical component in the diagnosis of female sexual dysfunction and should be carried out whenever possible. The results of the history, physical examination, laboratory testing, and the need for additional diagnostic testing should be reviewed in detail with the patient and her partner and, if indicated, appropriate referrals should be made. Patient and partner education not only facilitates physician–patient–partner communication, but also enhances patient compliance and treatment adherence.

Specialized diagnostic testing

Diagnostic modalities such as duplex Doppler ultrasound, vaginal and clitoral temperature, vibration sensory testing and selective pudendal arteriogram expand physician and patient understanding of the pathophysiologic mechanisms, but disadvantages such as invasiveness, cost, the associated risks and complications, and lack of normative data have limited the use of specialized testing.

Vaginal and clitoral warm, cold and vibratory sensory thresholds can be reliably measured with a thermal sensory analyzer/vibratory sensory analyzer system (TSA-3000 and VSA-3000; Medoc, Israel) and compared to currently available validated normograms, allowing quantitative neurologic assessment of the female genitalia.[34] This non-invasive valuable diagnostic tool has proved helpful in the management of women with sexual dysfunction.

Non-invasive vascular testing of women with sexual dysfunction has been reported by several investigators. These include vaginal photoplethysmography and genital duplex Doppler ultrasound.

Vaginal photoplethysmography

Vaginal photoplethysmography, the most widely used vascular testing technique, measures vaginal mucosal engorgement and vaginal blood volumes, providing quantitative data on the extent of vaginal vasocongestion.[31–34] The major drawbacks of this diagnostic tool are that it provides arbitrary rather than absolute units of measurement. In addition, it is susceptible to subject movement artifact and baseline drift.

Duplex Dopper ultrasound

The role of duplex Doppler ultrasonography in the management of women with sexual dysfunction remains to be determined. Although several investigators have reported small patient series using duplex Doppler ultrasound before and after stimulation (visual and vibratory) as a diagnostic

tool in females with sexual dysfunction, there is no standardized ultrasonographic technique to maximize diagnostic information. We routinely obtained volumetric and hemodynamic data before and after audiovisual sexual stimulation by placing an 11 MHz small parts probe on the side of the clitoris. Clitoral shaft diameter (Fig. 4.2a) is measured from the medial tunica albuginea of the corporal body across the septum to the lateral tunica albuginea of the contralateral corporal body. The angle of the clitoral shaft formed by the suspensory ligament is the sonographic landmark used for volumetric measurements. Maintaining this sonographic landmark, the small parts probe is then swept laterally to evaluate the hypoechoic, ill-defined, carrot-shaped corpus spongiosum that possesses a thin, occasionally visualized tunica, and a corpus spongiosum diameter is measured (Fig. 4.2b). Hemodynamic data (peak systolic, end diastolic and resistive index values) from the corpus spongiosum and cavernosal arteries are measured (Fig. 4.2c,d). We have found that the increase in pre- and postarousal clitoral and corpus spongiosum diameters directly correlated with an increase in both the pre- and postarousal clitoral and corpus spongiosum end diastolic velocity values, suggesting that end diastolic velocity values have an important physiologic implication as a direct determinant of genital engorgement. One of the limitations of the current ultrasonographic methodology is the lack of standardized use of topical vasoactive agents to maximize genital smooth muscle relaxation. Several investigators are performing genital duplex Doppler ultrasounds before and after audiovisual sexual stimulation in combination with topical application of 2% alprostadil with more consistent hemodynamic and volumetric data.[35,36]

Indications for referral

Physicians with appropriate training in sexual medicine should manage the vast majority of women with sexual dysfunction. However, there are several indications for referrals:

- Young patients with history of pelvic/perineal trauma
- Patients with anorgasmia due to traumatic pudendal neuropathy or hysterectomy

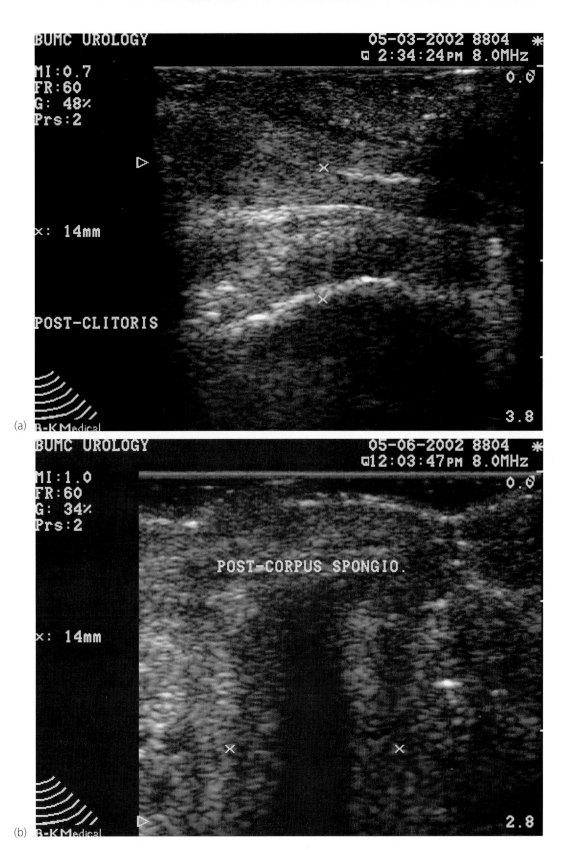

Figure 4.2 Clitoral and spongiosal volumetric and hemodynamic changes.

Continued

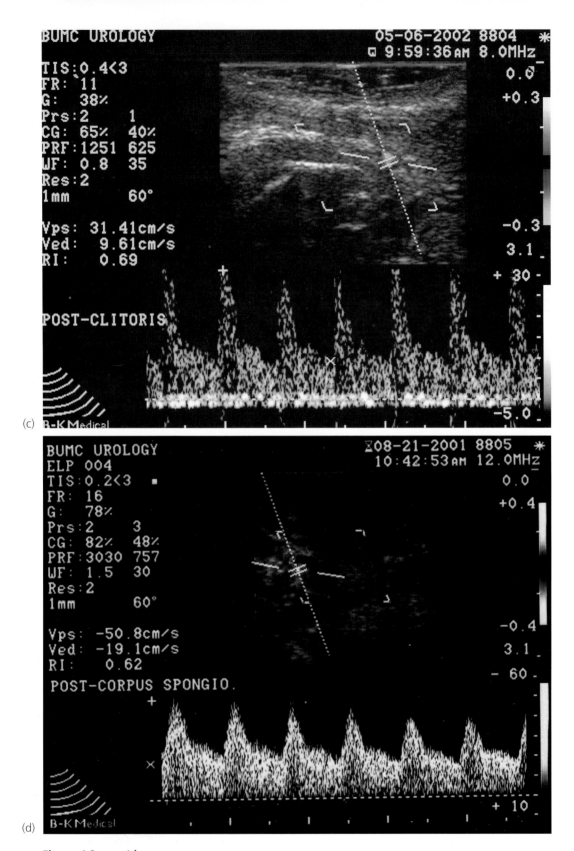

Figure 4.2, cont'd.

- Patients with genital pain due to neuromas, vestibular adenitis myofascial pain syndrome, etc.
- Patients with aortic aneurysm or bulbosacral disc disease that requires vascular or neurosurgical intervention
- Patients with complicated endocrinopathies
- Patients with complicated psychiatric or psychosexual disorders (e.g. refractory depression, transsexualism)
- Patient or physician request for specialized evaluation
- Medicolegal reasons (occupational or iatrogenic injuries).

Modifying reversible causes

Health care professionals should work with patients to modify reversible causes of female sexual dysfunction (FSD), such as psychogenic FSD, hormonal imbalances, hyperprolactinemia, specific drug-related FSD (e.g. selective serotonin reuptake inhibitors, SSRIs), vascular or neurologic sexual dysfunction secondary to blunt perineal trauma and anorgasmia due to pudendal neuropathy.

Sex steroid hormones

The role of sex steroid hormones in reproductive function has been extensively investigated and has significantly contributed to successful clinical management of women with infertility by sex hormones or hormone analogs. However, the role of sex steroid hormones in regulating vaginal arousal has been poorly investigated.

At present, there is no rationale for pharmacologic management of women with sexual dysfunction by sex hormones or hormone analogs. Bachmann et al[37] reported that estrogen deficiency associated with the postmenopausal state results in loss of collagen and adipose tissue in the vulva, attenuated maturation of vaginal epithelial cells, thinning and loss of elasticity of the vaginal wall with loss of premenopausal ridges, bleeding and ulceration of the vaginal epithelium after minor trauma, delayed onset of lubrication with sexual stimulation, and an increase in vaginal pH leading to heightened vulnerability to urogenital pathogens and flora. Sarrel[38–40] reported that women with plasma estradiol levels less than 50 pg/ml had significantly more complaints of vaginal dryness, frequency and intensity of dyspareunia and burning compared to women with estradiol values greater than 50 pg/ml. Several investigators have shown that treatment with estradiol increases vaginal blood flow and lubrication, improves epithelial maturation indices, normalizes vaginal pH, and prevents vaginal atrophy.[38,41,42]

Androgen insufficiency, in women who are adequately estrogenized, is also associated with sexual dysfunction.[39,43–45] Androgen replacement in women with sexual dysfunction is associated with changes in the external genitalia including increased sensitivity, engorgement and hypertrophy of the clitoris and vulvar hyperemia.[46–48] It has been reported that women with higher levels of testosterone had significantly greater levels of vaginal blood flow responses to erotic stimuli compared to those with lower levels of testosterone.[49,50] Exogenous administration of androgens has resulted in a significant increase in subjective ratings of sexual arousal in postmenopausal women.[51] In oophorectomized women treated with testosterone, those who had a higher ratio of testosterone to sex hormone binding globulin had higher sexual arousal.[43] Shifren et al[52] have shown that transdermal testosterone improved sexual function and psychologic well-being in women who had undergone oophorectomy and hysterectomy. Arlt et al[53] have shown that treatment of women with adrenal insufficiency with dehydroepiandrosterone (DHEA) improved overall well-being and sexual function. Munarriz et al[54] have shown that androgen replacement therapy with DHEA in women with sexual dysfunction and androgen insufficiency significantly decreased sexual distress, significantly increased sexual function in the domains of desire, arousal, lubrication, satisfaction and orgasm, and normalized androgen blood levels to values within the physiologic range.

Hyperprolactinemia

The treatment of hyperprolactinemia in women with sexual dysfunction consist of: the cessation of medication causing hyperprolactinemia (e.g. estrogens, alpha methyldopa); the administration of bromocriptine; or the surgical ablation or extirpation of a pituitary prolactin-secreting tumor.

Iatrogenic/drug-induced FSD

Psychotropic agents such as SSRIs, neuroleptics and antipsychotics have been associated with sexual dysfunction in women. In addition, luteinizing hormone-releasing hormone (LHRH) agonists and antiandrogens, commonly used in the treatment of endometriosis, infertility and uterine fibromas, are also associated with sexual dysfunction.

Psychogenic factors

Patients with destructive behaviors, alcoholism, cigarette smoking, and recreational drug use, should be counseled on the potential etiologic role of these factors in FSD.

Genital pain

Genital pain is a highly prevalent (14%), incapacitating and devastating condition associated with significant personal distress and diminished quality of life. Genital neuromas and vestibular adenitis may be successfully treated by excision of the affected area.

First-line therapy

First-line interventions, characterized by ease of administration, reversibility, non-invasive nature, and low cost, include oral erectogenic agents (e.g. sildenafil, apomorphine, oral phentolamine), vacuum erection devices, and psychosexual or couples therapy.

Oral vasoactive agents
Sildenafil

The introduction of sildenafil in 1998 revolutionized the management of men with erectile dysfunction[38] and empowered women with sexual dysfunction to seek medical attention. This potent and selective PDE-5 inhibitor, which blocks the hydrolysis of cGMP, enhances the accumulation of cGMP, and potentiates the relaxant effects of NO in the clitoris, it is not currently approved by the US Food and Drug Administration (FDA) for use in women. Sildenafil has been utilized in the treatment of women with sexual arousal disorders with mixed results.[55,56] Clinical studies evaluating efficacy and safety of this drug in women are currently in progress.

Phentolamine

Phentolamine is an alpha-1 and -2 adrenergic antagonist which decreases adrenergic tone, thus facilitating vasocongestion and delaying detumes-

cence. A pilot (single dose of oral phentolamine (40 mg) and placebo in a single-blind, dose-escalation) study of six postmenopausal women with a lack of lubrication and sexual arousal difficulties reported a mild, positive effect across all measures of arousal, with significant changes in self-reported lubrication and pleasurable sensations in the vagina.[57] Interestingly, Rubio-Aurioles et al[58] showed that physiologic readings and subjective reports were significantly different from placebo in the women using estrogen replacement therapy with 40 mg of phentolamine in vaginal solution. Further studies are needed to assess the potential value of phentolamine and other vasoactive agents in the treatment of female sexual dysfunction.

Apomorphine

Apomorphine is a central dopamine agonist known to induce mild to moderate penile erection in men. Its use in women with sexual dysfunction is experimental.

Prostaglandin E-1

The simplicity, non-invasiveness, and safety of topical administration of vasoactive agents are ideal for the treatment of women with sexual dysfunction. Preliminary reports on the use of topical alprostadil are encouraging, but further research is needed before this can be established as a first-line therapy agent.[59]

Vacuum devices

At the present time, EROS therapy is the only FDA-approved treatment of women with sexual dysfunction. EROS therapy is designed to increase blood flow to the clitoris facilitating clitoral engorgement and enhancing peripheral genital sexual arousal. It is generally accepted that clitoral stimulation and engorgement are important aspects of female sexual arousal. It is believed that the difficulty or inability to achieve maximal clitoral tumescence may be related to and associated with other symptoms of female sexual arousal disorder.[10]

During use in women with sexual arousal or orgasmic disorders, the EROS device is placed over the clitoris, providing three levels of gentle vacuum suction (low, medium, high). The postulated increase in blood flow to the clitoris is associated with increased sensation and enhanced sexual arousal including increased vaginal lubrication and labial engorgement. In women with sexual arousal disorder, use of the EROS therapy device has been shown to improve sexual function and satisfaction.[60,61]

Sexual therapy: individual or couples

Sexual therapy addressing relationship distress, sexual performance concerns and dysfunctional communication patterns is likely to enhance sexual functioning. It is recommended to involve both patient and partner in the sexual therapy. Sexual therapy is also indicated and beneficial in patients or couples who desire to resume sexual activity after a prolonged period of abstinence. Lastly, sexual therapy is effective in addressing psychologic reactions to the medical or surgical treatment.

Second- and third-line therapies

Unfortunately, there are no second- or third-line therapies available for the management of women with sexual dysfunction.

Conclusion

Despite the high prevalence of sexual dysfunction in women, studies concerning the anatomy, physiology and pathophysiology of female sexual function and dysfunction are limited. A collaborative and comprehensive psychologic and medical evaluation, continuous patient and partner education, modification of reversible causes, and individualized pharmacotherapy are strongly recommended.

References

1. Frank E, Anderson C, Rubinstein D. Frequency of sexual dysfunction in normal couples. N Engl J Med 1978; 299:111–115.
2. Spector I, Carey M. Incidence and prevalence of the sexual dysfunction: a critical review of the empirical literature. Arch Sex Behav 1990; 19:389–408.
3. Laumann EO, Paik A, Rosen RC. Sexual dysfunction in the United States. Prevalence and predictors. JAMA 1999; 281(6):537–544.
4. Basson R, Berman J, Burnett A, et al. Report of the international consensus development conference on female sexual dysfunction: definitions and classifications. J Urol 2000; 163(3):888–893.
5. O'Connell H, Hutson J, Anderson C, Plenter R. Anatomic relationship between urethra and clitoris. J Urol 1998; 159(6):1892–1897.
6. Palle C, Bredkjaer HE, Ottesen B, Fahrenkrug J. Vasoactive intestinal polypeptide and human vaginal blood flow: comparison between transvaginal and intravenous administration. J Clin Exp Pharm Physiol 1990; 17:61–68.
7. Giuliano F, Allard J, Compaigne S, et al. Vaginal physiological changes in a model of arousal in anesthetized rats. Am J Physiol Regul Integr Comp Physiol 2001; 281:R140–149.
8. Min K, O'Connell L, Munarriz R, et al. Sex steroid hormone modulation of vaginal hemodynamics in the female rabbit model. Female Sexual Function Forum, 2001.
9. Min K, Munarriz R, Kim NN, et al. Effects of ovariectomy and estrogen replacement on basal and pelvic nerve stimulated vaginal lubrication in an animal model. J Sex Marital Ther 2002; (in press).
10. Park K, Goldstein I, Andry C, et al. Vasculogenic female sexual dysfunction: the hemodynamic basis for vaginal engorgement insufficiency and clitoral erectile insufficiency. Int J Impot Res 1997; 9:27–37.
11. Park K, Ahn K, Lee S, et al. Decreased circulating levels of estrogen alter vaginal and clitoral blood flow and structure in the rabbit. Int J Impot Res 2001; 13:116–124.
12. Vachon P, Simmerman N, Zahran AR, Carrier S. Increases in clitoral and vaginal blood flow following clitoral and pelvic plexus nerve stimulations in the female rat. Int J Impot Res 2000; 12(1):53–57.
13. Min K, Munarriz R, Berman J, et al. Hemodynamic evaluation of the female sexual arousal response in an animal model. J Sex Marital Ther 2001; 27:557–565.
14. Min K, Kim NN, McAuley I, et al. Sildenafil augments pelvic nerve-mediated female genital arousal in the anesthetized rabbit. Int J Impot Res 2000; 12(suppl 3):S32–39.
15. Tarcan T, Siroky MB, Park K, et al. Systemic administration of apomorphine improves the hemodynamic mechanism of clitoral and vaginal engorgement in the rabbit. Int J Impot Res 2000; 12(4):235–240.
16. Cellek S, Moncada S. Nitrergic neurotransmission mediates the non-adrenergic non-cholinergic responses in the clitoral corpus cavernosum of the rabbit. Br J Pharmacol 1998; 125:1627–1629.
17. Vemulapalli S, Kurowski S. Sildenafil relaxes rabbit clitoral corpus cavernosum. Life Sci 2000; 67:23–29.
18. Ziessen T, Moncada S, Cellek S. Characterization of the non-nitrergic NANC relaxation responses in the rabbit vaginal wall. Br J Pharmacol 2002; 135:546–554.
19. Levin RJ. VIP, vagina, clitoral and periurethral glans – an update on human female genital arousal. Exp Clin Endocrinol 1991; 98:61–69.
20. Ottesen B, Ulrichsen H, Fahrenkrug J, et al. Vasoactive intestinal polypeptide and the female genital tract: relationship to reproductive phase and delivery. Am J Obstet Gynecol 1982; 43:414–420.
21. Otessen B. Vasoactive intestinal peptide as a neurotransmitter in the female genital tract. Am J Obstet Gynecol 1983; 147:208–224.

22. Ottesen B, Pedersen B, Nielsen J, et al. Vasoactive intestinal polypeptide (VIP) provokes vaginal lubrication in normal women. Peptides 1987; 8:797–800.

23. Palle C, Bredkjaer HE, Ottesen B, Fahrenkrug J. Vasoactive intestinal polypeptide and human vaginal blood flow: comparison between transvaginal and intravenous administration. J Clin Exp Pharm Physiol 1990; 17:61–68.

24. Meston CM, Heiman JR. Ephedrine-activated physiological sexual arousal in women. Arch Gen Psych 1998; 55:652–656.

25. Meston CM, Gorzalka BB, Wright JM. Inhibition of subjective and physiological sexual arousal in women by clonidine. Psychosom Med 1997; 59:399–407.

26. Riley AJ, Riley EJ. The effect of labetalol and propranolol on pressure response to sexual arousal in women. Br J Pharmacol 1981; 12:341–344.

27. Min K, Munarriz R, Kim NN, et al. Effects of ovariectomy and estrogen and androgen treatment on vaginal nitric oxide synthase activity and smooth muscle contractility. Female Sexual Function Forum; 2001 (Podium).

28. Park K, Moreland, RB, Atala A, et al. Characterization of phosphodiesterase activity in human clitoral corpus cavernosum smooth muscle cells in culture. Biochem Biophys Res Com 1998; 249:612–617.

29. Traish AM, Moreland RB, Huang YH, et al. Development of human and rabbit vaginal smooth muscle cultures: effects of vasoactive agents on intracellular levels of cyclic nucleotides. Mol Cell Biol Res Commun 1999; 2:131–137.

30. Berman JR, McCarthy MM, Kyprianou N. Effects of estrogen withdrawal on nitric oxide synthase expression and apoptosis in the rat vagina. Urology 1998; 51:650–656.

31. Al-Hijji J, Larsson B, Batra S. Nitric oxide synthase in the rabbit uterus and vagina: hormonal regulation and functional significance. Biol Reprod 2000; 62:1387–1392.

32. Batra S, Al-Hijji J. Characterization of NOS activity in the rabbit uterus and vagina: down regulation by estrogen. Life Sci 1998; 62:2093–2100.

33. Traish AM, Kim NN, Min K, et al. Role of androgens in female genital arousal: receptor expression, structure and function. Fertil Steril 2002; 77(suppl 4):11–18.

34. Vardi Y, Gruenwald I, Sprecher E, et al. Normative values for female genital sensation. Urology 2000; 56(6):1035–1040.

35. Becher E, Bechara A, Casabe A. Clitoral hemodynamic changes after a topical application of alprostadil. J Sex Marital Ther 2001; 27:405–410.

36. Bechara A, Bertolino M, Casabé A, et al. Duplex Doppler ultrasound assessment of clitoral hemodynamics after topical administration of alprostadil in women with arousal and orgasmic disorders. J Sex Marital Ther 2002; (in press)

37. Bachmann GA, Ebert GA, Burd ID. Vulvovaginal complaints. In: Lobo RA, ed. Treatment of the postmenopausal woman: basic and clinical aspects. Philadelphia: Lippincott Williams & Wilkins; 1999:195–201.

38. Sarrel PM. Sexuality in the middle years. Obstet Gynecol Clin North Am 1987; 14:49–62.

39. Sarrel PM. Ovarian hormones and vaginal blood flow: using laser Doppler velocimetry to measure effects in a clinical trial of post-menopausal women. Int J Impot Res 1998; 10(suppl 2):S91–93.

40. Sarrel PM. Effects of hormone replacement therapy on sexual psychophysiology and behavior in postmenopause. J Womens Health Gend Based Med 2000; 9(suppl 1):S25–32.

41. Semmens JP, Wagner G. Estrogen deprivation and vaginal function in postmenopausal women. JAMA 1982; 248:445–448.

42. Utian WH, Shoupe D, Bachmann G, et al. Relief of vasomotor symptoms and vaginal atrophy with lower doses of conjugated equine estrogens and medroxyprogesterone acetate. Fertil Steril 2001; 75:1065–1079.

43. Sherwin BB, Gelfand MM, Brender W. Androgen enhances sexual motivation in females: a prospective, crossover study of sex steroid administration in the surgical menopause. Psychosom Med 1985; 47:339–351.

44. Davis SR, Burger HG. The rationale for physiological testosterone replacement in women. Baillières Clin Endocrinol Metab 1998; 12:391–405.

45. Bachmann G, Bancroft J, Braunstein G, et al. Female androgen insufficiency: the Princeton consensus statement on definition, classification, and assessment. Fertil Steril 2002; 77:660–665.

46. Gebhart JB, Rickard DJ, Barrett TJ, et al. Expression of estrogen receptor isoforms alpha and beta messenger RNA in vaginal tissue of premenopausal and postmenopausal women. Am J Obstet Gynecol 2001; 185:1325–1330.

47. Carter AC, Cohen EJ, Shorr E. The use of androgens in women. Vitam Horm 1947; 5:317–391.

48. Salmon U. Rationale for androgen therapy in gynecology. J Clin Endocrinol 1941; 1:162–179.

49. Schreiner-Engel P, Schiavi RC, Smith H, White D. Sexual arousability and the menstrual cycle. Psychosom Med 1981; 43:199–214.

50. Schreiner-Engel P, Schiavi RC, White D, Ghizzani A. Low sexual desire in women: the role of reproductive hormones. Horm Behav 1989; 23:221–234.

51. Hackbert L, Heiman JR. Acute dehydroepiandrosterone (DHEA) effects on sexual arousal in postmenopausal women. J Womens Health Gend Based Med 2002; 11:155–162.

52. Shifren JL, Braunstein GD, Simon JA, et al. Transdermal testosterone treatment in women with impaired sexual function after oophorectomy. N Engl J Med 2000; 343:682–688.

53. Arlt W, Callies F, Allolio B. DHEA replacement in women with adrenal insufficiency – pharmacokinetics, bioconversion and clinical effects on well-being, sexuality and cognition. Endocrinol Res 2000; 26:505–511.

54. Munarriz R, Talakoub L, Flaherty E, et al. Androgen replacement therapy with dehydroepiandrosterone for androgen insufficiency and female sexual dysfunction: androgen and questionnaire results. J Sex Marital Ther 2002; 28(suppl 1):165–173.

55. Caruso S, Intelisano G, Lupo L, Agnello C. Premenopausal women affected by sexual disorder treated with sildenafil: a double blind, cross over, placebo controlled study. BJOG 2001; 108:623–628.

56. Kaplan SA, Reis RB, Kohn IJ, et al. Safety and efficacy of sildenafil in postmenopausal women with sexual dysfunction. Urology 1999; 53:481–486.

57. Rosen RC, Phillips NA, Gendrano NC 3rd, Ferguson DM. Oral phentolamine and female sexual arousal disorder: a pilot study. J Sex Marital Ther 1999; 25(2):137–144.

58. Rubio-Aurioles E, Lopez M, Lipezker M, et al. Phentolamine mesylate in postmenopausal women with female sexual arousal disorder: a psychophysiological study. J Sex Marital Ther 2002; 28(suppl 1):205–215.

59. Islam A, Mitchel J, Rosen R, et al. Topical alprostadil in the treatment of female sexual arousal disorder: a pilot study. J Sex Marital Ther 2001; 27(5):531–540.

60. Billups KL, Berman L, Berman J, et al. A new non-pharmacological vacuum therapy for female sexual dysfunction. J Sex Marital Ther 2001; 27(5):435–441.

61. Wilson SK, Delk JR 2nd, Billups KL. Treating symptoms of female sexual arousal disorder with the Eros-Clitoral Therapy Device. J Gend Specif Med 2001; 4(2):54–58.

5

Angiogenesis as a diagnostic and therapeutic tool in urological malignancy

Edward Streeter and Jeremy Crew

Angiogenesis

It is now three decades since the first demonstrations that tumors required a blood supply to grow beyond 2–3 mm³. These investigations, led by Judah Folkman, and summarized in 1990,[1] confirm what all surgeons know, that tumors often have extremely extensive vascular supplies, but it was the first suggestion that tumors interacted with their hosts in order to survive. This has been followed by a flurry of work describing the stimulatory factors and intermediaries involved, with those of particular relevance to the field of urological oncology discussed below. Additionally, greater understanding of the mechanisms of tumor development have led to an explosion of novel therapies currently under experimental and clinical trial, which will also be described.

What is angiogenesis?

An efficient circulatory system is mandatory to ensure the delivery of oxygen and nutrients, and aid the excretion of metabolic waste products. Low oxygen tension (hypoxia) for example, would occur beyond distances of 100–200 microns, the limit for extracellular fluid oxygen diffusion. Vasculogenesis is the process of major vessel formation de novo from mesenchymal tissues in embryonic development. Further branching vessels are developed from existing vessels via angiogenesis, while the established vessels mature and are pruned via angiogenic remodelling. Mechanisms of vessel development include vessel sprouting and bridge formation, which are dependent on endothelial cell migration and proliferation, and intussusception, where interstitial tissue columns expand and insert into the lumen of the existing vessel. New vessels may also develop from circulating endothelial progenitor cells,[2] derived from the bone marrow, and recruited to sites of active angiogenesis. An alternative mechanism is termed vascular mimicry, whereby vascular channels are formed without the presence of endothelial cells, by the tumor cells themselves organizing into a lumen.

Angiogenesis is seen physiologically in fetal development, the endometrial hyperplasia associated with the menstrual cycle, and in wound healing. Additionally, it is recognized to be involved in a diverse array of pathologic conditions, characterized by inflammation and tissue hypoxia. These include psoriasis, endometriosis, ischemic heart disease, rheumatoid arthritis, hepatitis, asthma, retinopathy associated with prematurity or diabetes, and most solid tumors.[3] Angiogenic vessels show several differences from mature vessels, with normal vascular architecture and a disorganized, irregular meshwork, with areas of relative hypoxia and acidosis. Endothelial cell membranes are more permeable than in normal vessels. Additionally, intercellular junctions are not tight, and the basement membrane may be incomplete. This results in angiogenic vessels being leaky, aiding extracellular matrix signaling and metabolism. Angiogenic endothelial cells exhibit variations in surface markers and cell adhesion molecules, reflecting their increased proliferation and protein expression and secretion. As discussed below, this factor may enable selective targeting of antiangiogenic therapy.

The potential advantages of antiangiogenic therapy

The majority of urological tumors may be treated using either traditional radio- and chemotherapeutic approaches or hormonal manipulation, but resistance and relapse occur even in those with complete response and with a dismal prognosis for patients with metastatic disease. Targeting the tumor neovasculature however offers an alternative therapeutic modality that may not be so susceptible to resistance. There are several reasons to support this:

- Cellular toxicity of radiotherapy depends on delivery of oxygen to the tumor, which as stated above is often hypoxic and necrotic in a number of solid tumors. In targeting the neovasculature however, the endothelial cell is easily reached by blood-borne therapies.
- Since the endothelial cell is non-neoplastic and thus genetically stable (in contrast to the labile nature of tumor cells), resistance to chemotherapy and hormonal manipulation is less likely to develop.
- Selectivity of the tumor-derived endothelium is possible since cell surface proteins, such as integrins expressed by angiogenic vessels, differ from those of the much more slowly dividing mature vascular endothelium.

These factors in combination theoretically promise a therapy of prolonged high efficacy, with few side effects. Additionally, antiangiogenic therapies may be used in combination with other existing modalities, with the potential for synergism of action.

How is angiogenesis assessed?

There are three principal ways of assessing tumor angiogenesis: direct measurement can be made histologically, indirect assessment performed radiographically, or alternatively surrogate markers of angiogenic activity obtained.

Histological assessment of angiogenesis

A commonly used histological measure of angiogenesis is microvessel density (MVD). This may be assessed as an average of counts over a number of randomly selected areas, termed the mean MVD. Alternatively the MVD may be quantified in the most dense area of neovascularization, called hotspots. Arguments can be made to support both methods, though both are clearly prone to sampling error. Different staining methods can be employed, often involving immunohistochemical techniques using antibodies to CD31, CD34 or factor VIII-related antigen. The inconsistency

within the published literature has often been partly blamed on the method of MVD assessment used. This is of particular relevance to prognostication using limited tissue specimens (e.g. prostatic needle biopsies) since the MVD has been shown to increase considerably from the peripheries towards the center of individual prostatic tumors.[4]

Radiological assessment of angiogenesis

A gross, non-invasive assessment of tumor microvascularity may be made using conventional imaging modalities, including Doppler ultrasound (USS), magnetic resonance imaging (MRI), computed tomography (CT) and positron emission tomography (PET) (reviewed in Anderson et al[5]). Intravascular enhancement may facilitate these imaging modalities.

Ultrasound may be enhanced using intravascular microbubble contrast material. This technique has recently been demonstrated to be sensitive in the identification of prostatic tumor,[6] and further refinement may lead to its use in more precise quantification of MVD.

MRI may be enhanced using gadolinium, with macromolecular contrast media, which are large enough to remain impermeable even in tumor neovasculature, aiming to improve the accuracy of MVD estimation. Conversely, measuring the changes in vascular permeability due to antiangiogenic therapy may be of use in assessing the efficacy of treatment. One interesting application is blood oxygenation level dependent (BOLD) MRI, which measures changes in T2 weighted signal due to variation in the concentration of deoxyhemoglobin. The signal of course depends not only on MVD, but also on oxygenation, blood volume and flow.

PET scanning measures overall perfusion rather than the fine resolution of the microvasculature, but has the advantages of being able to assess tumor metabolism and the distribution of labeled tumor endothelial-specific antibodies. PET scanning is however currently of very limited availability.

Like PET scanning, CT is insufficiently sensitive for directly assessing the microvasculature, but dynamic CT using an intravascular tracer may provide estimates of tumor perfusion. The ready availability of CT is likely to favor this modality for future development.

Surrogate markers of angiogenesis

A further way of assessing tumor angiogenesis indirectly is to measure the production of known angiogenic factors in blood or urine. This has been extensively investigated for its prognostic and monitory uses, as will be considered later. A further extension of this is to assess the biological activity of tissue or fluid, in their ability to induce or inhibit angiogenesis in vivo, or endothelial cell migration in vitro. This perhaps offers an ideal way of tailoring therapy to the individual patient.

Angiogenesis and prognosis in urological cancer

Prostate cancer

Carcinoma of the prostate is increasingly recognized as a major source of mortality in Western society, but persistent controversies in its management and the difficulty in predicting the course of the disease have led to a particular interest in the role of angiogenesis as a prognostic marker and therapeutic target. Table 5.1 shows published studies relating microvessel density to stage and grade at diagnosis, alongside outcome in terms of recurrence-free and disease-free survival.

The association between grade and MVD was first demonstrated in 1992 by Wakui et al,[17] with high MVD suggested to predict bone metastases. The correlation between MVD and stage at presentation was further described in 1993,[18,19] later claimed to be a more accurate predictor of extraprostatic extension or pelvic lymph node metastases than Gleason grading or serum prostate specific antigen (PSA) alone.[20] More recent studies have demonstrated the value of MVD based on transurethral prostatectomy specimens to predict survival following external beam radiotherapy,[8] of radical prostatectomy specimens to predict disease-free survival (of particular use in Gleason 5–7 tumors),[9] and of needle biopsies to predict overall survival in a watchful waiting population.[12] Thus the observational evidence weighs quite strongly in favor of high MVD being at least a marker of aggressive disease.

Table 5.1 Association between microvessel density and clinical parameters in carcinoma of the prostate

Series	Year	n (pts)	Tissue	Stained for	Stage association	Grade association	p (recurrence)	p (survival)	Uni/ multivariate	Comments
Vesalainen et al[7]	1994	88	TURP/ biopsy	Collagen IV	Not significant	Yes		0.027	Univariate	
Hall et al[8]	1994	25	TURP	Factor VIII		Yes	< 0.0001	0.0003	Univariate	Outcome post radiotherapy
Silberman et al[9]	1997	109/87	RP, Gn 5–7	CD31	No		< 0.0001		Multivariate	
Offersen et al[10]	1998	64	TURP	CD31				0.01	Multivariate	Mixed stages
Bettencourt et al[11]	1998	149	RP	CD34	Yes	Yes	0.03		Univariate	Correlated with serum PSA
Borre et al[12]	1998	221	Biopsy	Factor VIII	Yes	Yes		0.0001	Multivariate	Clinically localized
Rubin et al[13]	1999	87	RP	CD31	No	No	Not predictive		Univariate	
Strohmeyer et al[14]	2000	98	RP	Factor VIII	Yes	Yes	< 0.0001		Multivariate	
de la Taille et al[15]	2000	102	RP	CD34					Multivariate	
Halvorsen et al[16]	2000	66	RP, Gn 5–7	Factor VIII		Yes	0.0003		Multivariate	

Gn, Gleason grade; PSA, prostate specific antigen; RP, radical prostatectomy; TURP, transuretheral resection of prostate.

Bladder cancer

Identifying patients with superficial disease at highest risk of tumor progression is a priority in the management of bladder cancer. Angiogenesis is recognized as a marker of disease aggressiveness; however clinical data with regard to superficial bladder cancer remain controversial, possibly due to difficulties in microvessel quantification within a friable papillary tumor. The differing nature of histological methods of assessment, plus the comparison of transurethral resection versus cystectomy specimens may explain the inconsistencies between series.

The published literature regarding invasive tumors is more convincing. A number of series have demonstrated strong associations between high MVD and increased recurrence and reduced survival, both for assessment on the initial transurethral resection specimens, and following radical cystectomy (Table 5.2). Dickinson et al[21] measured MVD in 45 invasive bladder tumor specimens, obtained from transurethral resection, and showed a 2.5 times increase in mortality at 4 years associated with high MVD compared to those patients with less vascular tumors. Jaeger et al[22] related higher MVD in the primary tumor to lymph node metastases at radical cystectomy. In a series of 164 patients undergoing radical cystectomy, Bochner et al[23] demonstrated a decrease in 5-year patient survival relating to tumor MVD, being 68%, 44% and 34% for patients with low, medium and high MVD tumors, respectively. There

Table 5.2 Studies of microvessel density (MVD) and prognosis in bladder cancer

Study	Year	no	Stage	Stained for	p (recurrence-free survival)	p (overall survival)	Uni/multivariate	Comments
Dickinson et al[21]	1994	45	Invasive (TURBT)	CD31	N/A	0.026	Univariate	MVD not associated with stage and grade, but high MVD → 2.5× ↑ mortality
Jaeger et al[22]	1995	41	Invasive (cystectomy)	Factor VIII	N/A	N/A	N/A	↑ MVD correlates with lymph node metastases at presentation
Bochner et al[23]	1995	164	Invasive (cystectomy)	CD34	<0.0001	0.0007	Multivariate	↑ MVD correlates with stage at presentation, recurrence and survival
Philp et al[24]	1996	113	Superficial or invasive (TURBT)	CD31	N/A	0.01	Multivariate	MVD correlated with stage at presentation
Grossfeld et al[25]	1997	163	Invasive (cystectomy)	CD34	N/A	N/A	N/A	↑ MVD associated with ↓ survival and low thrombospondin-1
Bochner et al[26]	1997	161	Invasive (cystectomy)	CD34	<0.001	0.003	Multivariate	↑ MVD associated with progression, and loosely with ↑ p53
Dinney et al[27]	1998	54	T1 (TURBT and cystectomy)	Factor VIII	N/A	N/A	Univariate	No association between MVD and recurrence or progression
Hawke et al[28]	1998	42	Invasive (cystectomy)	Factor VIII	N/A	0.04	Univariate	MVD of no independent prognostic value
Chaudhary et al[29]	1999	88	Invasive (cystectomy)	CD31	0.03	0.02	Univariate	↑ MVD associated with nodal metastases at cystectomy, ↑ recurrence, ↓ survival.
Ozer et al[30]	1999	20	G3 T1 (TURBT)	Factor VIII	0.002	0.01	Univariate	↑ MVD associated with ↑ recurrence and ↓ survival.
Inoue et al[31]	2000	51	Invasive (cystectomy)	CD34	0.048	N/A	Multivariate	↑ MVD predicts recurrence in patients given neoadjuvant MVAC chemotherapy
Sagol et al 32	2001	80	Superficial (TURBT)	CD31	N/A	N/A	Univariate	MVD did not differ from Ta to T1, or predict recurrence. ↑ MVD associated with ↑ grade.

Invasive, stage T2 or greater; MVAC, methotrexate/vinblastine/doxorubicin/cisplatin; N/A, data not available; TURBT, transurethral resection of bladder tumour

was also a concomitant increase in recurrence, with figures of 19%, 56% and 68% with ascending MVD. In a series of 113 patients who had transurethral resection of newly diagnosed bladder cancer of various stages and grades, Philp et al[24] demonstrated an association between MVD and stage of tumor, the presence of vascular invasion, and the risk of death over a 12-year follow-up period. In solid bladder tumors therefore, MVD appears to be a powerful independent prognostic factor.

Renal cancer

The prognostic significance of MVD in relation to renal cell carcinoma is again slightly controversial, and is summarized in Table 5.3. In a series of 84 patients, low MVD (measured in vascular hotspots) was demonstrated to be a significant predictor of metastasis-free and overall survival in early stage adenocarcinoma.[33] Another study published the same year, of 97 cases, demonstrated no correlation between MVD and stage, grade or survival.[34] Delahunt et al,[35] assessing mean MVD in a series of 150 cases, conversely argued for a positive correlation between angiogenesis and survival, with low MVD cases having shorter survival. This would be in agreement with others who have reported higher histological grade to be associated with low MVD in T1 or T2 renal cancer.[39] Subsequent investigators have supported the favorable prognostic significance of low MVD, whilst others, with relatively small sample sizes, have been unable to reproduce this finding. The picture is thus far from clear when histological evidence is considered alone; however, as will be addressed later, experimental evidence strongly supports a key role of angiogenesis in the pathogenesis of renal cancer.

Testicular cancer

There have been relatively few data forthcoming on the role of angiogenesis in testicular tumors, possibly due to the effectiveness of conventional therapy in treating the majority of cases. In 1994 a small series was reported[40] which demonstrated an association between high MVD and occult metastatic disease.

The mechanisms underlying angiogenesis

Endothelial cells are normally quiescent, displaying a non-angiogenic phenotype. This state is the result of a dynamic balance of a vast number of pro- and antiangiogenic factors (Fig. 5.1). In the circumstances described previously, proangiogenic factors predominate, causing the endothelium to develop an angiogenic phenotype. This upregulation of cell division and motility has been termed the angiogenic switch, and it is this transformation which is thought to be crucial in enabling dormant or microscopic tumors to grow and become clinically apparent, and eventually metastasize. Stimuli which may promote this behavior include metabolic stresses, such as hypoxia, acidosis and hypoglycemia, as well as mechanical strain due to tissue growth, and inflammatory or immune cell activation. Genetic mutation, causing dysregulation of factors involved in angiogenesis, may affect the balance of angiogenic factors directly.

Table 5.3 The correlation between microvessel density and patient survival in renal cancer

Study	Year	n (patients)	Stage	Correlation with survival	p value	Uni/multivariate	Stained for
Yoshino et al[33]	1995	45	T1–2, M0	Negative	0.028	Multivariate	Factor VIII
MacLennan & Bostwick[34]	1995	97	Mixed	None	–		Factor VIII
Delathunt et al[35]	1997	150	Mixed	Positive		Univariate	Factor VIII
Gelb et al[36]	1997	52	T1–2, M0	None	–		Factor VIII and DC31
Ou et al[37]	1998	34	Mixed	None	–		Factor VIII
Nativ et al[38]	1998	36	T1–2, M0	Negative	0.0014	Multivariate	Factor VIII

Negative correlation indicates reduced survival with increasing MVD.

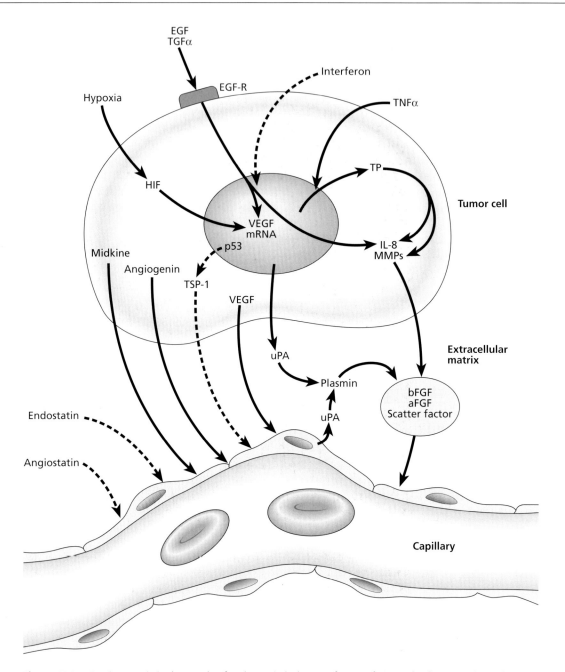

Figure 5.1 Angiogenesis is the result of a dynamic balance of many factors, both proangiogenic (solid arrows) and antiangiogenic (dashed arrows). Those best described in urological malignancy are shown. The extracellular matrix binds a number of factors (in circle) which are released under stimulation to further promote endothelial migration and division. aFGF, acidic fibroblast growth factor; bFGF, basic fibroblast growth factor; EGF, epidermal growth factor; EGF-R, epidermal growth factor receptor; HIF, hypoxia inducible factor; IL-8, interleukin-8; MMPs, matrix metalloproteinases; TGFα, transforming growth factor alpha; TNFα, tumour necrosis factor alpha; TP, thymidine phosphorylase; TSP-1, thrombospondin 1; uPA, urokinase plasminogen activator.

Table 5.4 Endogenous factors described in the regulation of angiogenesis in urological malignancy

Proangiogenic	Antiangiogenic
Vascular endothelial growth factor	Thrombospondin 1
Fibroblast growth factors	Angiostatin
Thymidine phosphorylase	Endostatin
Epidermal growth factor	Tissue inhibitors of matrix metalloproteinases
Tumour necrosis factor alpha	Interferon alpha
Transforming growth factor alpha	Interferon beta
Transforming growth factor beta	Maspin
Angiogenin	Prostate specific antigen
Hepatocyte growth factor/scatter factor	Interleukin-10
Angiopoietin-1	Angiopoietin-2
Interleukin-8	Cortisone
Interleukin-4	
Tissue factor	
Midkine	
Hyaluronic acid	
Cyclooxygenase 2	
Hypoxia inducible factors 1 and 2	
Eukaryotic initiation factor 4e	
Matrix metalloproteinases	
Urokinase plasminogen activator	
Platelet derived growth factor	
Mutant p53	
Prostaglandins E1 and E2	
Nuclear factor kappa B	

A list of pro- and antiangiogenic factors so far described in urological tumors is shown in Table 5.4. Although the list is extensive, most interest has focused on relatively few factors, which will be discussed in detail.

Vascular endothelial growth factor (VEGF)

There now exist six different growth factors with the names VEGF A to F. However, they bear only partial sequence homology to each other, and apart from VEGF A and VEGF C, the angiogenic effect of the others is yet to be proven. Few studies have related VEGF C to urological malignancies, so discussion will focus on VEGF A, generally referred to simply as VEGF.

Perhaps the most studied of all proangiogenic growth factors, VEGF is a potent chemoattractant and mitogenic stimulator of vascular endothelial cells. It exists in four forms of 121, 165, 189 and 206 amino acids in length, and binds to two receptors, Flt-1 and Flk-1/KDR, both of which have intracellular tyrosine kinase domains. A third VEGF receptor (VEGFR3) is thought to be related in adults more to lymphagenesis, in association with VEGF C. The expression of Flt-1 has been shown to correlate with VEGF production, suggesting an autocrine as well as a paracrine effect. The biochemical actions of VEGF have been investigated in a mouse mesentery model of microvessel growth where it led to increased intracellular calcium, activation of protein kinase C and the phosphorylation of several cellular proteins including both membrane VEGF receptors, phospholipase C-gamma, and phosphatidylinositol 3'-kinase.[41]

Perhaps stimulated downstream to VEGF is nitric oxide synthase (NOS). Increased nitric oxide (NO) associated with malignancy is seen in epithelial and endothelial cells. Once stimulated, endothelial cells produce urokinase-type and tissue-type plasminogen activators, their receptors and type IV collagenases. This leads to degradation of the extracellular matrix, enabling endothelial cell migration and invasion. It also causes increased endothelial cell permeability (hence its previous name vascular permeability factor), leading to an increase in interstitial plasminogen and plasmin. Inhibition of its effect in gene knockout mice, or via mutation or deletion of its two receptors Flt-1 and Flk-1/KDR, results in severe vascular anomalies and intrauterine or perinatal death.

VEGF is not confined to tumor cells, but is released by a wide variety of normal cells including lymphocytes and platelets. It is also seen in large quantities in semen, though its function here is unknown. Its distribution may be of particular relevance when studying tumor samples, where the presence of inflammatory cells overexpressing VEGF may influence its quantification overall. Though post-transcriptional regulation by eukaryotic transcription factor 4e may also enhance its levels,[42] the chief regulator of VEGF is hypoxia inducible factor 1 (HIF-1), itself a dimer of alpha and beta subunits. HIF-1 is normally rapidly degraded under conditions of normal oxygen tension, via the ubiquitin–proteasome pathway in conjunction with the von Hippel–Lindau protein (pVHL) (see Fig. 5.2). However, in hypoxia the protein is stabilized and binds to promoter regions of genomic DNA to stimulate the transcription of a large number of target proteins involved in angiogenesis, vascular hemostasis, glycolysis, erythropoiesis, cell proliferation and apoptosis among other functions. The role of pVHL in this pathway is particularly interesting in reference to the pathogenesis of renal cancer. As part of the von Hippel–Lindau (VHL) syndrome, characterized by mutation of the VHL gene on chromosome 3, patients develop renal adenocarcinomas at unusually young ages, as well as cerebellar hemangiomas, pheochromocytomas and retinal angiomas. Mutant VHL leads to constitutive upregulation of HIF-1 alpha in normoxia, due to reduced breakdown via the pathway illustrated in Figure 5.2. VHL mutation is found in the majority of

clear cell renal carcinomas, though not commonly in the relatively avascular papillary variant.[43] It is thus likely that increased HIF-1 alpha plays a crucial role in the early development of these tumors.

The role of VEGF in urological malignancy is perhaps best exemplified in bladder cancer, where it is particularly associated with high grade superficial disease, predicting recurrence and stage progression.[44] Similarly, increased levels of VEGF in the urine of bladder cancer patients have been demonstrated to be a sign of recurrent disease, though not sensitive enough as a stand-alone screening test. Urine VEGF can also be used to predict future recurrence.[45]

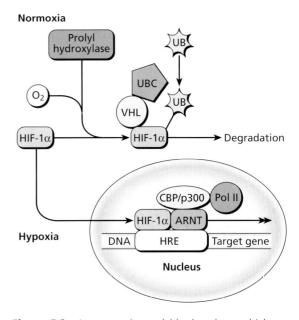

Figure 5.2 In normoxia, prolyl hydroxylase, which contains an oxygen-binding heme moiety, modifies hypoxia inducible factor-1α (HIF-1α), leading to its binding to the von Hippel–Lindau protein (VHL). This is followed by ubiquitinylation by the ubiquitinylation complex (UBC) and HIF degradation by the proteasome. In hypoxia, prolyl hydroxlyase cannot act on HIF-1α, which is thus free to translocate to the nucleus where it binds to specific sequences in DNA named hypoxic response elements (HRE), and in association with the aryl hydrocarbon nuclear transporter (ARNT – also known as HIF-2) stimulates target gene expression in association with Creb binding protein (CBP/p300) and DNA polymerase II (Pol II).

Its association with renal cell carcinoma (RCC) was first demonstrated in 1993.[46] Using in situ hybridization and immunohistochemistry, both VEGF mRNA and protein levels were shown to be upregulated in clear cell carcinoma, though not in the relatively avascular papillary variant. The correlation between VEGF mRNA and proximity to areas of necrosis was noted. mRNA for both receptors was upregulated only in endothelial cells, thus demonstrating its probable paracrine effect. Recently, VEGF has been described to be an independent predictor of outcome in 74 cases of RCC.[47] In that study, VEGF staining was also correlated with areas of high microvessel density. Raised serum VEGF is seen in patients with renal tumors versus controls, and it may also predict early progression in patients with metastatic disease.[48,49]

Angiogenesis and VEGF production in the prostate are under the influence of testosterone.[50] Its expression is not confined to malignant tissue, but it is upregulated in hypoxic areas.[51] Plasma levels are increased in metastatic disease,[52] and urinary levels may predict outcome in patients with advanced disease.[53] Anti-VEGF antibodies inhibited growth of established subcutaneous DU-145 prostate carcinoma cell tumors and prevented metastases in immunodeficient mice.[54]

Epidermal growth factor (EGF)

Immunohistochemistry has shown an association between the presence of the EGF receptor (EGF-R) and increasing grade and stage of bladder tumor. Its presence is an independent predictor of stage progression and reduced survival in superficial bladder cancer,[55] with 93% sensitivity and 81% specificity for predicting stage progression in G3 T1 tumors in a series of 212 patients.[56] EGF in the urine of 54 patients with transitional cell carcinoma of the bladder was noted to be reduced relative to normal,[57] possibly due to increased EGF-R binding. EGF stimulates the production of VEGF in prostate cancer cells, mediated at least in part by an increase in HIF-1 alpha.[58] Antibodies directed against EGF-R inhibit human cell lines in vitro[59] and angiogenesis in an orthotopic mouse model of human bladder cancer.[60] The EGF receptor's intracellular domain has tyrosine kinase activity, similar to the VEGF and basic fibroblast growth factor (bFGF) receptors. Agents which inhibit this

enzyme have recently attracted clinical interest, as will be considered later.

Matrix metalloproteinases (MMPs)

MMPs are enzymes capable of proteolytic cleavage of a number of extracellular matrix components. Thus, rather than having a direct action on endothelial cells, their effect is to induce other angiogenic agents. Most studied are 72 kDa MMP-2 (gelatinase A) and 92 kDa MMP-9 (gelatinase B). Their presence in bladder cancer tissue and urine is associated with increasing stage and grade,[61,62] though no apparent association between tissue levels and outcome is noted,[62,63] which is perplexing given the strong association obvious between invasion and reduced survival.

The mechanistic association between MMPs, angiogenesis and tumor invasion has been demonstrated by the use of halofuginone, which inhibits MMP-2 and has been shown to inhibit angiogenesis and prevent bladder cancer cell line invasion.[64] The release of MMP is known to be stimulated by epidermal growth factor, among other pathways.

Endogenous inhibitors of MMPs are also seen, termed tissue inhibitors of MMP (TIMPs). Paradoxically, however, increased levels of TIMP-2 in tissue are associated with worse outcome.[63] Similarly, serum levels of TIMP-1 in bladder cancer patients rise by around 50%, correlating with increasing stage.[65] The TIMPs may have additional functions and also are involved in producing a controlled microenvironment of proteolysis. Intense proteolysis may destroy tissue excessively and prevent growth and it is a common paradigm for inhibitors to be secreted with proteases (e.g. urokinase and PAI 1). Investigations into the mechanisms underlying these endogenous inhibitors of MMPs have produced apparently conflicting results, and their significance remains unclear.

Clinical trials of agents inhibiting MMPs have yielded disappointing results, probably because MMPs may have a previously unrecognized role in the generation of antiangiogenic agents via cleavage of other extracellular matrix glycoproteins.

The role of the extracellular matrix (ECM)

The ECM plays a crucial role in tumor angiogenesis. As well as physically linking tumor cells to the endothelium, it serves as a pool for several angiogenic factors. These may lie dormant (bound to glycosaminoglycans), awaiting cleavage by enzymes such as heparinases, plasmin, cathepsin-D and urokinase, or may result from the cleavage of other molecules, resulting in endogenous anti-angiogenic agents. The former include acidic and basic growth factors, both powerful proangiogenic agents, whereas the latter include angiostatin and endostatin, which are derived from plasminogen and collagen XVIII, respectively.

Acidic and basic fibroblast growth factor (aFGF and bFGF) are members of a family of heparin binding proteins, sharing multiple fibroblast growth factor receptors, which have intrinsic tyrosine kinase activity. They act non-specifically on vascular endothelial cells as potent mitogens and chemotactic agents, inducing the production of plasminogen activator and collagenase, amongst other actions. Both are raised in the urine of patients with bladder cancer, though not specifically, as elevated levels are also seen in other malignancies and in benign prostatic hyperplasia.[66] Thus neither is likely to replace current urine screening tests.

Serum bFGF is raised in most patients with renal carcinoma and prostate carcinoma. No association with stage has been shown, so it is unlikely again to be of significant clinical use.

Thymidine phosphorylase

Thymidine phosphorylase (TP) is an enzyme normally involved in the nucleotide salvage pathway. High levels of TP have previously been reported in breast, ovarian and colonic cancer, predicting lymph node involvement and overall survival. The by-product of its action is 2-deoxy 1-ribose, a powerful reducing sugar which rapidly generates free radical species. Brown et al[67] demonstrated in vitro that transfection of TP into the superficial bladder cancer cell line RT112 induces interleukin-8 (IL-8), VEGF and matrix metalloproteinase-1 (MMP-1) production, which in turn induces an invasive phenotype.[68] IL-8 is a potent endothelial cell chemoattractant and enhances bladder cell line invasion; the roles of VEGF and MMP-1 in angiogenesis have been described above. TP has been shown to be strongly upregulated with invasion in carcinoma of the bladder.[69] A correlation between increased TP expression in superficial tumors and reduced time to first recurrence[70] and reduced survival has been

demonstrated. Raised TP has also been described in prostate cancer in comparison with normal adjacent prostate. TP may be of particular relevance when it is realized that it is within hypoxic solid tumors where thymidine levels are greatest due to the degradation of necrotic cellular DNA. Thus TP may prove to be of particular importance in the ability of solid tumors to withstand hypoxia, cause invasion and metastasize, the hallmark of stage progression.

Cyclooxygenase 2 (COX-2)

COX-2 has been shown to promote angiogenesis in a range of cell lines, including common urological cancer lines, via the induction of prostaglandin E2. By blocking COX-2 in vitro, pVHL is raised leading to the degradation of HIF-1 alpha as described above, and its proangiogenic activity is thus abated. The action of non-steroidal anti-inflammatory drugs in cancer therapy is considered below.

Antiangiogenic factors

Endogenous agents with antiangiogenic activity have attracted particular interest over the last few years due to their potential exploitation as anti-angiogenic therapies. The best studied of these are endostatin, a cleavage product of collagen XVIII, and angiostatin, cleaved from plasminogen. Both were initially described to have powerful antiangiogenic activity in animal models of lung carcinoma.[71,72] However neither has as yet produced the same effect in human trials.

Thrombospondin-1 (TSP-1)

TSP-1, a 430 kDa glycoprotein, has been shown to be a powerful antiangiogenic agent released by normal urothelial cells. It inhibits the angiogenesis induced by VEGF and bFGF in a corneal angiogenesis assay.[73] Decreasing levels of TSP-1 staining have been correlated with increased microvessel density, increasing p53 mutation, increased rate of recurrence and reduced survival in bladder cancer in 163 cystectomy patients,[25] but more recently no such associations were found for patients undergoing radical prostatectomy for T3 carcinoma of the prostate. However, a further recent paper did associate reduced TSP-1 with increasing stage of prostate cancer,[75] and transfection of the DU-145 prostate cancer cell line with TSP-1 led to tumor inhibition in a nude mouse xenograft model. TSP-1 has not yet entered clinical trials.

p53

p53 is a tumor suppressor gene, the loss of which is associated with stage progression in bladder and prostate cancer, and it has been additionally associated with angiogenesis in these tumors. Its exact mechanism of action is still poorly understood, though loss of p53 is thought to facilitate a tumor's survival under hypoxia, thus perhaps reducing its sensitivity to antiangiogenic therapy.[76]

Prostate specific antigen (PSA)

One interesting observation is the antiangiogenic activity of PSA,[77] which may cleave plasminogen to form angiostatin. This may explain the slow progression of low grade, PSA-expressing prostate tumors, and why some tumors that produce very little PSA behave so aggressively.

Clinical aspects of antiangiogenic therapy

When designing and interpreting clinical trials of antiangiogenic agents versus conventional adjuvant therapies, allowance must be made for the intrinsic differences in the nature of their effects. Patient selection dictates that only advanced cases, usually those who have failed conventional therapy, are entered into trials of new modalities. Thus prognoses are poor from the outset, and treatment times may be short, while antiangiogenic agents – by acting to stabilize disease – may be more useful when given over prolonged periods. This may complicate the quantification of trial endpoints, since conventional disease responses in terms of disease regression may be an inappropriate measure of efficacy. In addition, antiangiogenic agents often have less toxicity than other modalities, contributing to further difficulty in assigning optimal dosing regimens. An alternative to using the maximum tolerated dose may be to use the optimal biological dose, determined by the assessment of patient serum levels in the light of experimental knowledge of effective inhibitory concentrations.

The use of combination therapies, i.e. administering antiangiogenic modalities alongside conventional therapy, has aroused much interest recently. Antiangiogenic agents used alone may eventually encounter resistance in a fashion similar to that seen with conventional therapies, perhaps due to the multiple pathways that may be augmented in neovascularization or the antiapoptotic function of other growth factors. By targeting multiple angiogenic pathways, or by inducing tumor cell toxicity to reduce the production of angiogenic factors, it is proposed that the development of resistance may be offset or prevented entirely.

The future of antiangiogenic therapy will include managing patients with localized disease with adjuvant or neoadjuvant treatment. Bladder cancer is a particularly good model for testing antiangiogenic agents for a number of reasons:

- The intravesical route of administration is convenient and provides potential contact between agent and tumor for prolonged periods.
- Low systemic absorption leads to few side-effects.
- Surveillance of marker lesions is possible cystoscopically.
- The treatment of superficial disease to prevent recurrence and progression readily identifies a subgroup of patients with a relatively good prognosis who could nonetheless benefit from early adjuvant intervention.
- Patients with localized invasive disease, currently treated with radical surgery or radiotherapy may possibly benefit from adjuvant therapy, with outcome measured in terms of disease-free and overall survival.

It is unlikely that ablative surgery will be superseded as the primary therapy for renal cell carcinoma in the foreseeable future. Again however, since conventional adjuvant therapy has only limited benefit, there is urgent need for more effective complementary treatment.

The case for early treatment in prostate cancer is harder to prove, given the long natural history of the disease and the success of current radical and adjuvant therapy. Nonetheless, as radical treatments have significant, often major side effects, and the outlook for patients with hormone refractory disease is poor, there are potential roles for antiangiogenic therapies at all stages of the disease.

Therapeutic strategies

Strategies to inhibit angiogenesis include direct inhibition of angiogenic growth factors, blocking their receptors, or preventing their transcription from RNA with antisense therapy. Enhancement of antiangiogenic pathways, and targeting the endothelial cells directly, are other approaches that may be taken. These strategies are summarized in Figure 5.3.

Endogenous antiangiogenic agents
Angiostatin and endostatin

As mentioned above, clinical trials for angiostatin and endostatin have so far yielded disappointing results. The reasons for this failure, given the pre-

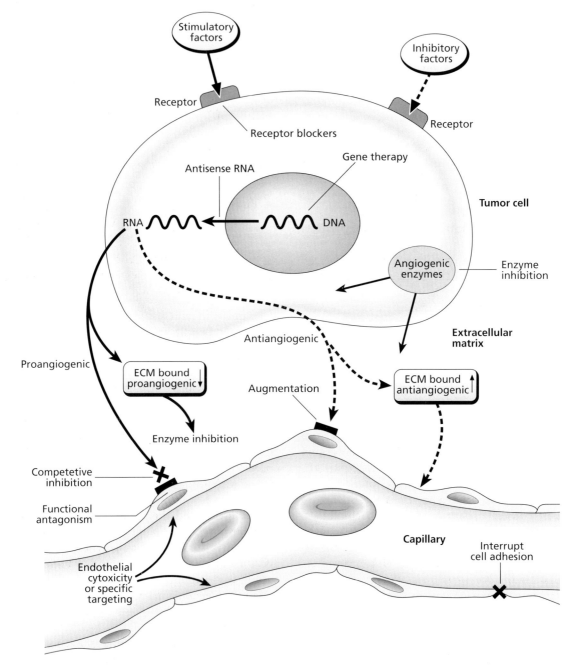

Figure 5.3 Antiangiogenic strategies offer a wide range of targets for therapy. ECM, extracellular matrix.

vious preclinical results, are not clear, but undoubtedly involve the increased complexity of patient tumor biology compared to xenograft models. Additionally, problems with dose adjustment and measuring therapeutic endpoints as discussed above will contribute to the confusion. Future trials should further define these problems. One suggestion with serious implications in the development of anti-angiogenic therapies is that in vitro and xenograft work looks at tumors where endothelial proliferation is extremely high when compared to human tumors. Thus the apparent sensitivity of model vasculature may be a gross overestimation of the clinical reality.

Interferon

Agents currently in widespread use for metastatic RCC include interferon and interleukin-2. Part of their mechanism again may be due to their anti-angiogenic properties, downregulating bFGF in vitro.[78] A recent Cochrane meta-analysis of all appropriately designed trials of interferon alpha (IFN-alpha) in metastatic RCC (4216 patients) demonstrated 3.2% complete response with a further 7% partial response.[79] Ongoing trials are using combinations of IFN-alpha with other antiangiogenic agents. A recent phase III trial of combined IFN-alpha and 13-*cis*-retinoic acid in metastatic RCC suggested a synergistic effect, with 19% progression-free at 2 years versus 10% in the interferon alone arm. Median survival however was not affected.[80] Ongoing trials are focusing on the combination of IFN-alpha with thalidomide (see Exogenous agents below).

The treatment of superficial bladder cancer already involves a potent antiangiogenic agent. Bacille Calmette-Guérin intravesically induces a range of cytokines with endogenous antiangiogenic action including interferon gamma and interferon-inducible protein-10, leading to the urine of responding patients being antiangiogenic in vitro.[81] A phase III trial of a single instillation of IFN-alpha versus epirubicin at the time of transurethral resection of primary superficial bladder tumors has however shown it to be ineffective in preventing recurrence.[82] Again longer courses and combination therapies may be more effective.

Exogenous agents

As shown in Figure 5.3, there are many stages at which the action of angiogenic factors can be interrupted. Although a myriad of agents have been tested, few have yielded promising results when transferred into the clinical setting. A few key agents in current trials will be used to illustrate this.

Thalidomide

Thalidomide was notorious for the limb abnormalities it produced in fetuses in the 1960s. This is a manifestation of its antiangiogenic effect, believed to be due to interruption of mRNA transcription, leading to downregulation of VEGF and tumor necrosis factor alpha (TNF-alpha).

A number of phase II trials have demonstrated partial response or disease stabilization in between 30 and 50% of patients with metastatic renal cell carcinoma, though this is not commonly of prolonged duration.[83,84] Similarly, early series have shown a significant fall in serum PSA in approximately 30% of patients with hormone escaped prostate cancer. Significant side effects included central and peripheral neuropathy, which is a feature common to a number of angiogenic inhibitors. Ongoing trials include a phase III trial of interferon alpha 2b in combination with thalidomide in metastatic or unresectable renal cell carcinoma, and a phase II trial of docetaxel plus thalidomide in androgen independent prostate cancer.

Suramin

Suramin was previously used for many decades as an antitrypanosomal drug. However it also possesses powerful affinity for heparin binding growth factors, including VEGF and bFGF, inhibiting their action. When given intravenously to patients with metastatic prostate cancer, it had wide ranging and severe dose limiting side effects in up to 50% of patients, though approximately one-third of patients exhibited a significant drop in serum PSA,[85,86] and in the group of responders survival was slightly increased. A phase III trial is underway to compare low, medium and high doses in hormone refractory prostate cancer in an attempt to reduce the toxicity of treatment.

A phase I dose escalation study of intravesical suramin in recurrent superficial bladder cancer is nearing completion in our unit. The benefit of intravesical administration is that systemic absorption is only slight, thus side effects have not yet been seen. In an orthotopic model of bladder cancer, intravesical suramin greatly reduced tumor development and metastasis.[87] A planned phase II study will compare suramin with conventional intravesical chemotherapy in its ability to prevent recurrence and progression.

Anti-VEGF antibodies

Antibodies binding VEGF directly, competitively inhibiting its interaction with its receptors, have been shown in animal models to inhibit the progression of bladder and renal tumors. Initial clinical data suggest the therapy is reasonably tolerated, though again concerns regarding neurological function have been raised. A phase III trial is underway recruiting patients with metastatic renal cell carcinoma.

Receptor tyrosine kinase inhibitors

The receptors for a number of angiogenic factors, including VEGF, FGFs and EGF have intrinsic tyrosine kinase activity as part of their signalling mechanism. Tyrosine kinase inhibitors thus have the potential to interrupt several angiogenic pathways simultaneously. Administered orally, animal trials in renal cancer models have confirmed efficacy, and clinical trials are anticipated eagerly.

Cyclooxygenase inhibitors

As described above, COX-2 produces the pro-angiogenic prostaglandin E2, and selective cyclooxygenase inhibitor celecoxib is in phase I trials in patients with localized prostate cancer with high risk of capsular spread as a neoadjuvant agent to prevent local recurrence. A phase III trial of celecoxib is also in progress to prevent recurrence of superficial transitional cell carcinoma of the bladder.

Other antiangiogenic agents

Halofuginone is an alkaloid coccidiostat that has been used to treat parasitic infections for many years. It has also been shown to downregulate MMP-2 expression and collagen type I deposition in mice when administered orally.[64] Early clinical trials of this drug in superficial bladder cancer are underway.

An interesting naturally occurring agent under trial is neovastat, derived from shark cartilage. Its action in vitro is to inhibit matrix metalloproteinases and VEGF receptor binding and tyrosine phosphorylation. A phase III trial is examining neovastat in patients with failure of first line immunotherapy for advanced renal cell carcinoma.

One further agent in phase II trial for metastatic RCC is IM862, a naturally occurring peptide.

Gene therapy

Gene therapy involves inserting genes into cells so as to alter the balance of angiogenic agents produced by the cell, or its response to other exogenous agents. This may be suited to superficial bladder cancer, since intravesical access may circumvent problems with tumor transfection evident with solid tumors. A phase I trial has encouragingly reported transfectional efficacy in four patients instilled with live vaccinia prior to cystectomy for invasive disease.[88]

Antisense therapy

Antisense RNA imported into cells aims to interrupt endogenous RNA transcription, and therapy with antisense RNA to prevent transcription of interleukin-8, bFGF and angiogenin have all demonstrated antiangiogenic potential preclinically.[89–91]

Endothelial cell specific targeting

Potentially the most promising aspect of angiogenic therapy is to target the endothelial cells directly, thus obviating the problems of resistance and multiple pathways described above. Endothelial cells are normally quiescent, and exhibit a number of physical changes upon angiogenic stimulation. Evidence is accumulating of cell surface proteins (e.g. integrin alpha v beta 3)[92] which could potentially act as selective markers, specific even for individual growth factors. A phase I trial of the anti-integrin alpha v beta 3 antibody, vitaxin, demonstrated disease stabilization or partial response in 8 out of 17 patients with a range of metastatic solid organ tumors.[93] Further trials are awaited.

Conventional drugs may be tailored to affect tumor endothelium selectively. Pulsed chemotherapeutic regimens are thought to have antiangiogenic activity in this way. Other agents, such as microtubule inhibitors, may be able to target dividing endothelial cells only. Razoxane, a topoisomerase II inhibitor, appeared to stabilize tumor vasculature in early preclinical trials, but a phase II trial in patients with metastatic RCC showed only modest effects.[94]

Cell adhesion molecules offer a further target to disrupt endothelial cell function. Rather than targeting cell proliferation, endothelial cell functions such as adhesion and migration, may be a more profitable approach in future. This will avoid the previously mentioned problem of relatively low cell turnover in human compared with animal tumors.

The prospect of developing a vaccine against tumor endothelium has been suggested recently by the use of xenografted endothelial cells to induce autoimmunity against angiogenic endothelial cells, with resultant powerful effects on solid tumor models in mice.[95]

One further agent in development is TNP-470, an analog of fumagillin. Early experimental work on fumagillin, which has non-specific toxicity towards endothelial cells, demonstrated antiangiogenic activity in animal models. However a phase II trial in 33 patients with previously treated metastatic RCC produced only one partial response of short duration, though six patients had stable disease for at least 6 months.[96] The relative non-specificity and toxicity of fumagillin may thus limit its usefulness in a significant proportion of patients.

Conclusion

Angiogenesis is undoubtedly a key step in tumor development. Despite encouraging preclinical data, the struggle to produce truly effective anti-angiogenic agents goes on. The failure of conventional chemotherapies demands continued efforts to develop novel therapies and, with increasing understanding of the complex biology underlying malignancy, comes fresh hope of improving this situation.

References

1. Folkman J. What is the evidence that tumors are angiogenesis dependent? [editorial]. J Natl Cancer Inst 1990; 82(1):4–6.
2. Asahara T, Murohara T, Sullivan A, et al. Isolation of putative progenitor endothelial cells for angiogenesis. Science 1997; 275(5302):964–967.
3. Carmeliet P, Jain RK. Angiogenesis in cancer and other diseases. Nature 2000; 407(6801):249–257.
4. Siegal JA, Yu E, Brawer MK. Topography of neovascularity in human prostate carcinoma. Cancer 1995; 75(10):2545–2551.
5. Anderson H, Price P, Blomley M, et al. Measuring changes in human tumour vasculature in response to therapy using functional imaging techniques. Br J Cancer 2001; 85(8):1085–1093.
6. Strohmeyer D, Frauscher F, Klauser A, et al. Contrast-enhanced transrectal color doppler ultrasonography (TRCDUS) for assessment of angiogenesis in prostate cancer. Anticancer Res 2001; 21(4B):2907–2913.
7. Vesalainen S, Lipponen P, Talja M, et al. Tumor vascularity and basement membrane structure as prognostic factors in T1-2MO prostatic adenocarcinoma. Anticancer Res 1994; 14(2B):709–714.
8. Hall MC, Troncoso P, Pollack A, et al. Significance of tumor angiogenesis in clinically localized prostate carcinoma treated with external beam radiotherapy. Urology 1994; 44(6):869–875.
9. Silberman MA, Partin AW, Veltri RW, Epstein JI. Tumor angiogenesis correlates with progression after radical prostatectomy but not with pathologic stage in Gleason sum 5 to 7 adenocarcinoma of the prostate. Cancer 1997; 79(4):772–779.
10. Offersen BV, Borre M, Overgaard J. Immunohistochemical determination of tumor angiogenesis measured by the maximal microvessel density in human prostate cancer. APMIS 1998;106(4):463–469.
11. Bettencourt MC, Bauer JJ, Sesterhenn IA, et al. CD34 immunohistochemical assessment of angiogenesis as a prognostic marker for prostate cancer recurrence after radical prostatectomy. J Urol 1998; 160(2):459–465.
12. Borre M, Offersen BV, Nerstrom B, Overgaard J. Microvessel density predicts survival in prostate cancer patients subjected to watchful waiting. Br J Cancer 1998; 78(7):940–944.
13. Rubin MA, Buyyounouski M, Bagiella E, et al. Microvessel density in prostate cancer: lack of correlation with tumor grade, pathologic stage, and clinical outcome. Urology 1999; 53(3):542–547.
14. Strohmeyer D, Rossing C, Strauss F, et al. Tumor angiogenesis is associated with progression after radical prostatectomy in pT2/pT3 prostate cancer. Prostate 2000; 42(1):26–33.
15. de la Taille A, Katz AE, Bagiella E, et al. Microvessel density as a predictor of PSA recurrence after radical prostatectomy. A comparison of CD34 and CD31. Am J Clin Pathol 2000; 113(4):555–562.
16. Halvorsen OJ, Haukaas S, Hoisaeter PA, Akslen LA. Independent prognostic importance of microvessel density in clinically localized prostate cancer. Anticancer Res 2000; 20(5C):3791–3799.
17. Wakui S, Furusato M, Itoh T, et al. Tumour angiogenesis in prostatic carcinoma with and without bone marrow metastasis: a morphometric study. J Pathol 1992; 168(3):257–262.
18. Fregene TA, Khanuja PS, Noto AC, et al. Tumor-associated angiogenesis in prostate cancer. Anticancer Res 1993; 13(6B):2377–2381.
19. Weidner N, Carroll PR, Flax J, et al. Tumor angiogenesis correlates with metastasis in invasive prostate carcinoma. Am J Pathol 1993; 143(2):401–409.
20. Brawer MK, Deering RE, Brown M, et al. Predictors of pathologic stage in prostatic carcinoma. The role of neovascularity. Cancer 1994; 73(3):678–687.

21. Dickinson AJ, Fox SB, Persad RA, et al. Quantification of angiogenesis as an independent predictor of prognosis in invasive bladder carcinomas. Br J Urol 1994; 74(6):762–766.

22. Jaeger TM, Weidner N, Chew K, et al. Tumor angiogenesis correlates with lymph node metastases in invasive bladder cancer. J Urol 1995; 154(1):69–71.

23. Bochner BH, Cote RJ, Weidner N, et al. Angiogenesis in bladder cancer: relationship between microvessel density and tumor prognosis. J Natl Cancer Inst 1995; 87(21):1603–1612.

24. Philp EA, Stephenson TJ, Reed MW. Prognostic significance of angiogenesis in transitional cell carcinoma of the human urinary bladder [see comments]. Br J Urol 1996; 77(3):352–357.

25. Grossfeld GD, Ginsberg DA, Stein JP, et al. Thrombospondin-1 expression in bladder cancer: association with p53 alterations, tumor angiogenesis, and tumor progression. J Natl Cancer Inst 1997; 89(3):219–227.

26. Bochner BH, Esrig D, Groshen S, et al. Relationship of tumor angiogenesis and nuclear p53 accumulation in invasive bladder cancer. Clin Cancer Res 1997; 3(9):1615–1622.

27. Dinney CP, Babkowski RC, Antelo M, et al. Relationship among cystectomy, microvessel density and prognosis in stage T1 transitional cell carcinoma of the bladder. J Urol 1998; 160(4):1285–1290.

28. Hawke CK, Delahunt B, Davidson PJ. Microvessel density as a prognostic marker for transitional cell carcinoma of the bladder. Br J Urol 1998; 81(4):585–590.

29. Chaudhary R, Bromley M, Clarke NW, et al. Prognostic relevance of micro-vessel density in cancer of the urinary bladder. Anticancer Res 1999; 19(4C):3479–3484.

30. Ozer E, Mungan MU, Tuna B, et al. Prognostic significance of angiogenesis and immunoreactivity of cathepsin D and type IV collagen in high-grade stage T1 primary bladder cancer. Urology 1999; 54(1):50–55.

31. Inoue K, Slaton JW, Karashima T, et al. The prognostic value of angiogenesis factor expression for predicting recurrence and metastasis of bladder cancer after neoadjuvant chemotherapy and radical cystectomy. Clin Cancer Res 2000; 6(12):4866–4873.

32. Sagol O, Yorukoglu K, Sis B, et al. Does angiogenesis predict recurrence in superficial transitional cell carcinoma of the bladder? Urology 2001; 57(5):895–899.

33. Yoshino S, Kato M, Okada K. Prognostic significance of microvessel count in low stage renal cell carcinoma. Int J Urol 1995; 2(3):156–160.

34. MacLennan GT, Bostwick DG. Microvessel density in renal cell carcinoma: lack of prognostic significance. Urology 1995; 46(1):27–30.

35. Delahunt B, Bethwaite PB, Thornton A, et al. Prognostic significance of microscopic vascularity for clear cell renal cell carcinoma. Br J Urol 1997; 80(3):401–404.

36. Gelb AB, Sudilovsky D, Wu CD, et al. Appraisal of intratumoral microvessel density, MIB-1 score, DNA content, and p53 protein expression as prognostic indicators in patients with locally confined renal cell carcinoma. Cancer 1997; 80(9):1768–1775.

37. Ou YC, Chen JT, Yang CR, et al. Tumor angiogenesis and metastasis: correlation in invasive renal cell carcinoma. Chung Hua I Hsueh Tsa Chih (Taipei) 1998; 61(8):441–447.

38. Nativ O, Sabo E, Reiss A, et al. Clinical significance of tumor angiogenesis in patients with localized renal cell carcinoma. Urology 1998; 51(5):693–696.

39. Kohler HH, Barth PJ, Siebel A, et al. Quantitative assessment of vascular surface density in renal cell carcinomas. Br J Urol 1996; 77(5):650–654.

40. Olivarez D, Ulbright T, DeRiese W, et al. Neovascularization in clinical stage A testicular germ cell tumor: prediction of metastatic disease. Cancer Res 1994; 54(10):2800–2802.

41. Mukhopadhyay D, Nagy JA, Manseau EJ, Dvorak HF. Vascular permeability factor/vascular endothelial growth factor-mediated signaling in mouse mesentery vascular endothelium. Cancer Res 1998; 58(6):1278–1284.

42. Crew JP, Fuggle S, Bicknell R, et al. Eukaryotic initiation factor-4E in superficial and muscle invasive bladder cancer and its correlation with vascular endothelial growth factor expression and tumour progression. Br J Cancer 2000; 82(1):161–166.

43. Gnarra JR, Tory K, Weng Y, et al. Mutations of the VHL tumour suppressor gene in renal carcinoma. Nat Genet 1994; 7(1):85–90.

44. Crew JP, O'Brien T, Bradburn M, et al. Vascular endothelial growth factor is a predictor of relapse and stage progression in superficial bladder cancer. Cancer Res 1997; 57(23):5281–5285.

45. Crew JP, O'Brien T, Bicknell R, et al. Urinary vascular endothelial growth factor and its correlation with bladder cancer recurrence rates. J Urol 1999; 161(3):799–804.

46. Brown LF, Berse B, Jackman RW, et al. Increased expression of vascular permeability factor (vascular endothelial growth factor) and its receptors in kidney and bladder carcinomas. Am J Pathol 1993; 143(5):1255–1262.

47. Paradis V, Lagha NB, Zeimoura L, et al. Expression of vascular endothelial growth factor in renal cell carcinomas. Virchows Arch 2000; 436(4):351–356.

48. Dirix LY, Vermeulen PB, Pawinski A, et al. Elevated levels of the angiogenic cytokines basic fibroblast growth factor and vascular endothelial growth factor in sera of cancer patients. Br J Cancer 1997; 76(2):238–243.

49. Dosquet C, Coudert MC, Lepage C, et al. Are angiogenic factors, cytokines, and soluble adhesion molecules prognostic factors in patients with renal cell carcinoma? Clin Cancer Res 1997; 3(12 Pt 1):2451–2458.

50. Joseph IB, Isaacs JT. Potentiation of the antiangiogenic ability of linomide by androgen ablation involves down-regulation of vascular endothelial growth factor in human androgen-responsive prostatic cancers. Cancer Res 1997; 57(6):1054–1057.

51. Cvetkovic D, Movsas B, Dicker AP, et al. Increased hypoxia correlates with increased expression of the angiogenesis marker vascular endothelial growth factor in human prostate cancer. Urology 2001; 57(4):821–825.

52. Duque JL, Loughlin KR, Adam RM, et al. Plasma levels of vascular endothelial growth factor are increased in patients with metastatic prostate cancer. Urology 1999; 54(3):523–527.

53. Bok RA, Halabi S, Fei DT, et al. Vascular endothelial growth factor and basic fibroblast growth factor urine

levels as predictors of outcome in hormone-refractory prostate cancer patients: a cancer and leukemia group B study. Cancer Res 2001; 61(6):2533–2536.

54. Melnyk O, Zimmerman M, Kim KJ, Shuman M. Neutralizing anti-vascular endothelial growth factor antibody inhibits further growth of established prostate cancer and metastases in a pre-clinical model. J Urol 1999; 161(3):960–963.

55. Lipponen P, Eskelinen M. Expression of epidermal growth factor receptor in bladder cancer as related to established prognostic factors, oncoprotein (c-erbB-2, p53) expression and long-term prognosis. Br J Cancer 1994; 69(6):1120–1125.

56. Mellon K, Wright C, Kelly P, et al. Long-term outcome related to epidermal growth factor receptor status in bladder cancer. J Urol 1995; 153(3 Pt 2):919–925.

57. Messing EM, Murphy-Brooks N. Recovery of epidermal growth factor in voided urine of patients with bladder cancer. Urology 1994; 44(4):502–506.

58. Zhong H, Chiles K, Feldster D, et al. Modulation of hypoxia-inducible factor 1 alpha expression by the epidermal growth factor/phosphatidylinositol 3-kinase/PTEN/AKT/FRAP pathway in human prostate cancer cells: implications for tumor angiogenesis and therapeutics. Cancer Res 2000; 60(6):1541–1545.

59. Gleave ME, Hsieh JT, Wu HC, et al. Epidermal growth factor receptor-mediated autocrine and paracrine stimulation of human transitional cell carcinoma. Cancer Res 1993; 53(21):5300–5307.

60. Perrotte P, Matsumoto T, Inoue K, et al. Anti-epidermal growth factor receptor antibody C225 inhibits angiogenesis in human transitional cell carcinoma growing orthotopically in nude mice. Clin Cancer Res 1999; 5(2):257–265.

61. Ozdemir E, Kakehi Y, Okuno H, Yoshida O. Role of matrix metalloproteinase-9 in the basement membrane destruction of superficial urothelial carcinomas. J Urol 1999; 161(4):1359–1363.

62. Papathoma AS, Petraki C, Grigorakis A, et al. Prognostic significance of matrix metalloproteinases 2 and 9 in bladder cancer. Anticancer Res 2000; 20(3B):2009–2013.

63. Grignon DJ, Sakr W, Toth M, et al. High levels of tissue inhibitor of metalloproteinase-2 (TIMP-2) expression are associated with poor outcome in invasive bladder cancer. Cancer Res 1996; 56(7):1654–1659.

64. Elkin M, Ariel I, Miao HQ, et al. Inhibition of bladder carcinoma angiogenesis, stromal support, and tumor growth by halofuginone. Cancer Res 1999; 59(16):4111–4118.

65. Naruo S, Kanayama H, Takigawa H, et al. Serum levels of a tissue inhibitor of metalloproteinases-1 (TIMP-1) in bladder cancer patients. Int J Urol 1994; 1(3):228–231.

66. Nguyen M, Watanabe H, Budson AE, et al. Elevated levels of the angiogenic peptide basic fibroblast growth factor in urine of bladder cancer patients. J Natl Cancer Inst 1993; 85(3):241–242.

67. Brown NS, Jones A, Fujiyama C, et al. Thymidine phosphorylase induces carcinoma cell oxidative stress and promotes secretion of angiogenic factors. Cancer Res 2000; 60(22):6298–6302.

68. Jones A, Fujiyama C, Turner K, et al. Role of thymidine phosphorylase in an in vitro model of human bladder cancer invasion. J Urol 2002; 167(3):1482–1486.

69. O'Brien T, Cranston D, Fuggle S. et al. Different angiogenic pathways characterize superficial and invasive bladder cancer. Cancer Res 1995; 55(3):510–513.

70. Mizutani Y, Okada Y, Yoshida O. Expression of platelet-derived endothelial cell growth factor in bladder carcinoma. Cancer 1997; 79(6):1190–1194.

71. O'Reilly MS, Holmgren L, Chen C, Folkman J. Angiostatin induces and sustains dormancy of human primary tumors in mice. Nat Med 1996; 2(6):689–692.

72. O'Reilly MS, Boehm T, Shing Y, et al. Endostatin: an endogenous inhibitor of angiogenesis and tumor growth. Cell 1997; 88(2):277–285.

73. Campbell SC, Volpert OV, Ivanovich M, Bouck NP. Molecular mediators of angiogenesis in bladder cancer. Cancer Res 1998; 58(6):1298–1304.

74. Grossfeld GD, Carroll PR, Lindeman N, et al. Thrombospondin-1 expression in patients with pathologic stage T3 prostate cancer undergoing radical prostatectomy: association with p53 alterations, tumor angiogenesis, and tumor progression. Urology 2002; 59(1):97–102.

75. Kwak C, Jin RJ, Lee C, et al. Thrombospondin-1, vascular endothelial growth factor expression and their relationship with p53 status in prostate cancer and benign prostatic hyperplasia. BJU Int 2002; 89(3):303–309.

76. Yu JL, Rak JW, Coomber BL, et al. Effect of p53 status on tumor response to antiangiogenic therapy. Science 2002; 295(5559):1526–1528.

77. Fortier AH, Nelson BJ, Grella DK, Holaday JW. Antiangiogenic activity of prostate-specific antigen. J Natl Cancer Inst 1999; 91(19):1635–1640.

78. Singh RK, Gutman M, Bucana CD, et al. Interferons alpha and beta down-regulate the expression of basic fibroblast growth factor in human carcinomas. Proc Natl Acad Sci USA 1995; 92(10):4562–4566.

79. Coppin C, Porzsolt F, Kumpf J, et al. Immunotherapy for advanced renal cell cancer (Cochrane review). Cochrane Database Syst Rev 2000; 3:CD001425.

80. Motzer RJ, Murphy BA, Bacol K, et al. Phase III trial of interferon alfa-2a with or without 13-cis-retinoic acid for patients with advanced renal cell carcinoma. J Clin Oncol 2000; 18(16):2972–2980.

81. Pavlovich CP, Kraling BM, Stewart RJ, et al. BCG-induced urinary cytokines inhibit microvascular endothelial cell proliferation. J Urol 2000; 163(6):2014–2021.

82. Rajala P, Liukkonen T, Raitanen M, et al. Transurethral resection with perioperative instillation of interferon-alpha or epirubicin for the prophylaxis of recurrent primary superficial bladder cancer: a prospective randomized multicenter study – Finnbladder III. J Urol 1999; 161(4):1133–1135; discussion 1135–1136.

83. Eisen T, Boshoff C, Mak I, et al. Continuous low dose thalidomide: a phase II study in advanced melanoma, renal cell, ovarian and breast cancer. Br J Cancer 2000; 82(4):812–817.

84. Motzer RJ, Berg W, Ginsberg M, et al. Phase II trial of thalidomide for patients with advanced renal cell carcinoma. J Clin Oncol 2002; 20(1):302–306.

85. Eisenberger MA, Reyno LM, Jodrell DI, et al. Suramin, an active drug for prostate cancer: interim observations in a phase I trial [see comments] [published erratum appears in J Natl Cancer Inst 1994; 86(8):639–640]. J Natl Cancer Inst 1993; 85(8):611–621.

86. Rosen PJ, Mendoza EF, Landaw EM, et al. Suramin in hormone-refractory metastatic prostate cancer: a drug with limited efficacy. J Clin Oncol 1996; 14(5):1626–1636.

87. Graham SD Jr, Napalkov P, Oladele A, et al. Intravesical suramin in the prevention of transitional cell carcinoma. Urology 1995; 45(1):59–63.

88. Gomella LG, Mastrangelo MJ, McCue PA, et al. Phase I study of intravesical vaccinia virus as a vector for gene therapy of bladder cancer. J Urol 2001; 166(4):1291–1295.

89. Inoue K, Perrotte P, Wood CG, et al. Gene therapy of human bladder cancer with adenovirus-mediated antisense basic fibroblast growth factor. Clin Cancer Res 2000; 6(11):4422–4431.

90. Inoue K, Wood CG, Slaton JW, et al. Adenoviral-mediated gene therapy of human bladder cancer with antisense interleukin-8. Oncol Rep 2001; 8(5):955–964.

91. Olson KA, Byers HR, Key ME, Fett JW. Prevention of human prostate tumor metastasis in athymic mice by antisense targeting of human angiogenin. Clin Cancer Res 2001; 7(11):3598–3605.

92. Brooks PC, Clark RA, Cheresh DA. Requirement of vascular integrin alpha v beta 3 for angiogenesis. Science 1994; 264(5158):569–571.

93. Gutheil JC, Campbell TN, Pierce PR, et al. Targeted antiangiogenic therapy for cancer using Vitaxin: a humanized monoclonal antibody to the integrin alphavbeta3. Clin Cancer Res 2000; 6(8):3056–3061.

94. Braybrooke JP, O'Byrne KJ, Propper DJ, et al. A phase II study of razoxane, an antiangiogenic topoisomerase II inhibitor, in renal cell cancer with assessment of potential surrogate markers of angiogenesis. Clin Cancer Res 2000; 6(12):4697–4704.

95. Wei YQ, Wang QR, Zhao X, et al. Immunotherapy of tumors with xenogeneic endothelial cells as a vaccine. Nat Med 2000; 6(10):1160–1166.

96. Stadler WM, Kuzel T, Shapiro C, et al. Multi-institutional study of the angiogenesis inhibitor TNP-470 in metastatic renal carcinoma. J Clin Oncol 1999; 7(8):2541–2545.

6

Chemoprevention of prostate cancer

Wade J Sexton and Ian M Thompson

Prostate cancer chemoprevention is defined as the administration of dietary supplements, micronutrients, biologic agents, drugs, etc., to prevent or delay the initiation, promotion, or progression of prostate cancer precursors (dysplasia and prostatic intraepithelial neoplasia) to invasive and metastatic prostate adenocarcinoma.[1] It is believed that precursor lesions such as high grade prostatic intraepithelial neoplasia (HGPIN) develop at least 10 years prior to the development of localized carcinomas and it is this prolonged process of carcinogenesis that lends itself well to opportunities for chemoprevention.[2]

Chemoprevention has attracted widespread interest and is rapidly gaining momentum as a priority in the field of prostate cancer research. This is in part due to the controversy surrounding prostate cancer screening. For a large percentage of patients with clinically localized disease, physicians have limited indicators to determine which patients will experience morbidity or mortality from prostate cancer, as opposed to those who have inconsequential cancers. Phase III studies including the Prostate, Lung, Colorectal, and Ovarian cancer (PLCO) screening study of the National Cancer Institute and the European Randomized Study of Screening for Prostate Cancer (ERSPC) are designed to examine the morbidity and mortality of prostate cancer in screened versus unscreened men. However, the results of these two prospective studies will not be available until 2010 and 2008 respectively. Thus, it is of utmost importance to determine which agents or drugs will prevent the development of invasive prostate cancers, and to develop strategies whereby these potential agents can be tested for their chemopreventive capabilities in population-based studies or in cohorts of

men felt to be at high risk for developing this disease (Table 6.1).

Also critical is the need to identify biological markers to serve as intermediate endpoints to measure treatment efficacy as the natural history of prostate cancer development and progression is one of a slowly progressive malignancy – often requiring many years for patients to succumb to the disease even following definitive localized treatment.[3] Without doubt, important information will be gained from ongoing clinical trials measuring the effectiveness of various chemopreventive agents in altering not only prostate cancer incidence and detection, but also slowing prostate cancer progression. The focus of this chapter will be to review the most promising agents for the prevention of prostate cancer including hormonal therapies, phytoestrogens, micronutrients, carotenoids, retinoids, vitamin D analogs, non-steroidal anti-inflammatory drugs (NSAIDs), and farnesyl protein transferase inhibitors (Table 6.2).

Table 6.1 Suitable patient populations for chemoprevention trials

Age > 55 years, normal DRE, normal PSA
Positive family history (at least two first-degree relatives)
Abnormal PSA with previously negative prostate biopsy
Biopsy proven HGPIN or atypia
Watchful waiting patients
Favourable cancers (PSA < 10, biopsy GL sum < 7, stage < cT2b)
High risk for recurrence following definitive local therapy
PSA recurrence following definitive local therapy

DRE, digital rectal examination; GL, Gleason's; HGPIN, high grade prostatic intraepithelial neoplasia; PSA, prostate specific antigen

Table 6.2 Promising agents for prostate cancer chemoprevention

Hormonal therapies
    5-alpha reductase inhibitors
    Antiandrogens
    Antiestrogens
    SERMs

Phytoestrogens
    Isoflavones/isoflavenoids (soy proteins, genistein, BBI)
    Lignans

Micronutrients/antioxidants
    Selenium
    Tocopherols (vitamin E)

Carotenoids (lycopene)
Vitamin D analogs

Non-steroidal anti-inflammatory drugs
    Cyclooxygenase inhibitors
    Lipooxygenase inhibitors
    cGMP phosphodiesterase inhibitors

Farnesyl protein transferase inhibitors

BBI, Bowman-Birk inhibitor; cGMP, cyclic guanosine monophosphate phosphodiesterase; SERM, selective estrogen receptor modulator

Hormonal therapies

Androgens

Evidence that androgens play a critical role in prostate embryogenesis is a basis for attempting to modulate the androgenic milieu in both treating and preventing prostate cancers. Testosterone, which is produced by the Leydig interstitial cells of the testis, is converted intracellularly to dihydro-testosterone (DHT) by 5-alpha reductase. DHT is 100 times more potent an androgen compared to testosterone. Together, testosterone and DHT are responsible for regulating the normal development and function of the prostate gland. Men born deficient in 5-alpha reductase or castrated prior to the onset of puberty do not develop prostate cancer.[4,5] It is not known if a lack of androgens following puberty will affect the incidence of prostate cancer, but there is a suggestion that a higher cumulative exposure to androgens might increase the development of clinically detected prostate cancer. For instance, higher levels of androgens and metabolites of DHT have been found in US African–Americans and Caucasians (high risk populations) compared to Japanese (low risk population).[6] African–Americans have been demonstrated to have polymorphisms of the androgen receptor (i.e. a shorter CAG repeat in the trans-

activation domain) that makes the receptor more active.[7] Variations in other genes such as the CYP3A4 gene responsible for testosterone degradation and the SRD5A2 gene which codes for 5-alpha reductase have also been associated with a higher risk of prostate cancer.[8,9]

Huggins and Hodges published their pioneering work regarding the effects of androgens on prostate cancer in 1941.[10] Since their initial report, many series have demonstrated the benefits of treating patients with luteinizing hormone-releasing hormone (LHRH) agonists designed to alter the normal function of the hypothalamic–pituitary–gonadal axis. These agents have been primarily used for the treatment of locally advanced or metastatic prostate cancer.[11–13] Non-steroidal antiandrogens (flutamide, bicalutamide, and nilutamide) that function as androgen receptor antagonists are approved for the treatment of prostate cancer either as single agent therapy or more commonly as combination therapy with LHRH agonists for advanced prostate cancer.[14,15] These antiandrogens share the same mechanism of action. While they most commonly function as androgen receptor antagonists, in the presence of mutated androgen receptors they may function as receptor agonists.[16] However, while the side effect profile of non-steroidal antiandrogens might be more appealing than those of LHRH analogs, their role for younger patients in prostate cancer prevention strategies is limited. Instead, these agents may be better utilized in preventing cancer recurrence following definitive local therapy or in patients (such as those with HGPIN) determined to be at high risk for disease development.[17]

Finasteride

The 5-alpha reductase inhibitor, finasteride (Proscar, Merck) has potential chemoprevention capabilities via its inhibitory effect on the production of DHT from testosterone. Finasteride leads to the regression of prostatic hyperplasia and inhibits prostate growth.[18] In men treated with finasteride, serum and prostatic levels of DHT drop considerably whereas serum and tissue levels of testosterone are slightly higher. As demonstrated in the PLESS study (Proscar Long Term Efficacy and Safety Study) the side effect profile of Proscar is very favorable with no significant difference in the rates of impotence, altered libido, and ejaculatory disturbances between patients taking finasteride versus those taking placebo.[19] Preliminary small, randomized, yet non-blinded studies of finasteride use have had mixed outcomes with regard to the incidence of prostate cancer. Men randomized to take finasteride in the PLESS study demonstrated a non-significant decrease in the incidence of prostate cancer. A smaller study of 52 men with elevated prostate specific antigens (PSAs) and negative prostate biopsies revealed no reduction in prostate cancer rates between those men randomized to receive finasteride versus men randomized to observation. Conversely, this smaller study revealed an actual increase in the detection of prostatic intraepithelial neoplasia (PIN) in men receiving finasteride.[20] However, these studies lacked sufficient power to determine whether 5-alpha reductase inhibitors exerted any true effect on the overall rates of prostate cancer development and may not have actually provided a placebo for the non-treated group. There is a suggestion that finasteride can delay the progression of prostate cancer in men with a detectable PSA post prostatectomy and no clinical or radiographic evidence of metastases. Men were randomized to treatment for 12 months with either finasteride or placebo. The group receiving finasteride had a delay in PSA rise by 8 months, compared with the placebo group. Those men with a PSA ≤ 1 ng/dl appeared to derive greater benefit as no patient in this group experienced a PSA elevation at 24 months.[21]

Based on finasteride's chemoprevention potential and its favorable toxicity profile, in 1993 the Southwest Oncology Group (SWOG) supported by the National Cancer Institute (NCI) sought to overcome the constraints of earlier underpowered preliminary studies and initiated the Prostate Cancer Prevention Trial (PCPT).[22] The objective of this study is to determine if finasteride can decrease the cumulative incidence (period prevalence) of prostate cancer. In this large prospective, double-blind study, 18 881 men were randomized to receive placebo versus 5 mg finasteride. The study design enabled investigators to detect a 25% reduction in prostate cancers in men taking finasteride compared to those taking placebo. Eligibility criteria included men ≥ 55 years of age with a normal digital rectal examination (DRE) and an initial PSA of ≤ 3 ng/dl. Patient accrual lasted exactly 3 years and after 7 years on the study,

patients are scheduled to undergo end of study prostate biopsies. Although the majority of prostate biopsies were completed by the end of 2001, results of the PCPT study will not be available until 2004, when the last participants undergo their prostate biopsy.

Estrogens

There is increasing evidence that estrogens play important roles in prostate growth, development, and carcinogenesis. Estrogen stimulates prostate cellular growth through the local production of stimulatory peptide growth factors including transforming growth factor alpha (TGF-alpha), insulin-like growth factor (IGF), and epidermal growth factor (EGF), and by inhibiting the expression of growth inhibitory factors like transforming growth factor beta (TGF-beta).[23] Prostate stroma and epithelium express estrogen receptors (ER) that may modulate prostate epithelial proliferation.[24] While both ER-alpha and ER-beta subtypes are present in prostate tissue,[23] ER-alpha appears to be more predominant in cases of HGPIN and invasive carcinomas.[25] This finding supports the rationale for evaluating antiestrogens in early prostate cancer, as well as the development of selective antiestrogens that might decrease associated side effects of therapy. More work is required to elucidate the estrogen receptor's role in prostate cancer development and its potential for cancer chemoprevention.

Selective estrogen receptor modulators (SERMs) have partial agonist and antagonist properties depending on the tissue type studied. One of the best-known SERMs is tamoxifen, an important adjunct in the treatment and prevention of breast cancer. Other SERMs include toremifene, raloxifene, and SERM-3. SERMs have effects on various growth factors such as TGF-beta and IGF-1, and may ameliorate side effects of antiandrogens (e.g. gynecomastia).[1] Animal models and in vitro studies using LNCaP cell lines suggest that SERMs may slow the progression or decrease the incidence of prostate cancer. In addition to possible chemoprevention capabilities, SERMs could benefit patients by decreasing cardiovascular risks, preventing osteoporosis, and suppressing benign prostatic hyperplasia (BPH) formation.[23] Human prostate cancer clinical trials using SERMs for chemoprevention are underway.

Phytoestrogens (soy proteins/isoflavenoids, lignans)

Phytoestrogens are non-steroidal substances with weak estrogenic properties, and like SERMs, they have partial estrogen receptor agonist and antagonist activity. Although phytoestrogens are 1000 times less potent than estradiol, their affinity for estrogen receptors is equivalent to that of tamoxifen and other SERMs.[26] Phytoestrogens may prevent prostate cancer by lowering 5-alpha reductase activity, by increasing the serum levels of sex hormone binding globulin or lowering the serum levels of free testosterone, and by decreasing the enzymatic activities of both tyrosine-specific protein kinase and P450 aromatase.[26] Phytoestrogens might adversely affect angiogenesis or function as antioxidants.

There are two major classes of phytoestrogens: isoflavenoids and lignans. Genistein is one of the most well known plant-derived isoflavenoids, and it is a major component of soybeans. Soy products are vegetable sources of dietary protein and are largely deficient in Western diets. However, soy products are consumed in much larger quantities in Asian countries such as China and Japan. The typical Asian diet contains 10–20 times more genistein than the standard western diet,[27–29] and there appears to be an inverse correlation between isoflavenoid consumption and prostate cancer incidence.[26] Furthermore, isoflavenoids (including daidzein and equol) concentrate in the prostate and prostatic secretions when compared to plasma concentrations.[27] While autopsy studies show that the incidence of latent prostate cancers is similar in both Asian and Western populations of patients, Asian males have a lower age-adjusted incidence of clinically evident and advanced staged prostate cancer (i.e. cT3–cT4). Epidemiological studies also reveal a lower incidence of metastatic prostate cancer in individuals consuming soy-based diets compared to traditional Western diets.[30] The epidemiological evidence suggests that isoflavenoids may prevent or slow the transformation of latent adenocarcinomas into more malignant phenotypes of prostate cancer.

Genistein has been reported to inhibit 5-alpha reductase, P450 aromatase, and 17-beta hydroxysteroid oxidoreductase – an important enzyme in estrogen metabolism. Other possible mechanisms for genistein's anticancer effects include in vitro evidence for increased cell adhesion in prostate cancer cell lines (including the highly metastatic PC3 cell line), growth inhibition of non-adherent cells through apoptotic pathways, and protein tyrosine kinase inhibition (important enzymes for regulating cellular growth and differentiation).[31–33] Other soy-derived substances such as the serine protease Bowman-Birk inhibitor have detrimental effects on the growth and survival of LNCaP and PC3 cell lines and may be important in the design of future chemoprevention trials.[34] Currently, soy products are being evaluated in dose escalation trials in normal healthy volunteers and in clinical phase I and II studies of patients with hormone refractory cancer, in patients at risk for prostate cancer recurrence, and in patients with early stage prostate cancer.[35,36]

Lignans are other natural sources of dietary estrogenic compounds and are derived from seeds, cereals and grains. Two of the most common lignans are enterolactone and enterodiol. Like genistein, enterolactone can inhibit several steroid metabolizing enzymes such as aromatase, 5-alpha reductase and 17-beta hydroxysteroid dehydrogenase. Vegetarians have high urinary and plasma concentrations of lignans. However, at least in some patient populations, vegetarian diets have not correlated with lower cancer-related mortality rates (including prostate cancer mortality).[37] Together with isoflavones, these types of phytoestrogen require further prospective testing as prostate cancer chemopreventive agents.

Micronutrients/antioxidants

Considerable evidence points to reactive oxygen species (ROS) and the oxidative damage they cause as etiologic agents in the development and progression of various malignancies including prostate cancer. ROS may damage cellular components including lipids, proteins and DNA. As DNA mutations accumulate, there is an increased risk for altered gene function and for the transcription of various factors involved in neoplastic transformation. ROS also might affect the P53 gene, which has been associated with the progression of various human malignancies.[38]

Selenium

Selenium is a non-metallic trace mineral and an integral component of glutathione peroxidase – a selenium-dependent enzyme that protects the cell from oxidative damage by catalyzing the reduction of lipid hydroperoxides.[39] Selenium is found in varying concentrations in the soil throughout the world. Dietary selenium comes from grains, meat, yeast, and some vegetables. Onions and garlic are good dietary sources of this element but reflect the soil concentrations where grown. Selenium's role in cancer chemoprevention is unknown, but it may act as an antioxidant, an anticarcinogen, through antiproliferation, or through apoptotic events. Interestingly, there is opposing evidence that selenium interacts with thiols, including L-cysteine and reduced glutathione to form compounds that result in the production of reactive oxygen species. These free radicals may in turn result in cellular apoptosis.[40]

In vitro data demonstrate selenium's effects on cell line and animal models of prostate cancer. In the DU145 prostate cancer cell line, seleno-methionine inhibited prostate cancer cells in a dose-dependent fashion in doses ranging from 45 to 130 μm while growth inhibition of normal diploid fibroblasts required 1 mM selenomethio-nine, an approximately 1000-fold higher concentration than for the cancer cells. The addition of selenomethionine to the cell cultures resulted in apoptotic cell death and aberrant mitoses.[41,42] Selenium has also been shown to inhibit cadmium-induced growth of prostate cancer epithelial cells in vitro.[43]

Numerous studies have demonstrated inverse correlations between selenium intake or selenium tissue levels and various malignancies.[44,45] Evidence from the Health Professionals Follow-Up Study suggested that there was a two-thirds reduction in prostate cancer risk in men with the highest quartile of selenium measured in toenail clippings.[46] However, some of the most promising evidence for selenium's potential as a prostate cancer preventive agent resulted from a secondary observation in a phase III clinical trial comparing selenium and placebo to prevent dermatologic malignancies. In this study, conducted in several regions of the US where selenium intake is lower, 1312 patients were randomized to either selenium (200 μg as 0.5 g of brewer's yeast tablet) or placebo. While there was no difference in skin cancer risk, study investigators reported a two-thirds reduction in prostate cancer risk.[47]

Vitamin E

The best known and the primary intracellular anti-oxidant is vitamin E. Vitamin E is the collective name for a group of naturally occurring, essential, fat-soluble vitamins called tocopherols and toco-trienols. Vitamin E functions as the major lipid-soluble antioxidant in cell membranes. The most common hypothesis for the cancer prevention activity of vitamin E is a reduction of oxidative injury. Vitamin E may enhance immune functions and limit cellular growth. Finally, vitamin E may diminish the activity of protein kinases – cellular signal transducers that regulate cell proliferation.[48,49]

Cumulative data from both in vitro (DU145 and PC3) and in vivo prostate cancer models (LNCaP xenografts in athymic mice) reveal that vitamin E has the potential to alter prostate cancer proliferation and growth.[50,51] Epidemiological evidence for vitamin E's role in prostate cancer chemoprevention evolved from a study of plasma vitamin levels and the risk of cancer-related mortality in nearly 3000 males in Basel, Switzerland. In this prospective study, Eichholzer and colleagues found an inverse relationship between low vitamin E levels in smokers and an increased risk of prostate cancer.[52] However, conflicting data from a prospective trial analyzing vitamin E supplementation was reported in the Health Professionals Follow-Up Study, in which a total of 1896 men with prostate cancer were identified out of 47 780 males. Men who supplemented with at least 100 IU of vitamin E daily had a multivariate relative risk of 1.07 for all prostate cancers and 1.14 for metastatic or fatal prostate cancer. Only among current smokers or recent quitters was the risk reduced (RR of 0.44; 95% CI = 0.18–1.07).[53] Some of the most intriguing data surrounding vitamin E stem from the Alpha-Tocopherol, Beta-Carotene (ATBC) trial. In this double-blind clinical trial, more than 29 000 male Finnish smokers were randomized in a 2×2 factorial design to receive the study agents over 5–8 years. Secondary findings revealed a 32% reduction in prostate cancer incidence and a 41% reduction in prostate cancer mortality among the men who received supplemental vitamin E. Interestingly, the authors suggested that vitamin E had no effect on advanced prostate cancers as the time from diagnosis until death in vitamin E recipients was unchanged compared to non-recipients. Rather, supplementation with vitamin E was hypothesized to diminish the transformation of latent prostate cancers into clinical cancers, a point supported by the overall reduction in prostate cancer mortality.[54]

To determine the efficacy of selenium and vitamin E alone, and in combination for preventing clinical prostate cancers, the Selenium and Vitamin E Cancer Prevention Trial (SELECT) has recently been initiated.[55] SELECT is an intergroup phase III, randomized, double-blind, placebo-controlled clinical trial that began accruing patients in 2001. Over 32 000 men with a normal digital rectal examination and a PSA < 4.0 ng/ml will be randomized in a 2 × 2 manner to 400 IU vitamin E, 200 µg selenium, both, or neither with each participant receiving two capsules. Participant enrolment will last for approximately 5 years and the duration of therapy will be from a minimum of 7 years to a maximum of 12 years. Study results will not be available at least until 2012.

Other prospective randomized studies of selenium and vitamin E are also underway. These studies are crucial to identify potential intracellular biomarkers affected by the administration of supplements such as selenium and vitamin E, and may further serve to identify intermediate endpoints for measuring the success of these supplements as chemopreventive agents. Validated intermediate endpoints would make large, prolonged and expensive studies like the PCPT and SELECT trials unnecessary. One SWOG-sponsored study is designed to examine the effects of selenium supplementation to patients with biopsy-proven, high grade prostatic intraepithelial neoplasia on the clinical development of invasive prostate cancer. Through special frozen section biopsy techniques, other investigators are examining the effects of selenium and vitamin E on intracellular markers and reactive oxygen species in the prostates of patients scheduled to undergo prostate biopsies or radical prostatectomies. Overall, the potential for these specific micronutrients to delay or prevent the induction, promotion or progression of prostate cancer precursors to invasive or metastatic prostate cancers is very encouraging and the ensuing research should provide very interesting data in the area of prostate cancer chemoprevention.

Carotenoids/retinoids

Carotenoids are naturally occurring compounds found in carrots, green leafy vegetables and tomato-based products. They have a variety of proposed actions including an antioxidant effect and apoptosis.[56] Two of the most commonly studied carotenoids for cancer chemoprevention are beta-carotene (the precursor of vitamin A) and lycopene. However, multiple other carotenoids have been studied in both laboratory and clinical settings for their roles in modifying prostate carcinogenesis including: neoxanthin, fucoxanthin, phytoene, phytofluene, canthaxanthin, beta-cryptoxanthin, zeta-carotene and zeaxanthin.[56,57]

Carotenoids

The cancer prevention data from studies involving beta-carotene and most of the other carotenoids have been controversial. While in vitro, 5,6-mono-epoxy carotenoids such as neoxanthin (found in spinach) and acyclic carotenoids such as phytofluene, zeta-carotene and lycopene (all present in tomatoes) reduced the viability of PC3, DU145 and LNCaP prostate cancer cell lines, other carotenoids including phytoene, canthaxanthin, beta-cryptoxanthin and zeaxanthin had no apparent effect on cell viability.[56] While some preclinical data and epidemiological observations suggest that carotenoids reduce the risk of prostate cancer, more recent studies do not support a beneficial association. In the Physicians' Health Study, over 22 000 male physicians were randomized to 50 mg beta carotene on alternate days and, after long-term follow-up, the incidence of prostate cancer among the supplement group compared to the control group was unchanged except for a reduction in patients with the highest body mass index (RR = 0.8, 95% CI 0.6–1.0).[58] Furthermore, there was no significant inverse relationship between low plasma beta-carotene levels and death from prostate cancer compared to prostate cancer survivors in the prospective study from Basel, Switzerland.[52] However, in the ATBC trial, the incidence of prostate cancer in male smokers receiving daily supplements of 20 mg beta-carotene actually increased 23% while the prostate cancer-related mortality increased 15% compared to patients not supplementing with beta-carotene.[54] As a result of these findings, most physicians in the field of cancer chemoprevention are no longer recommending routine supplementation with beta-carotene.

Recently, there has been significant interest with regard to lycopene as a preventive agent for prostate cancer. Lycopene is one of the carotenoids found in tomato products, watermelon and other vegetables. It is released during the cooking process and absorbed in the presence of fat. Tomato sauce is the primary source of bioavailable lycopene. Imaida and colleagues reported that there was no identifiable chemopreventive effect of lycopene in prostate carcinogenesis in their animal model.[59] However, multiple other studies have demonstrated a positive association between lycopene consumption and a reduced prostate cancer risk. Population-based case control studies have found inverse relationships between plasma lycopene concentrations and the risk of developing prostate cancer.[57,60] Giovannucci and associates updated previous epidemiological data regarding dietary lycopene intake and reduced prostate cancer risk. Their most recent report using data from the Health Professionals Follow-Up Study once again identified lycopene or tomato product consumption as associated with a reduced risk of prostate cancer (RR of high versus low quintiles = 0.84, 95% CI 0.73–0.96).[61] In their phase II randomized study, Kucuk and colleagues administered 15 mg lycopene or placebo twice daily to a small group of patients with clinically localized prostate cancer prior to radical prostatectomy. They demonstrated favorable clinicopathological markers in the group receiving lycopene including lower pre-prostatectomy serum PSAs, lower rates of positive margins and extracapsular disease, and decreased tumor volumes. However, the biomarkers connexin 43, Bcl-2 and Bax were not significantly different between the two groups.[62] Currently, it is difficult to form sound conclusions regarding lycopene consumption or supplementation and any association with prostate cancer chemoprevention. Like many dietary supplements, lycopene's potential as a chemopreventive agent will only be determined through further phase II and phase III randomized, controlled clinical trials.

Retinoids

The metabolites of vitamin A and its synthetic analogs are called retinoids. Retinoids influence cell growth, differentiation and apoptosis through activation of retinoid X receptors and retinoic acid receptors in the cell nucleus.[63] Early investigator experience with retinoic acid suggested that retinoids might be beneficial for both preventing and treating prostate cancer.[64,65] However, results from clinical studies were not as promising. Pienta and colleagues administered 4-hydroxyphenyl retinamide to 22 men at high risk for developing prostate cancer and, following biopsy, found prostate cancer in eight patients. These results led to the early termination of this study.[66] Furthermore, case control studies pointed to an association between vitamin A intake and higher rates of prostate cancer. These clinical results combined with the secondary results from the ATBC trial[54] and the Physicians' Health Study[58] which revealed either an increased risk or no change in the risk of developing prostate cancer when supplementing with beta-carotene (the precursor of vitamin A), have dampened earlier enthusiasm for using retinoids as prostate cancer chemoprevention supplements.

Vitamin D and analogs

Calcitriol (vitamin D3 or $1,25(OH)_2D_3$) is an active metabolite of vitamin D. The majority of vitamin D3 in humans comes from the sunlight conversion of 7-dehydrocholesterol in the skin to vitamin D. Vitamin D is converted to 25 hydroxy-vitamin D in the liver, and then to 1,25 dihydroxy-vitamin D in the kidneys. In 1990, Schwartz and Hulka noted that several clinical prostate cancer risk factors including older age, African–American race and residence in more sun-deprived northern latitudes, were associated with low serum levels of vitamin D.[67] These observations stemmed from the knowledge that older men are relatively vitamin D deficient, and that the pigment melanin (increased in African–Americans) inhibits vitamin D synthesis through a reduction in sunlight exposure. Hanchette and Schwartz later reported their intriguing data linking prostate cancer to vitamin D by correlating the prostate cancer mortality with the distribution of ultraviolet radiation exposure in 3073 contiguous counties within the United States. They found a significant north–south trend, with lower rates of prostate cancer in the southern regions.[68] More recently, researchers in the

Physicians' Health Study found an association between higher dietary calcium intake and an increased risk of prostate cancer. These higher risks were hypothesized to be due to calcium's lowering of circulating $1,25(OH)_2D_3$. These same researchers reported that higher fruit consumption (specifically fructose intake) directly correlated with a reduced risk of prostate cancer as fructose transiently reduces plasma phosphate which, in turn, stimulates vitamin D production.[69,70] On the heels of these reports, there has been much interest and much effort in defining vitamin D's effects on prostate cancer cells and its role in prostate cancer chemoprevention.

Presently, vitamin D's mechanism of action regarding prostate cancer cell inhibition is not clearly understood. Vitamin D receptors (VDRs) are present within each of the three major prostate cancer cell lines (LNCaP, PC3, DU145) and in vitro treatment of these cancer cells with vitamin D or a non-calcemic analog (1,25-dihydroxy-16-ene-23-yne-cholecalciferol) inhibits cellular proliferation and limits cellular invasiveness.[71,72] Other potential mechanisms of action for vitamin D include an interaction with the androgen receptor. Treatment of androgen-dependent LNCaP cells with $1,25(OH)_2D_3$ appears to upregulate the androgen receptor and, in the presence of dihydrotestosterone, leads to decreased cellular proliferation.[73] However, recent evidence from studies using human leukemia cells (HL60) suggests that vitamin D may have antiproliferative activity through cell cycle arrest in G_1 via induction of p27.[74] In an androgen-independent line of LNCaP cells (LNCaP-104R1), $1,25(OII)_2D_3$ inhibited cellular growth in the absence of androgen and in the presence of the antiandrogen casodex. These findings correlated with the G_1 phase cell cycle accumulation of the cyclin-dependent kinase inhibitor (CKI) p27 and suggest that the antiproliferation effects of vitamin D3 do not require an androgen-activated receptor. Thus, p27-induced cell cycle arrest may be the downstream result of vitamin D's action on prostate cancer cells.[75] Finally, additional research suggests that $1,25(OH)_2D_3$ upregulates insulin-like growth factor binding protein 3 (IGFBP-3). Together, vitamin D and IGFBP-3 resulted in growth inhibition of LNCaP cells possibly through the induction of another cyclin-dependent kinase inhibitory protein p21/WAF1.[76]

The efficacy of vitamin D administration for the prevention of prostate cancer has yet to be defined. Only prospective studies will clearly answer this question and allow clinicians to determine which patients will derive such a benefit. However, vitamin D has been used in clinical trials of patients with hormone refractory prostate cancer and early results suggest that treatment with vitamin D is generally safe and well tolerated. This treatment has also been associated with significant PSA responses suggesting a potential therapeutic benefit for patients with advanced prostate cancer.[77] In future trials of patients with hormone refractory disease, vitamin D will likely be combined with other established treatments to take advantage of possible synergistic activities.[78]

An undesired side effect of supplementing or treating patients with vitamin D is hypercalcemia. Less calcemic analogs of vitamin D are currently being studied in various clinical settings and in animal models have demonstrated antimetastatic and antiproliferative activities.[79,80] Analogs of vitamin D include paricalcitol, calcitriol, and doxercalciferol. 1-Alpha hydroxy vitamin D2 (1-alpha OHD2) is a less calcemic analog that was tested in phase I dose escalation trials in hormone refractory prostate cancer and was well tolerated at doses five times that of vitamin D. Therapeutic benefits were achieved as determined by soft tissue responses and PSA decreases (although there were initial PSA increases). The outcome of a phase II study with this drug is pending.[1]

Non-steroidal anti-inflammatory drugs

Other encouraging agents at the forefront of cancer chemoprevention strategies include the non-steroidal anti-inflammatory drugs (NSAIDs). NSAIDs have shown promise as chemoprevention agents in various cancer cell lines including bladder, lung, breast and prostate. However, much of the laboratory and clinical success with NSAIDs has been achieved with colorectal carcinomas where more selective NSAIDs are now indicated for the prevention and treatment of familial polyposis, a disorder that almost always progresses to invasive colorectal cancer.

Arachidonic acid is an omega-6 fatty acid found in meat and animal products, but not in plant sources. NSAIDs block the conversion of arachidonic acid to a variety of products (including the prostaglandins) by inhibiting cyclooxygenase (COX) and lipoxygenase enzymes. Both of these enzymes have important isoforms. COX-1 is constitutively expressed in platelets, in the stomach and in the intestines, whereas COX-2 is an inducible form of the enzyme associated with inflammatory responses. COX-2 inhibitors are more specific and less ulcerogenic than their counterpart NSAIDs such as ibuprofen. There is evidence that COX-1 and COX-2 expression is higher in the prostate than in any other organ[81] and that prostate cancers show selective overexpression of COX-2.[82] Together, these enzyme isomers as well as lipoxygenase enzymes lead to the production of eicosanoids, which are believed to have important roles in the biology of prostate cancer by increasing cellular proliferation, cellular invasion, neoangiogenesis, metastasis rates and hormonal responsiveness.[83] While the exact mechanisms for prostate cancer prevention have not been discerned, it is possible that the NSAIDs and their derivatives have several mechanisms of action that include direct inhibition of eicosanoid formation, indirect inhibition of eicosanoid formation by inhibiting expression of enzymes involved in eicosanoid synthesis, or by interfering with the function of cyclic guanosine monophosphate phosphodiesterase.[84]

Eicosanoids include 12-hydroxyeicosatetraenoic acid (12-HETE), 5-HETE and prostaglandin E2 (PGE2). Evidence suggests that these eicosanoids modulate the behavior of prostate cancer cells. Gao and colleagues added 12-HETE to human prostate cancer cells and noted an increase in tumor motility and invasiveness. When they examined human tumor specimens with matched normal prostate specimens, they found statistically significant higher mRNA levels of the 12-lipoxygenase enzyme that converts arachidonic acid to 12-HETE, in advanced stage, high-grade prostate cancers.[85] Ghosh and Meyers determined that 5-HETE was critical for prostate cancer cell survival. The addition of an inhibitor of 5-lipoxygenase to LNCaP and PC3 cell cultures resulted in dramatic cellular apoptosis, whereas cell survival (in the presence of the inhibitor) could only be salvaged by the addition of 5-HETE, and not by the addition of androgen. Interestingly, the addition of arachidonic acid to both LNCaP and PC3 cell lines markedly increased cellular growth. However,

apoptosis only occurred in the presence of an inhibitor of 5-lipoxygenase, and not with inhibitors of 12-lipoxygenase or cyclooxygenase.[86] Finally, PGE2 is found in higher concentrations in cancerous tissue from radical prostatectomy specimens compared to normal surrounding prostate tissue.[87] When exogenous PGE2 is added to PC3 and LNCaP cells, there is an increase in cellular proliferation and cellular growth, as well as an increase in the mRNA levels of COX-2.[81] In the presence of exogenous PGE2, the NSAID flurbiprofen inhibited cellular growth as well as the upregulation of COX-2 mRNA.[81] Liu and associates inoculated nude mice with PC3 cells. Compared to controls, the tumors in the mice treated with intraperitoneal injections of a COX-2 inhibitor demonstrated increased apoptosis, decreased angiogenesis as measured by microvessel density, and a decreased expression of vascular endothelial growth factor (VEGF).[88]

Generally, case control studies support the hypothesis that NSAIDs decrease prostate cancer incidence. In New Zealand, Norrish and colleagues identified 317 newly diagnosed prostate cancers over a 13-month period (including 192 patients with advanced disease) and compared NSAID and aspirin use to 480 age-matched control patients. Controlling for dietary fat intake and socioeconomic status, these researchers demonstrated a trend towards a reduced risk of advanced prostate cancer in regular users of NSAIDs (RR = 0.73; 95% CI 0.5–1.07) and aspirin (RR = 0.71; 95% CI 0.47–1.08).[89] These results were strengthened by two more recent case control studies that demonstrated significant differences in prostate cancer incidence between regular users of over-the-counter or prescription NSAIDs and non-users. Nelson and Harris studied 417 prostate cancer patients and 420 age-matched control patients. They found a 66% reduction in prostate cancer risk among regular users of over-the-counter NSAIDs, aspirin and ibuprofen (OR = 0.34; 95% CI 0.23–0.58; p < 0.01). Prostate cancer risk was also reduced in men taking prescription NSAIDs (OR = 0.35; 95% CI 0.15–0.84; p < 0.05).[90] Roberts and associates[91] also reported an overall risk reduction for the development of clinical prostate cancer in users of prescription or over-the-counter NSAIDs compared to non-users (OR = 0.45; 95% CI 0.28–0.73). These same authors found that the inverse association associated with NSAID use was stronger in older groups of patients at study onset suggesting an effect of NSAIDs on the transformation of latent cancers into clinically detected cancers.[91] However, data from one recent case control study suggest that NSAID use might increase the risk of prostate cancer. Researchers from the UK reported that the odds of developing prostate cancer were greater in patients who received at least seven prescriptions for NSAIDs in a 36-month period prior to the diagnosis of prostate cancer (OR 1.33; CI 1.07–1.64). While the increased risk was not dose related, the authors recognized that their findings were based on prescription data and not on actual consumption of the NSAIDs.[92]

Currently, there is a broad array of novel NSAIDs being tested for their cancer prevention capabilities. Sulindac is an NSAID used in the treatment of patients with arthritic conditions. Sulindac sulfone (Exisulind, Cell Pathways) is a metabolite of sulindac that may have significant anticancer activity. Sulindac sulfone's mechanism of action does not appear to be via inhibition of the COX enzyme isomers, but through inhibition of a cyclic guanosine monophosphate (cGMP) phosphodiesterase-5 which permits the activation of protein kinase G by cGMP, and the activation of apoptosis-associated caspases.[84] Derivatives of sulindac (sulindac sulfone, sulindac sulfide) and an analog of sulindac sulfone (CP248) were demonstrated to inhibit cellular growth in PrEC (normal human prostate epithelial cell line), BPH-1, LNCaP and PC3 cell lines. The sulindac derivatives also induced apoptosis in all of the cell lines except for the PrEC cells, suggesting that apoptosis was linked to malignant transformation.[93] Exisulind has recently been evaluated in a prospective, randomized, placebo-controlled, multi-institutional study of 96 patients with PSA-only recurrence following radical prostatectomy. In the patients who received 250 mg Exisulind twice daily compared to placebo, there was a significant suppression in the increase in PSA compared to baseline, beginning after approximately 2 months on therapy. In addition, the median PSA doubling time was increased in patients classified at high risk for developing metastases (2.12 month increase) compared to high risk patients on placebo (3.37 month decrease, p = 0.048).[94]

Encouraging results from these preclinical and clinical studies have prompted further prospective evaluation of combination therapies incorporating Exisulind with docetaxel in patients with hormone refractory prostate cancer.[95] R-flurbiprofen is a single enantiomer of a racemic NSAID that does not inhibit cyclooxygenases, but appears to decrease COX-2 mRNA levels.[81] In the transgenic adenocarcinoma mouse prostate (TRAMP) model, mice fed R-flurbiprofen were found to have a significantly lower incidence of metastases and a reduction in the primary tumor incidence.[96] Finally, future trials might also involve the 5-lipoxygenase inhibitor zileutin (Zyflo, Abbott). This agent has been approved for the treatment of chronic asthma. Based on its in vitro effects on prostate cancer cells, this drug could have indications for prostate cancer treatment and prevention.[86]

Farnesyl protein transferase inhibitors

Ras proteins play a central role in signal transduction pathways that are important in ontogenesis. Farnesyl protein transferase (FPT) inhibitors prevent the plasma membrane localization and activation of Ras thereby disconnecting the signals between the plasma membrane and the downstream nuclear effectors. It is hypothesized that the inhibition of Ras proteins interferes with cellular growth and proliferation.[97] There are potential problems using FPT inhibitors in prostate cancer chemoprevention strategies. Ras mutations are more common in pancreatic and colon cancers. However, in prostate cancer, Ras mutations are much less common with the exception of higher mutation rates reported in some Japanese populations. In preclinical models of FPT inhibitors, there is regrowth of tumors after therapy is stopped, and there may be some myelosuppressive side effects of therapy.[36] Nevertheless, there are some non-specific plant derived inhibitors of FPT that are being studied for their cancer chemoprevention capabilities. Perillyl alcohol (POH) is a monoterpene isolated from the oils of several plants including lavendin, peppermint, spearmint, cherries and celery seeds. Few trials have been accomplished with POH and its metabolites (dihydroperillic acid and perillic acid). Thus far, safe doses of these natural substances have demonstrated limited effects on p21ras expression in

DU145 prostate carcinoma cells.[98] More work is required to determine if treatment or supplementation with FPT inhibitors (including POH or other monoterpenes) will be beneficial for patients with prostate cancer or for patients at high risk for developing a prostate malignancy.

Conclusions

Prostate cancer places a significant burden on patients, their relatives, on health care providers, and on society. This burden mandates that new strategies be investigated to meet the growing challenges and costs of diagnosing and treating patients with prostate cancer. In this regard, finding the means to prevent or modulate the natural development of prostate cancer is certainly a worthy goal and will continue to be a top research priority. There are various molecular pathways by which chemoprevention might be accomplished, and some of these mechanisms for prevention or for slowing cancer progression could be synergistic. Only prospective randomized studies will identify the best agents or combination of agents for chemoprevention, and to which populations of patients these agents should be administered. Results from ongoing clinical trials including the PCPT and SELECT studies may not only identify possible efficacious chemopreventive agents, but these studies and other trials might also provide avenues into identifying cancer biomarkers and surrogate endpoints for measuring the effects these agents have on prostate cancer initiation, promotion and progression.

Disclaimer

The views expressed in this publication are those of the authors and do not reflect the official policy or position of the Department of the Air Force, Department of Defense, or the United States Government.

References

1. Lieberman R, Bermejo C, Greenwald P, et al. Progress in prostate cancer chemoprevention: modulators of promotion and progression. Urology 2001; 58(6):835–842.
2. Sakr WA, Haas GP, Cassin BJ, et al. The frequency of carcinoma and intraepithelial neoplasia of the prostate in young male patients. J Urol 1993; 150(2 Pt 1):379–385.
3. Pound CR, Partin AW, Eisenberger MA, et al. Natural history of progression after PSA elevation following radical prostatectomy. JAMA 1999; 281(17):1591–1597.
4. Imperto-McGinley J, Guerrero L, Gautier T, et al. Steroid 5α-reductase deficiency in man: an inherited form of male pseudohermaphroditism. Science 1974; 186:1213–1215.
5. Wilding G. Endocrine control of prostate cancer. Cancer Surv 1995; 23:43–62.
6. Ross RK, Bernstein L, Lobo RA, et al. 5-alpha-reductase activity and risk of prostate cancer among Japanese and US white and black males. Lancet 1992; 339(8798):887–889.
7. Sartor O. Molecular factors in the assessment of prostate cancer risk. In: Resnick MI, Thompson IM, eds. Advanced therapy of prostate disease. Hamilton, Ontario: BC Decker; 2000:44–49.
8. Rebbeck TR, Jaffe JM, Walker AH, et al. Modification of clinical presentation of prostate tumors by a novel genetic variant in CYP3A4. J Natl Cancer Inst 1998; 90(16):1225–1229.
9. Makridakis NM, Ross RK, Pike MC, et al. Association of mis-sense substitution in SRD5A2 gene with prostate cancer in African–American and Hispanic men in Los Angeles, USA. Lancet 1999; 354(9183):975–978.
10. Huggins C, Hodges CV. Studies in prostatic cancer: I. The effects of castration, of estrogen, and of androgen injection on serum phosphatases in metastatic carcinoma of the prostate. Cancer Res 1941; 1:293–297.
11. Messing EM, Manola J, Sarosdy M, et al. Immediate hormonal therapy compared with observation after radical prostatectomy and pelvic lymphadenectomy in men with node-positive prostate cancer. N Engl J Med 1999; 341(24):1781–1788.
12. Bolla M, Gonzalez D, Warde P, et al. Improved survival in patients with locally advanced prostate cancer treated with radiotherapy and goserelin. N Engl J Med 1997; 337(5):295–300.
13. The Leuprolide Study Group. Leuprolide versus diethylstilbestrol for metastatic prostate cancer. The Leuprolide Study Group. N Engl J Med 1984; 311(20):1281–1286.
14. Iversen P, Tyrrell CJ, Kaisary AV, et al. Bicalutamide monotherapy compared with castration in patients with nonmetastatic locally advanced prostate cancer: 6.3 years of followup. J Urol 2000; 164(5):1579–1582.
15. Chodak G, Sharifi R, Kasimis B, et al. Single-agent therapy with bicalutamide: a comparison with medical or surgical castration in the treatment of advanced prostate carcinoma. Urology 1995; 46(6):849–855.
16. Tsukamoto S, Akaza H, Onozawa MA, et al. Five-alpha reductase inhibitor or an antiandrogen prevents the progression of microscopic prostate carcinoma to macroscopic carcinoma in rats. Cancer 1998; 82(3):531–537.
17. Alberts SR, Blute ML. Chemoprevention for prostatic carcinoma: the role of flutamide in patients with prostatic intraepithelial neoplasia. Urology 2001; 57(4 suppl 1):188–190.
18. Gormley GJ, Stoner E, Bruskewitz RC, et al. The effect of finasteride in men with benign prostatic hyperplasia. The Finasteride Study Group. N Engl J Med 1992; 327(17):1185–1191.

19. McConnell JD, Bruskewitz R, Walsh P, et al. The effect of finasteride on the risk of acute urinary retention and the need for surgical treatment among men with benign prostatic hyperplasia. Finasteride Long-Term Efficacy and Safety Study Group. N Engl J Med 1998; 338(9):557–563.

20. Cote RJ, Skinner EC, Salem CE, et al. The effect of finasteride on the prostate gland in men with elevated serum prostate-specific antigen levels. Br J Cancer 1998; 78(3):413–418.

21. Andriole G, Lieber M, Smith J, et al. Treatment with finasteride following radical prostatectomy for prostate cancer. Urology 1995; 45(3):491–497.

22. Thompson IM, Coltman CA Jr, Crowley J. Chemoprevention of prostate cancer: the Prostate Cancer Prevention Trial. Prostate 1997; 33(3):217–221.

23. Steiner MS, Raghow S, Neubauer BL. Selective estrogen receptor modulators for the chemoprevention of prostate cancer. Urology 2001; 57(4 suppl 1):68–72.

24. Krege JH, Hodgin JB, Couse JF, et al. Generation and reproductive phenotypes of mice lacking estrogen receptor beta. Proc Natl Acad Sci USA 1998; 95(26):15677–15682.

25. Bonkhoff H, Fixemer T, Hunsicker I, et al. Estrogen receptor expression in prostate cancer and premalignant prostatic lesions. Am J Pathol 1999; 155(2):641–647.

26. Denis L, Morton MS, Griffiths K. Diet and its preventive role in prostatic disease. Eur Urol 1999; 35(5–6):377–387.

27. Morton MS, Chan PS, Cheng C, et al. Lignans and isoflavonoids in plasma and prostatic fluid in men: samples from Portugal, Hong Kong, and the United Kingdom. Prostate 1997; 32(2):122–128.

28. Messina MJ, Persky V, Setchell KD, et al. Soy intake and cancer risk: a review of the in vitro and in vivo data. Nutr Cancer 1994; 21(2):113–131.

29. Griffiths K, Morton MS, Denis L. Certain aspects of molecular endocrinology that relate to the influence of dietary factors on the pathogenesis of prostate cancer. Eur Urol 1999; 35(5–6):443–455.

30. Adlercreutz H. Western diet and Western diseases: some hormonal and biochemical mechanisms and associations. Scand J Clin Lab Invest 1990; 201(suppl):3–23.

31. Bergan R, Kyle E, Nguyen P, et al. Genistein-stimulated adherence of prostate cancer cells is associated with the binding of focal adhesion kinase to beta-1-integrin. Clin Exp Metastasis 1996; 14(4):389–398.

32. Kyle E, Neckers L, Takimoto C, et al. Genistein-induced apoptosis of prostate cancer cells is preceded by a specific decrease in focal adhesion kinase activity. Mol Pharmacol 1997; 51(2):193–200.

33. Akiyama T, Ishida J, Nakagawa S, et al. Genistein, a specific inhibitor of tyrosine-specific protein kinases. J Biol Chem 1987; 262(12):5592–5595.

34. Kennedy AR, Wan XS. Effects of the Bowman-Birk inhibitor on growth, invasion, and clonogenic survival of human prostate epithelial cells and prostate cancer cells. Prostate 2002; 50(2):125–133.

35. Kennedy AR. Chemopreventive agents: protease inhibitors. Pharmacol Ther 1998; 78(3):167–209.

36. Bergan RC, Waggle DH, Carter SK, et al. Tyrosine kinase inhibitors and signal transduction modulators: rationale and current status as chemopreventive agents for prostate cancer. Urology 2001; 57(4 suppl 1):77–80.

37. Key TJ, Fraser GE, Thorogood M, et al. Mortality in vegetarians and nonvegetarians: detailed findings from a collaborative analysis of 5 prospective studies. Am J Clin Nutr 1999; 70(3 suppl):516S–524S.

38. Fleshner NE, Kucuk O. Antioxidant dietary supplements: rationale and current status as chemopreventive agents for prostate cancer. Urology 2001; 57(4 suppl 1):90–94.

39. El-Bayoumy K. The role of selenium in cancer prevention. In: Devita VT, Hellman S, Rosenberg S, eds. Cancer prevention. Philadelphia: JB Lippincott, 1991:1–15.

40. Yan L, Spallholz JE. Generation of reactive oxygen species from the reaction of selenium compounds with thiols and mammary tumor cells. Biochem Pharmacol 1993; 45(2):429–437.

41. Redman C, Scott JA, Baines AT, et al. Inhibitory effect of selenomethionine on the growth of three selected human tumor cell lines. Cancer Lett 1998; 125(1–2):103–110.

42. Webber MM, Perez-Ripoll EA, James GT. Inhibitory effects of selenium on the growth of DU145 human prostate carcinoma cells in vitro. Biochem Biophys Res Commun 1985; 130(2):603–609.

43. Webber MM. Selenium prevents the growth stimulatory effects of cadmium on human prostatic epithelium. Biochem Biophys Res Commun 1985; 127(3):871–877.

44. Helzlsouer KJ, Comstock GW, Morris JS. Selenium, lycopene, alpha-tocopherol, beta-carotene, retinol, and subsequent bladder cancer. Cancer Res 1989; 49(21):6144–6148.

45. Hunter DJ, Morris JS, Stampfer MJ, et al. A prospective study of selenium status and breast cancer risk. JAMA 1990; 264(9):1128–1131.

46. Yoshizawa K, Willett WC, Morris SJ, et al. Study of prediagnostic selenium level in toenails and the risk of advanced prostate cancer. J Natl Cancer Inst 1998; 90(16):1219–1224.

47. Clark LC, Combs GF Jr, Turnbull BW, et al. Effects of selenium supplementation for cancer prevention in patients with carcinoma of the skin. A randomized controlled trial. Nutritional Prevention of Cancer Study Group. JAMA 1996; 276(24):1957–1963.

48. Das S. Vitamin E in the genesis and prevention of cancer. A review. Acta Oncol 1994; 33(6):615–619.

49. Meydani M. Vitamin E. Lancet 1995; 345(8943):170–175.

50. Pastori M, Pfander H, Boscoboinik D, et al. Lycopene in association with alpha-tocopherol inhibits at physiological concentrations proliferation of prostate carcinoma cells. Biochem Biophys Res Commun 1998; 250(3):582–585.

51. Fleshner N, Fair WR, Huryk R, Heston WD. Vitamin E inhibits the high-fat diet promoted growth of established human prostate LNCaP tumors in nude mice. J Urol 1999; 161(5):1651–1654.

52. Eichholzer M, Stahelin HB, Ludin E, et al. Smoking, plasma vitamins C, E, retinol, and carotene, and fatal prostate cancer: seventeen-year follow-up of the prospective Basel study. Prostate 1999; 38(3):189–198.

53. Chan JM, Stampfer MJ, Ma J, et al. Supplemental vitamin E intake and prostate cancer risk in a large cohort of men in the United States. Cancer Epidemiol Biomarkers Prev 1999; 8(10):893–899.

54. Heinonen OP, Albanes D, Virtamo J. Prostate cancer and supplementation with alpha-tocopherol and beta-carotene: incidence and mortality in a controlled trial. J Natl Cancer Inst 1998; 90(6):440–446.

55. Klein EA, Thompson IM, Lippman SM, et al. SELECT: the next prostate cancer prevention trial. Selenium and Vitamin E Cancer Prevention Trial. J Urol 2001; 166(4):1311–1315.

56. Kotake-Nara E, Kushiro M, Zhang H, et al. Carotenoids affect proliferation of human prostate cancer cells. J Nutr 2001; 131(12):3303–3306.

57. Lu QY, Hung JC, Heber D, et al. Inverse associations between plasma lycopene and other carotenoids and prostate cancer. Cancer Epidemiol Biomarkers Prev 2001; 10(7):749–756.

58. Cook NR, Le IM, Manson JE, et al. Effects of beta-carotene supplementation on cancer incidence by baseline characteristics in the Physicians' Health Study (United States). Cancer Causes Control 2000; 11(7):617–626.

59. Imaida K, Tamano S, Kato K, et al. Lack of chemopreventive effects of lycopene and curcumin on experimental rat prostate carcinogenesis. Carcinogenesis 2001; 22(3):467–472.

60. Norrish AE, Jackson RT, Sharpe SJ, et al. Prostate cancer and dietary carotenoids. Am J Epidemiol 2000; 151(2):119–123.

61. Giovannucci E, Rimm EB, Liu Y, et al. A prospective study of tomato products, lycopene, and prostate cancer risk. J Natl Cancer Inst 2002; 94(5):391–398.

62. Kucuk O, Sarkar FH, Sakr W, et al. Phase II randomized clinical trial of lycopene supplementation before radical prostatectomy. Cancer Epidemiol Biomarkers Prev 2001; 10(8):861–868.

63. de Vos S, Dawson MI, Holden S, et al. Effects of retinoid X receptor-selective ligands on proliferation of prostate cancer cells. Prostate 1997; 32(2):115–121.

64. Reese DH, Gordon B, Gratzner HG, et al. Effect of retinoic acid on the growth and morphology of a prostatic adenocarcinoma cell line cloned for the retinoid inducibility of alkaline phosphatase. Cancer Res 1983; 43(11):5443–5450.

65. Peehl DM, Wong ST, Stamey TA. Vitamin A regulates proliferation and differentiation of human prostatic epithelial cells. Prostate 1993; 23(1):69–78.

66. Pienta KJ, Esper PS, Zwas F, et al. Phase II chemoprevention trial of oral fenretinide in patients at risk for adenocarcinoma of the prostate. Am J Clin Oncol 1997; 20(1):36–39.

67. Schwartz GG, Hulka BS. Is vitamin D deficiency a risk factor for prostate cancer? (Hypothesis). Anticancer Res 1990; 10(5A):1307–1311.

68. Hanchette CL, Schwartz GG. Geographic patterns of prostate cancer mortality. Evidence for a protective effect of ultraviolet radiation. Cancer 1992; 70(12):2861–2869.

69. Chan JM, Giovannucci E, Andersson SO, et al. Dairy products, calcium, phosphorus, vitamin D, and risk of prostate cancer (Sweden). Cancer Causes Control 1998; 9(6):559–566.

70. Chan JM, Stampfer MJ, Ma J, et al. Dairy products, calcium, and prostate cancer risk in the Physicians' Health Study. Am J Clin Nutr 2001; 74(4):549–554.

71. Skowronski RJ, Peehl DM, Feldman D. Vitamin D and prostate cancer: 1,25 dihydroxyvitamin D3 receptors and actions in human prostate cancer cell lines. Endocrinology 1993; 132(5):1952–1960.

72. Schwartz GG, Oeler TA, Uskokovic MR, et al. Human prostate cancer cells: inhibition of proliferation by vitamin D analogs. Anticancer Res 1994; 14(3A):1077–1081.

73. Zhao XY, Ly LH, Peehl DM, et al. 1-alpha,25-dihydroxyvitamin D3 actions in LNCaP human prostate cancer cells are androgen-dependent. Endocrinology 1997; 138(8):3290–3298.

74. Wang QM, Jones JB, Studzinski GP. Cyclin-dependent kinase inhibitor p27 as a mediator of the G1-S phase block induced by 1,25-dihydroxyvitamin D3 in HL60 cells. Cancer Res 1996; 56(2):264–267.

75. Yang ES, Maiorino CA, Roos BA, et al. Vitamin D-mediated growth inhibition of an androgen-ablated LNCaP cell line model of human prostate cancer. Mol Cell Endocrinol 2002; 186(1):69–79.

76. Boyle BJ, Zhao XY, Cohen P, et al. Insulin-like growth factor binding protein-3 mediates 1 alpha,25-dihydroxyvitamin d(3) growth inhibition in the LNCaP prostate cancer cell line through p21/WAF1. J Urol 2001; 165(4):1319–1324.

77. Beer TM, Hough KM, Garzotto M. Weekly high-dose calcitriol and docetaxel in advanced prostate cancer. Semin Oncol 2001; 28(4 suppl 15):49–55.

78. Peehl DM, Seto E, Feldman D. Rationale for combination ketoconazole/vitamin D treatment of prostate cancer. Urology 2001; 58(2 suppl 1):123–126.

79. Getzenberg RH, Light BW, Lapco PE, et al. Vitamin D inhibition of prostate adenocarcinoma growth and metastasis in the Dunning rat prostate model system. Urology 1997; 50(6):999–1006.

80. Blutt SE, Polek TC, Stewart LV, et al. A calcitriol analog, EB1089, inhibits the growth of LNCaP tumors in nude mice. Cancer Res 2000; 60(4):779–782.

81. Tjandrawinata RR, Dahiya R, Hughes-Fulford M. Induction of cyclo-oxygenase-2 mRNA by prostaglandin E2 in human prostatic carcinoma cells. Br J Cancer 1997; 75(8):1111–1118.

82. Gupta S, Srivastava M, Ahmad N, et al. Over-expression of cyclooxygenase-2 in human prostate adenocarcinoma. Prostate 2000; 42(1):73–78.

83. Lupulescu A. Prostaglandins, their inhibitors and cancer. Prostaglandins Leukot Essent Fatty Acids 1996; 54(2):83–94.

84. Myers C, Koki A, Pamukcu R, et al. Proapoptotic anti-inflammatory drugs. Urology 2001; 57(4 suppl 1):73–76.

85. Gao X, Grignon DJ, Chbihi T, et al. Elevated 12-lipoxygenase mRNA expression correlates with advanced stage and poor differentiation of human prostate cancer. Urology 1995; 46(2):227–237.

86. Ghosh J, Myers CE. Inhibition of arachidonate 5-lipoxygenase triggers massive apoptosis in human prostate cancer cells. Proc Natl Acad Sci USA 1998; 95(22):13182–13187.

87. Chaudry AA, Wahle KW, McClinton S. Arachidonic acid metabolism in benign and malignant prostatic tissue in vitro: effects of fatty acids and cyclooxygenase inhibitors. Int J Cancer 1994; 57(2):176–180.

88. Liu XH, Kirschenbaum A, Yao S, et al. Inhibition of cyclooxygenase-2 suppresses angiogenesis and the growth of prostate cancer in vivo. J Urol 2000; 164(3 Pt 1):820–825.

89. Norrish AE, Jackson RT, McRae CU. Non-steroidal anti-inflammatory drugs and prostate cancer progression. Int J Cancer 1998; 77(4):511–515.

90. Nelson JE, Harris RE. Inverse association of prostate cancer and non-steroidal anti-inflammatory drugs (NSAIDs): results of a case-control study. Oncol Rep 2000; 7(1):169–170.

91. Roberts RO, Jacobson DJ, Girman CJ, et al. A population-based study of daily nonsteroidal anti-inflammatory drug use and prostate cancer. Mayo Clin Proc 2002; 77(3):219–225.

92. Langman MJ, Cheng KK, Gilman EA, et al. Effect of anti-inflammatory drugs on overall risk of common cancer: case-control study in general practice research database. BMJ 2000; 320(7250):1642–1646.

93. Lim JT, Piazza GA, Han EK, et al. Sulindac derivatives inhibit growth and induce apoptosis in human prostate cancer cell lines. Biochem Pharmacol 1999; 58(7):1097–1107.

94. Goluboff ET, Prager D, Rukstalis D, et al. Safety and efficacy of exisulind for treatment of recurrent prostate cancer after radical prostatectomy. J Urol 2001; 166(3):882–886.

95. Ryan CW, Stadler WM, Vogelzang NJ. Docetaxel and exisulind in hormone-refractory prostate cancer. Semin Oncol 2001; 28(4 suppl 15):56–61.

96. Wechter WJ, Leipold DD, Murray ED Jr, et al. E-7869 (R-flurbiprofen) inhibits progression of prostate cancer in the TRAMP mouse. Cancer Res 2000; 60(8):2203–2208.

97. Gibbs JB, Kohl NE, Koblan KS, et al. Farnesyltransferase inhibitors and anti-Ras therapy. Breast Cancer Res Treat 1996; 38(1):75–83.

98. Hudes GR, Szarka CE, Adams A. Phase I pharmacokinetic trial of perillyl alcohol (NSC 641066) in patients with refractory solid malignancies. Clin Cancer Res 2000; 6(8):3071–3080.

7

Apoptosis in the prostate

*Colm Morrissey, R William G Watson and
John M Fitzpatrick*

Introduction

The prostate is an androgen-dependent gland. Androgens maintain the differentiated phenotype and drive proliferation of the epithelium within the prostate. While organ-confined, androgen-dependent prostate cancer can be treated with antiandrogens such as cyproterone acetate, hydroxy-flutamide and bicalutamide, treatment for metastatic androgen-independent prostate cancer remains elusive. This has led to a variety of well-established and novel therapeutic approaches that have one underlying principle – to target and induce apoptosis or programmed cell death. While apoptosis ultimately results in cell death it is quite clear that the activation of this mechanism is dependent upon the phenotype of the cell and the therapy used.

This chapter will address the hormonal dependence of the prostate and the physiologic changes that occur after androgen ablation, the effects of antiandrogens and novel compounds on apoptosis in the prostate and finally give an overview of the molecular aspects of apoptosis as they may relate to the prostate.

Androgens, metabolism and action

The prostate requires androgens for development and glandular maintenance. Within the gland testosterone is metabolized to 5-alpha dihydro-testosterone (5-alpha DHT) by 5-alpha reductase (3-oxo-5 alpha-steroid delta 4-reductase) and subsequently less active metabolites such as 3-alpha androstanediol and 3-beta androstanediol, by 3-alpha hydroxysteroid dehydrogenase and 3-beta hydroxysteroid dehydrogenase respectively. Thus 5-alpha DHT is not transported systemically to its target tissues as are most classical steroid hormones,

but is generated intracellularly in target organs. 5-Alpha DHT preferentially binds to the androgen receptor and is most probably the only active androgen in the prostate.[1,2] The binding of 5-alpha DHT to the nuclear androgen receptor initiates the androgenic effects of the steroid by binding to the androgen response element (ARE) as a homodimer[3] (Fig. 7.1). A number of AREs have been identified; however unlike other hormone response elements the consensus sequence varies quite considerably. In the rat, the probasin promoter is ATAGCAtctTGTTCT,[4] the C3 (1) gene promoter is AGTACCtgaTGTTCT,[5] and the tyrosine aminotransferase gene promoter is TGTACAggaTGTTCT.[6] This variation in AREs may lead to substantially different binding characteristics that in turn may lead to significant variation in the response.

Hormonal dependence of the prostate

The rat prostate represents a good model for the study of apoptosis, since the secretory epithelial cells are critically dependent on androgens for survival and die by apoptosis after their withdrawal, induced by castration or antiandrogen treatment. The reduction in prostate size is due to the selective loss of the secretory luminal epithelial cells in the distal and intermediate regions of the ducts, resulting in the complete obliteration of many of the ducts while maintaining the proximal segments of the ducts. The luminal epithelial cells in the intermediate and distal regions of the ducts are highly differentiated and die extensively due to their critical dependence on androgens. However, the luminal epithelial cells in the proximal regions of the ducts are cuboidal in morphology and have no secretory activity. Neither these cells nor the basal epithelial cells that predominate in the

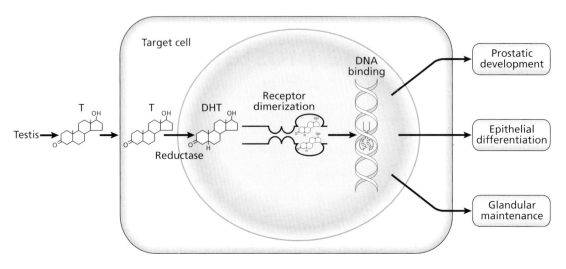

Figure 7.1 The mechanism of androgen action in the prostate. Testosterone enters the prostate cells. Testosterone is metabolized to 5-alpha DHT by 5-alpha reductase (3-oxo-5 alpha-steroid delta 4-reductase), then binds to the androgen receptor, which then translocates to the nucleus. The 5-alpha DHT–androgen receptor complex binds to androgen response elements in the chromatin to mediate gene expression responsible for prostate development, epithelial differentiation and maintenance of the prostate gland.

proximal region are androgen dependent.[7] The loss of the androgen-dependent tall columnar epithelial cells occurs via apoptosis.

The stroma of the prostate also does not require androgens for survival. Castration results in the atrophy of the prostatic epithelium alone, the stromal compartment appearing to remain relatively unaffected except for tissue remodeling. The morphology of prostates excised from long-term castrates clearly indicates that a subpopulation of androgen-independent luminal epithelial cells are far less affected by androgen ablation than the tall columnar epithelial cells in the inter-mediate and distal regions.[8]

There are a number of prostate-specific secre-tory and non-secretory proteins that are androgen dependent and downregulated after castration. One of these is prostate steroid binding protein, a marker of androgenic control that consists of three different subunits: C1, C2 and C3. The synthesis of each subunit is completely dependent on androgens.[9] Secretory prostatic acid phosphatase activity is androgen regulated and downregulated after castration in the prostate and has been used as an indicator of the androgenic status of the rat ventral prostate.[10] Human prostatic acid phospha-tase and rat prostatic acid phosphatase are glyco-

proteins synthesized by the epithelial cells of the prostate gland and released into the lumen as part of the prostatic secretion.[11] Androgens also regulate the synthesis and secretion of human prostate specific antigen (PSA or hK1) and human prostate specific glandular kallikrein (hK2).[12] The expression of these genes diminishes very substan-tially after castration.

In addition to the loss of expression of these secretory proteins, the synthesis and expression of several other gene products also decreases after hormonal ablation, including RNA polymerases I and III,[13] spermine binding protein,[14] ornithine decarboxylase,[15] and the beta-2 adrenergic recep-tor.[16] However, it should be noted that even though there is a loss of expression of these proteins after hormonal ablation this does not mean that these gene products are androgen regulated. Their expres-sion would also appear to decrease if they are con-stitutively expressed by the androgen-dependent cells that die during the regression process.

In contrast, a number of proteins are induced during regression of the rat ventral prostate including HSP 27, poly(ADP)ribose polymerase, cathepsin B,[17] cathepsin D,[18] c-fos, c-myc, HSP 70,[19] tissue transglutaminase,[20] DNase 1,[21] matri-lysin, tissue inhibitors of matrix metalloproteinases

1 (TIMP-1), and urokinase-type plasminogen activators.[22,23] The steady state levels of clusterin also increase significantly after castration or administration of antiandrogen in the rat ventral prostate.[24]

Androgen replacement in castrated rats results in luminal epithelial cell proliferation, without significant proliferation of either basal or stromal cells. This cycle of androgen withdrawal and replacement can be repeated several times with constant repopulation of the stroma by the epithelial cells and the restoration of a fully functional gland.[25,26] This suggests that there is a precursor epithelial, stem-like, androgen-independent cell in the prostate that will replace the lost luminal secretory epithelium after androgen replacement.

Aspects of apoptosis in the prostate

Background

Much of the underlying research on apoptosis in the prostate has relied on the use of a variety of animal, cell culture and to a lesser extent primary culture models. The cellular events that occur during apoptosis in the prostatic epithelium have yet to be fully elucidated. However, it is clear that apoptosis in the glandular epithelial cells of the human prostate shares many features of apoptosis seen in other cell types (Fig. 7.2).

Cell death, or apoptosis, is not a single phenomenon but a series of morphologically and biochemically related processes.[27] Cell death of lymphocytes and other cells of reticuloendothelial origin is dominated by changes in nuclear morphology[28] and mitochondrial biology,[29] while apoptotic death of glandular epithelial cells, such as those of the prostate, also requires profound cytoplasmic changes and alterations in the cell–cell and cell–substratum interactions.[30] The cytoplasmic changes that occur in epithelial cells undergoing apoptosis that lead to the release of the dying cell from the underlying in the extracellular matrix (ECM) occurs through the upregulation and action of proteins such as tissue transglutaminase and the activation of caspases.[20] Cell death in the prostate is known to be an active process as the rapid rate of prostatic cell death following castration can be inhibited by actinomycin D or cycloheximide, inhibitors of RNA and protein synthesis, respectively.[31]

The caspases

The central molecules involved in apoptotic events within the cell are the caspase family of cysteine proteases. Caspases normally exist in cells as inactive proenzymes and can be activated by proteolytic cleavage. All caspases have similar cleavage specificity and may be activated by other previously activated caspase molecules. The activation of the 'caspase cascade' occurs initially by the initiator caspases (e.g. caspase-8 and 9), which then activate downstream effector caspases (e.g. caspase-3, 6 and 7).[32] The caspase cascade is activated by receptor and mitochondrial mediated pathways. A number of caspase-independent mechanisms of cell death also exist, including Bin1, the serine protease Omi and the ceramide pathway.[33–35]

Receptor mediated cell death

Receptor mediated cell death involves death receptors, i.e. cell surface receptors that transmit apoptotic signals initiated by specific ligands.[36] Death receptors belong to the tumor necrosis factor (TNF) receptor gene superfamily, which is defined by similar, cysteine-rich extracellular domains. The most characterized death receptors are CD95/Fas/Apo1 and TNFRI/p55/CD120a.[37–39] In the case of Fas mediated apoptosis, the Fas receptor molecules trimerize into a membrane bound complex. This complex recruits procaspase-8 molecules through the adaptor protein FADD (FAS associated death domain). This is followed by recruitment of procaspase-8 to the DISC (death inducing signaling complex) and its subsequent autocatalytic activation.[32,36] Fas may also recruit receptor-interacting protein (RIP), which may recruit an adaptor molecule RIP-associated ICH-1/CED-3-homologous protein with a death domain (RAIDD). RAIDD may recruit and activate procaspase-2 through its caspase recruitment domain (CARD).[40] TNF similarly trimerizes tumor necrosis factor receptor I (TNFRI) upon binding.[37,38] This induces association of the receptor's death domains and subsequently an adaptor protein TNFR-associated death domain (TRADD).[41] TRADD recruits several signaling molecules to the activated receptor: TNFR-associated factor-2 (TRAF-2) and RIP.[41–43] These proteins stimulate pathways leading to the activation of nuclear factor kappa B (NF-kappa B) and c-Jun N-terminal kinase/activator protein-1

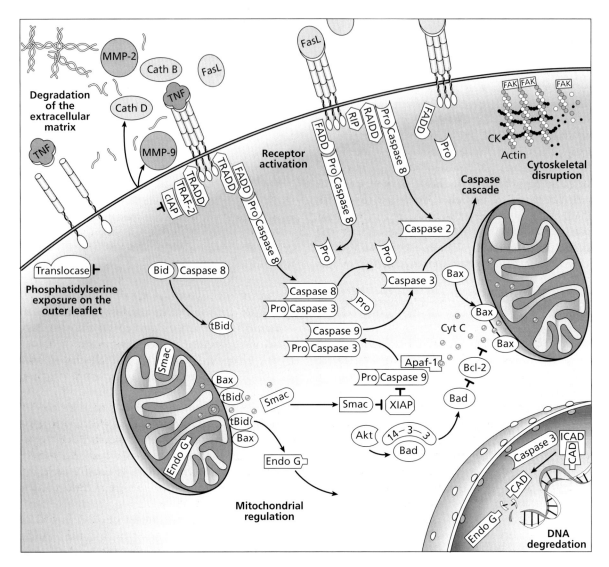

Figure 7.2 Signaling cascades involved in apoptosis. 14-3-3, adaptor protein; Akt, serine/threonine protein kinase; Apaf-1, apoptotic protease-activating factor 1; Bax/Bid, proapoptotic proteins of the Bcl-2 family; CAD, caspase-activated DNase; Cath B, cathepsin B; cIAP, an inhibitor of apoptosis protein; CK, cytokeratins; Cyt C, cytochrome c; ENDO G, endonuclease G; FADD, FAS associated death domain; FAK, focal adhesion kinase; FasL, fas ligand; ICAD, inhibitor of caspase-activated DNase; MMP, matrix metalloproteinase; RAIDD, RIP-associated ICH-1/CED-3-homologous protein with a death domain; RIP, receptor-interacting protein; Smac, secondary mitochondria-derived activator of caspase; tBid, truncated Bid; TNF, tumor necrosis factor; TNFR, tumor necrosis factor receptor; TRADD, TNFR-associated death domain; TRAF-2, TNFR-associated factor-2; Translocase, phosphatidylserine translocase; XIAP, X-linked inhibitor of apoptosis protein.

(JNK/AP-1). However, they may also recruit FADD, mediating the activation of apoptosis.[41,44,45]

Mitochondrial regulation of cell death

Receptor mediated cell death is not the only orchestrated form of apoptosis in mammalian cells.

The signal induced by the engagement of the Fas receptor proceeds primarily through the adaptor FADD, which directly activates caspase-8 and may bypass the Bcl-2 family.[46] Although mitochondrial involvement and cytochrome c release may not be universal aspects of apoptosis, the Bcl-2 family reacts to signals from diverse cytotoxic stimuli, for example cytokine deprivation and exposure to glucocorticoids, DNA damage, or staurosporine.[47] Many, but not all Bcl-2 family proteins reside on the cytoplasmic face of the mitochondrial outer membrane, endoplasmic reticulum and nuclear envelope. The Bcl-2 family has been implicated in regulating mitochondrial permeability transition through the permeability transition pore. This permeability transition during apoptosis through an opening of the permeability pore would lead to the release of cytochrome c from the mitochondria, resulting in mitochondrial dysfunction and caspase activation. This release is inhibited by the presence of Bcl-2 or Bcl-xL in excess of Bax; however when Bax is in excess it will initiate the apoptotic process.[48,49]

Bid and Bad are proapoptotic members of the Bcl-2 family of proteins. In the presence of survival factors Bad is phosphorylated by Akt and sequestered by binding to the 14-3-3 protein. This leaves Bcl-2 and Bcl-xL free to promote survival.[50,51] The activation of Bax through the binding of Bid results in the initiation of apoptosis through cytochrome c release. The activation of Bid and cleavage into a truncated (tBid) form may occur through caspase-8 cleavage, which results in the relaying of an apoptotic signal from the cytoplasm to the mitochondria.[52,53] These and many other Bcl-2 family members are involved in a complex set of interactions that may initiate or inhibit membrane permeability transition via a variety of signaling mechanisms.

Cytosolic cytochrome c forms an essential part of the 'apoptosome', which is composed of cytochrome c, apoptotic protease-activating factor 1 (Apaf-1), and procaspase-9.[54] Apaf-1 binds and hydrolyses ATP or dATP. The hydrolysis of ATP/dATP and the binding of cytochrome c promote Apaf-1 oligomerization, forming a large multimeric Apaf-1/cytochrome c complex, which is sufficient to recruit and activate procaspase-9. The result is the activation of caspase-9, which then processes and activates other downstream caspases, including caspase-3, leading to apoptotic cell death.[55]

While the members of the inhibitors of apoptosis proteins (IAP) family of antiapoptotic proteins (cIAP-1, cIAP-2 and XIAP) can inhibit caspase-9 activation by blocking formation of the apoptosome, two other proapoptotic proteins

(Smac/Diablo and Omi) are released from the mitochondria after the stimulation of mitochondria with truncated Bid (tBid). Smac/Diablo and Omi can bind IAPs and prevent them from inhibiting caspase activation promoting apoptosis.[35,56,57]

The IAPs

The inhibitors of apoptosis proteins (IAPs) are a group of proteins known to inhibit caspase activation during apoptosis. So far five members have been described in the human: NAIP, cIAP-1, cIAP-2, XIAP and survivin.

Structurally the IAPs contain three N-terminal BIR (Baculovirus inhibitory repeat) sequences that are responsible for the inhibition of caspase activity except survivin which has only one repeat sequence. A single BIR domain is sufficient for binding and inhibiting caspases in XIAP.[58,59] cIAP-1 and cIAP-2 also contain a caspase recruitment domain, a protein–protein motif first identified in the caspases and their adaptor molecules.[60] At the C-terminal end of the protein XIAP, cIAP-1 and cIAP-2 also have a zinc RING (really interesting new gene) finger domain that confers ubiquitin protein ligase activity to IAPs that may confer auto-ubiquitination.[61,62] This RING structure is not present in the survivin protein; instead it contains a coiled-coil motif that may be involved in association with the microtubules of the mitotic spindle that is necessary for survivin's antiapoptotic function during mitosis.[63]

All the IAPs except NAIP have been shown to inhibit the activity of activated caspases-3 and 7. Furthermore cIAP-1, cIAP-2 and XIAP can inhibit the cytochrome c induced activation of procaspase-9, which activates caspases-3 and 7.[65,65] Central to this theme, Smac released from the mitochondria during apoptosis has been shown to bind to XIAP, possibly acting as a neutralizer of the caspase inhibitor leading to apoptosis in LNCaP cells.[57]

TNF-alpha signaling induces apoptosis mainly through the TNFRI. TNF-alpha signaling may upregulate cIAP-1, cIAP-2, TRAF-1 and TRAF-2 (TNF receptor associated factor) through NF-kappa B activation. cIAP-1 and cIAP-2 can bind to TRAF-1 and TRAF-2 which associate with the cytosolic death domain of the receptor, thereby blocking caspase-8 activation in response to the cell death signal.[66] However, TNF-alpha signaling may also act through the TNFRII. This interaction can induce ubiquitination and proteasomal degradation of TRAF-2 through cIAP-1 ubiquitin protein ligase activity potentiating TNF-induced apoptosis and may play a proapoptotic role in TNF-alpha signaling.[67] IAP expression in the prostatic epithelium has been assessed in the LNCaP, PC3 and DU145 cell lines.[68]

Caspase-independent pathways

Cell death may also be activated by a number of caspase-independent mechanisms. One example is Bin1, a c-Myc interacting adaptor protein that activates a pathway that is p53, Rb and caspase independent. The apoptotic cells lack nucleosomal DNA cleavage and nuclear lamina degradation.[33] Another possible mechanism involves the use of a synthetic retinoid CD437 in DU145, PC3 and LNCaP cells; while DU145 and LNCaP cell death are caspase dependent the PC3 cells display a caspase-independent mechanism of cell death.

Omi is also released from the mitochondria after the mitochondrial membrane is disrupted by tBid. As mentioned above, Smac/Diablo and Omi can bind IAPs and prevent them from inhibiting caspase activation. However Omi also appears to act independently of the caspases through its serine protease activity.[35,56,57]

Ceramide-induced cell death in MCF-7 and Fas-resistant Hodgkin's disease cells has been shown to act through a caspase-independent mechanism. Ceramide treatment does not result in caspase-3 or poly (ADP-ribose) polymerase cleavage in Fas-resistant Hodgkin's disease cells and apoptosis is not inhibited by pan-caspase inhibitors.[34,69] While there are many papers detailing caspase-independent cell death pathways, many of these papers base their hypothesis on the premise that the mechanism of cell death is caspase independent solely on the inability of the pan-caspase inhibitor z-VAD-fmk to block the cell death process.

Characteristics of apoptosis

The plasma membrane

Plasma membrane phospholipids are asymmetrically distributed across the plasma membrane with phosphatidylserine found in the inner leaflet and sphingomyelin on the outer leaflet of the lipid bilayer. Plasma membrane asymmetry is maintained by aminophospholipid translocase that redistributes phosphatidylserine and phosphatidylethanolamine from the outer leaflet to the inner leaflet.[70] The loss of plasma membrane asymmetry results in the exposure of phosphatidylserine groups on the surface of the plasma membrane. During apoptosis phosphatidylserine is presented on the outer leaflet of the plasma membrane and may be observed using the phosphatidylserine binding protein annexin V.[71,72] This may occur for several reasons including a calcium-dependent mechanism involving the scramblases, the caspases and tissue transglutaminase.[73-77] While this is generally considered to be an early event, morphological alterations have been shown to occur before phosphatidylserine exposure depending upon the inductive mechanism involved.[78,79]

The cytoskeleton, cell–cell and cell–substratum interactions

The caspases are responsible for the proteolytic cleavage of cadherins,[80] cytokeratins,[81] pp125[FAK] which is involved in focal adhesion formation,[82] and gelsolin, a protein that severs actin filaments, which upon cleavage is constitutively active.[83] Truncation of the beta-catenin binding domain of E-cadherin has also been shown to precede apoptosis in the epithelium of the regressing prostate underlying the important role cell–cell contact plays in maintaining cell survival.[84]

The cell–cell and cell–substratum interactions may also be altered through the expression and activation of proteases such as cathepsin B,[17] cathepsin D,[18] and matrix metalloproteinases resulting in the degradation of specific components of the ECM, including fibronectin, collagen, laminin and vitronectin.[22,85,86] This may also occur through the upregulation and action of proteins such as tissue transglutaminase on the integrins at the cell surface.[20]

DNA fragmentation

One of the principal morphological features of apoptosis is chromatin condensation. In the rat prostate castration results in the sequential activation of a Ca^{2+} and Mg^{2+} dependent nuclease leading to the fragmentation of the genome into nucleosomal sized fragments of DNA 180–200 bp in size.[87] DNA fragmentation during apoptosis involves the cleavage of high molecular weight

DNA fragments and finally the production of oligonucleosomal fragments that are characterized by DNA laddering. There are a number of different DNase enzymes involved in degrading the DNA into high molecular weight fragments and the classical nucleosomal units seen in apoptotic DNA laddering.

Caspase-activated DNase (CAD, CPAN or DFF40) is a DNase that can be activated by a caspase-3 dependent pathway.[88] CAD is required for oligonucleosomal fragmentation in caspase-dependent apoptosis.[89] CAD is found in an inactive state complexed with its inhibitor ICAD, this complex residing predominantly in the nucleus of non-apoptotic cells.[90] Activated caspase-3 cleaves ICAD, releasing CAD facilitating DNA degradation within the nucleus.

While CAD relies on a caspase-dependent mechanism of action there are apoptotic pathways that are caspase independent. One of these pathways is a serine–protease dependent pathway. LEI (leukocyte elastase inhibitor) is a serine–protease inhibitor that may be post-translationally modified, either by a change in pH or by other proteases, conferring an endonuclease activity on the protein called L-DNase II. When activated L-DNase II may induce pycnosis and oligonucleosomal ladders.[91]

Another DNase involved in apoptosis is endonuclease G, which normally resides in the mitochondria and translocates to the nucleus during apoptosis. Its primary function is to cleave DNA into nucleosomal fragments. Interestingly endonuclease G has been shown to be caspase independent and may be released through tBid activity.[92,93]

The mechanism of antiandrogens

Apoptosis is a fundamental part of the events that occur in the regressing prostate after androgen ablation. How this process is activated following androgen withdrawal remains unknown. A number of antiandrogens have been developed including: cytoproterone acetate, a steroidal antiandrogen; and hydroxyflutamide and bicalutamide, two non-steroidal antiandrogens. These compounds bind to the steroid binding hydrophobic pocket of the androgen receptor blocking its action.

The most widely used antiandrogen in the world is bicalutamide, which inhibits gene expression and cell growth stimulated by androgens. However very little is known about the exact cellular events that occur during apoptosis in the prostate epithelial cells after bicalutamide administration.[94] Bicalutamide induces regression in the prostate after administration and can limit the growth of the transplantable androgen-responsive Dunning rat tumor. When bound to the androgen receptor, bicalutamide causes the rapid degradation of the receptor in the nucleus of prostate epithelial cells.[95]

Insulin-like growth factor (IGF) is important for the suppression of apoptosis in the prostate.[96] The IGF-1 pathway has been implicated in the mechanism of cell death induced by bicalutamide. The IGF binding proteins 2, 3, 4 and 5 are up-regulated in the rat ventral prostate after treatment with bicalutamide and may attenuate the IGF-1 receptor interaction, with IGF-1 leading to apoptosis in the hormone-dependent secretory epithelial cells.[97]

Survival mechanisms in prostate cancer

While the antiandrogens and androgen ablation result in apoptosis in androgen-dependent prostate cancer, a number of factors have been associated with the survival of androgen-dependent and androgen-independent prostate cancer cells. As mentioned above, IGF and testosterone are two of the growth factors that protect against apoptosis in prostate cancer.

IGF-1 can induce survival signals through PI3 kinase to activate Akt. IGF-1 interaction with the IGF receptor may be regulated by the IGF binding proteins in the prostate, in particular IGFBP-5 (which may block apoptosis) and IGFBP-3 (which may induce apoptosis by sequestering IGF-1).[98,99]

In the absence of androgen, PI3 kinase and Akt represent important cell survival pathways that may be potentiated by IGFBP-5 overexpression, the loss of IGFBP-3 or HER-2/neu activation of Akt.[100,101]

The overexpression of antiapoptotic and stress response proteins may also play a role in cell survival. Bcl-2 overexpression has been implicated as a marker for poor prognosis in prostate cancer and HSP-72 overexpression inhibits apoptosis in prostate cancer cells.[102,103]

Alternative therapies for prostate cancer

While antiandrogens block androgen action, clearly this therapy is not effective for the treatment of androgen-independent disease, leading to the development of alternative therapies. One target is cyclooxygenase 2 (COX-2), which converts arachidonic acid to prostaglandins and other eicosanoids. COX-2 is highly expressed in prostate tumors and inhibition of the enzyme decreases tumor microvessel density and angiogenesis. Inhibiting COX-2 may represent a treatment strategy as it has been shown to induce apoptosis in vitro and in vivo.[104]

Vitamin D deficiency has been suggested as a risk factor for prostate cancer. A number of groups have treated prostate cancer cell lines with $1,25(OH)_2D_3$, resulting in growth inhibitory effects and an increase in apoptosis in vitro and in vivo. A variety of vitamin D analogs are currently under investigation to alleviate the hypercalcemic effects of vitamin D.[105]

Antioxidants may also play a role in prostate cancer chemoprevention or therapy in the future. Selenium, vitamin E, lycopene and epigallocatechin-3-gallate (EGCG) all fall into this category. EGCG is found at high levels in green tea. Epidemiologic studies suggest that green tea has chemopreventative properties.[106] Much of the literature regarding green tea and the inhibition of prostate cancer have used EGCG and other catechins found in green tea to treat cell lines in culture resulting in cell cycle disruption and apoptosis.[107,108] Animal studies include the use of EGCG on athymic mice inoculated with PC3 and LNCaP 104-R cells and more recently the treatment of TRAMP mice with a polyphenolic fraction isolated from green tea. Both studies showed an inhibition of tumor growth after treatment.[109,110]

The phytoestrogens are another group of diverse plant-derived compounds that have estrogenic and in some cases antioxidant action. A number of studies have shown that neonatal estrogenization results in prostatic dysplasia in animal models.[111] Genistein is one of the phytoestrogens that is a strong inhibitor of protein tyrosine kinase and DNA topoisomerase II activities. Genistein is the predominant isoflavone found in soy and may decrease estrogen receptor alpha and estrogen receptor beta in the prostate after administration and reduce the incidence of prostate adenocarcinoma in vitro and in vivo.[112,113] While the phytoestrogens are grouped according to their estrogenic activity, a variety of phytoestrogens have antioxidant activity as well as antiandrogenic activity (e.g. resveratrol, curcumine and luteolin).[114]

Conclusions

Androgens are required to maintain the integrity of the prostate and the survival of androgen-dependent epithelial cells within the gland. While tissue remodeling occurs within the prostate, apoptosis is central to the regression process after androgen ablation.

Many of the receptor and mitochondrial mediated apoptotic pathways have been clearly defined in a variety of model systems; however the cell death pathway induced within the epithelial portion of the prostate after hormonal ablation in vivo remains to be elucidated. It is clear that the cell death pathways induced by the antiandrogens, currently used in treating androgen-dependent prostate cancer, are poorly understood and require further investigation.

There has been a focus in prostate cancer research on the use and design of better antiandrogens to induce apoptosis in prostate cancer cells. Most of this research is based on the physiologic observation that the majority of prostate epithelial cells are androgen dependent.

However, this therapeutic approach does not work in the long term and leads to androgen-independent prostate cancer. One possible reason is that this therapeutic approach may only activate a specific cell death pathway within the prostate epithelial cell. Therefore, through a selection process, the cells may use survival signals like Akt, IGFBPs or Bcl-2 to block the cell death pathway induced by androgen withdrawal, ultimately leading to androgen independence and disease progression.

Another reason may be that the tumor is only androgen sensitive not androgen dependent. While a proportion of the cells will die after androgen ablation, the majority of the cells do not require androgen for survival, making this therapeutic strategy useful for palliative treatment, but ultimately useless as a tool to improve long-term survival.

Either way, alternative treatment modalities that may induce apoptosis in the prostatic epithelium should be investigated using a number of different cell death pathways to induce apoptosis within the same cell type.

Understanding the pro- and antiapoptotic mechanisms that exist in the prostatic epithelium may ultimately lead to the design and use of therapeutic strategies that will target a variety of apoptotic pathways in prostate cancer.

Acknowledgment

Colm Morrissey was funded by an EU (E)UROESTROGEN(E)S grant contract no. QLK6-CT-2000-00565.

References

1. Mainwaring WI. The binding of (1,2-3H) testosterone within nuclei of the rat prostate. J Endocrinol 1969; 44:323–333.
2. Tenniswood M, Abrahams P, Winterton V, et al. Binding of testosterone, 5 alpha-dihydrotestosterone and 5 alpha-androstane (3 alpha- and 3 beta-), 17 beta-diols to serum proteins in the rat. J Steroid Biochem 1982; 16:617–620.
3. Wong CI, Zhou ZX, Sar M, Wilson EM. Steroid requirement for androgen receptor dimerization and DNA binding. Modulation by intramolecular interactions between the NH2-terminal and steroid binding domains. J Biol Chem 1993; 268:19004–19012.
4. Rennie PS, Bruchovsky N, Sheppard PC, et al. Characterization of two cis-acting DNA elements involved in the androgen regulation of the probasin gene. Mol Endocrinol 1993; 7:23–26.
5. Claessens F, Celis L, Peeters B, et al. Functional characterization of an androgen response element in the first intron of the C3(1) gene of prostatic binding protein. Biochem Biophys Res Commun 1989; 164:833–840.
6. Amero SA, Kretsinger RH, Moncrief ND, et al. The origin of nuclear receptor proteins: a single precursor distinct from other transcription factors. Mol Endocrinol 1992; 6:3–7.
7. Rouleau M, Leger JG, Tenniswood MP. Ductal heterogenicity of cytokeratins, gene expression and cell death in the rat ventral prostate. Mol Endocrinol 1990; 4:2003–2013.
8. Moore CR, Price D, Gallagher TF. Rat-prostate cytology as a testis hormone indicator and the prevention of castration changes by testis-extract injections. Am J Anat 1930; 45:71–107.
9. Parker MG, Scrace GT, Mainwaring WI. Testosterone regulates the synthesis of major proteins in rat ventral prostate. Biochem J 1978; 170:115–121.
10. Tenniswood M, Bird CE, Clark AF. Acid phosphatases: androgen dependent markers of rat prostate. Can J Biochem 1976; 54:350–357.
11. Vanha-Perttula T, Niemi R, Helminen HJ. Separate lysosomal and secretory acid phosphatases in the ventral prostate. Investig Urol 1972; 9:345–352.
12. Wolf DA, Schulz P, Fittler F. Transcriptional regulation of prostate kallikrein-like genes by androgen. Mol Endocrinol 1992; 6:753–762.
13. Mainwaring WI, Mangan FR, Peterken BM. Studies on the solubilized ribonucleic acid polymerase from rat ventral prostate gland. Biochem J 1971; 123:619–628.
14. Hiipakka RA, Chen C, Schilling K, et al. Immunochemical characterization of the androgen-dependent spermine-binding protein of the rat ventral prostate. Biochem J 1984; 218:563–571.
15. Piik K, Rajamaki P, Guha SK, Janne J. Regulation of L-ornithine decarboxylase and S-adenosyl-L-methionine decarboxylase in rat ventral prostate and seminal vesicle. Biochem J 1977; 168:379–385.
16. Collins S, Quarmby VE, French FS, et al. Regulation of the beta 2-adrenergic receptor and its mRNA in the rat ventral prostate by testosterone. FEBS Lett 1988; 233:173–176.
17. Guenette RS, Mooibroek M, Wong K, et al. Cathepsin B, a cysteine protease implicated in metastatic progression, is also expressed during regression of the rat prostate and mammary glands. Eur J Biochem 1994; 226:311–321.
18. Sensibar JA, Liu XX, Patai B, et al. Characterization of castration-induced cell death in the rat prostate by immunohistochemical localization of cathepsin D. Prostate 1990; 16:263–276.
19. Buttyan R, Zakari Z, Lockshin R, Wogemuth D. Cascade induction of c-fos, c-myc, and heat shock 70 transcripts during regression of the rat ventral prostate gland. Mol Endocrinol 1988; 2:650–657.
20. Cummings M. Apoptosis of epithelial cells in vivo involves tissue transglutaminase upregulation. J Pathol 1996; 179:288–293.
21. Rauch F, Polzar B, Stephan H, et al. Androgen ablation leads to an upregulation and intranuclear accumulation of deoxyribonuclease 1 in the rat prostate epithelial cells paralleling their apoptotic elimination. J Cell Biol 1997; 137:909–923.
22. Powell WC, Domann FE, Mitchen JM, et al. Matrilysin expression in the involuting rat ventral prostate. Prostate 1996; 29:159–168.
23. Freeman SN, Rennie PS, Chao J, et al. Urokinase- and tissue-type plasminogen activators are suppressed by cortisol in the involuting prostate of castrated rats. Biochem J 1990; 269:189–193.
24. Léger JG, Montpetit ML, Tenniswood MP. Characterization and cloning of androgen-repressed mRNAs from rat ventral prostate. Biochem Biophys Res Commun 1987; 147:196–203.
25. Lesser B, Bruchovsky N. The effects of testosterone, 5-dihydrotestosterone and adenosine 3′,5′-monophosphate on cell proliferation and differentiation in rat prostate. Biochim Biophys Acta 1973; 308:426–437.
26. Berry SJ, Isaacs JT. Comparative aspects of prostatic growth and androgen metabolism with aging in the rat versus dog. Endocrinology 1984; 114:511–520.
27. Clarke PG. Developmental cell death: morphological diversity and multiple mechanisms. Anat Embryol 1990; 181:195–213.

28. Cohen JJ. Apoptosis. Immunol Today 1993; 14:126–130.

29. Zamzami N, Susin SA, Marchetti P, et al. Mitochondrial control of nuclear apoptosis. J Exp Med 1996; 183:1533–1544.

30. Sandford N, Searle JW, Kerr JFR. Successive waves of apoptosis in the rat prostate after repeated withdrawal of testosterone stimulation. Pathology 1984; 16:406–410.

31. Stanisic T, Sadlowski R, Lee C, Grayhack JT. Partial inhibition of castration induced ventral prostate regression with actinomycin D and cycloheximide. Investig Urol 1978; 16:19–22.

32. Thornberry NA, Lazebnik Y. Caspases: enemies within. Science 1998; 281:1312–1316.

33. Elliott K, Ge K, Du W, Prendergast GC. The c-Myc-interacting adaptor protein Bin1 activates a caspase-independent cell death program. Oncogene 2000; 19:4669–4684.

34. Pirianov G, Colston KW. Interactions of vitamin D analogue CB1093, TNFalpha and ceramide on breast cancer cell apoptosis. Mol Cell Endocrinol 2001; 172:69–78.

35. Hegde R, Srinivasula SM, Zhang Z, et al. Identification of Omi/HtrA2 as a mitochondrial apoptotic serine protease that disrupts inhibitor of apoptosis protein–caspase interaction. J Biol Chem 2002; 277:432–438.

36. Ashkenazi A, Dixit VM. Death receptors: signaling and modulation. Science 1998; 281:1305–1308.

37. Smith CA, Farrah T, Goodwin G. The TNF receptor superfamily of cellular and viral proteins: activation, constimulation, and death. Cell 1994; 76:959–962.

38. Gruss H, Dower SK. Tumor necrosis factor ligand superfamily: involvement in the pathology of malignant lymphomas. Blood 1995; 85:3378–3404.

39. Nagata S. Apoptosis by death factor. Cell 1997; 88:355–365.

40. Duan H, Dixit VM. RAIDD is a new 'death' adaptor molecule. Nature 1997; 385:86–89.

41. Hsu H, Xiong J, Goeddel DV. The TNF receptor 1-associated protein TRADD signals cell death and NF-KB activation. Cell 1995; 81:495–504.

42. Rothe M, Pan M, Henzel WJ, et al. The TNFR2-TRAF signaling complex contains two novel proteins related to baculoviral inhibitor of apoptosis proteins. Cell 1995; 83:1243–1252.

43. Ting AT, Pimental-Muinos FX, Seed B. RIP mediates tumor necrosis factor receptor 1 activation of NF-αB but not Fas/APO-1-initiated apoptosis. EMBO J 1996; 15:6189–6196.

44. Chinnaiyan AM, O'Rourke K, Tewari M, Dixit VM. FADD, a novel death domain-containing protein, interacts with the death domain of Fas and initiates apoptosis. Cell 1995; 81:505–512.

45. Varfolomeev EE, Boldin MP, Goncharov TM, Wallach D. A potential mechanism of 'cross-talk' between the p55 tumor necrosis factor receptor and Fas/APO1: proteins binding to the death domains of the two receptors also bind to each other. J Exp Med 1996; 183:1271–1275.

46. Adams JM, Corry S. The Bcl-2 protein family: arbiters of cell survival. Science 1998; 281:1322–1326.

47. Green DR, Reed JC. Mitochondria and apoptosis. Science 1998; 281:1309–1312.

48. Yang J, Liu X, Bhalla K, et al. Prevention of apoptosis by Bcl-2: release of cytochrome c from mitochondria blocked. Science 1997; 275:1129–1132.

49. Kluck RM, Bossy-Wetzel E, Green DR, Newmeyer DD. The release of cytochrome c from mitochondria: a primary site for Bcl-2 regulation of apoptosis. Science 1997; 275:1132–1137.

50. Yano S, Tokumitsu H, Soderling TR. Calcium promotes cell survival through CaM-K kinase activation of the protein-kinase-B pathway. Nature 1998; 396:584–587.

51. Korsmeyer SJ. Bcl-2 gene family and the regulation of programmed cell death. Cancer Res 1999; 59:1693–1700.

52. Desagher S, Osen-Sand A, Nichols A, et al. Bid-induced conformational change of Bax is responsible for mitochondrial cytochrome c release during apoptosis. J Cell Biol 1999; 144:891–901.

53. Luo X, Budihardjo I, Zou H, et al. Bid, a Bcl2 interacting protein, mediates cytochrome c release from mitochondria in response to activation of cell surface death receptors. Cell 1998; 94:481–490.

54. Li P, Nijhawan D, Budihardjo I, et al. Cytochrome C and dATP-dependent formation of apaf-1/caspase-9 complex initiates an apoptotic protease cascade. Cell 1997; 91:479–489.

55. Zou H, Li Y, Liu X, Wang X. An Apaf-1 cytochrome c multimeric complex is a functional apoptosome that activates procaspase-9. J Biol Chem 1999; 274:11549–11556.

56. Du C, Fang M, Li Y, et al. Smac, a mitochondrial protein that promotes cytochrome c-dependent caspase activation by eliminating IAP inhibition. Cell 2000; 102:33–42.

57. Carson JP, Behnam M, Sutton JN, et al. Smac is required for cytochrome c-induced apoptosis in prostate cancer LNCaP cells. Cancer Res 2002; 62:18–23.

58. Ambrosini G, Adida C, Altieri DC. A novel anti-apoptosis gene, survivin, expressed in cancer and lymphoma. Nat Med 1997; 8:917–921.

59. Takahashi R, Deveraux Q, Tamm I, et al. A single BIR domain of XIAP sufficient for inhibiting caspases. J Biol Chem 1998; 273:7787–7790.

60. Hofmann K, Bucher P, Tschopp J. The CARD domain: a new apoptotic signalling motif. Trends Biochem Sci 1997; 5:155–156.

61. Miller LK. An exegesis of IAPs: salvation and surprises from BIR motifs. Trends Cell Biol 1999; 9:323–328.

62. Yang Y, Fang S, Jensen JP, et al. Ubiquitin protein ligase activity of IAPs and their degradation in proteosomes in response to apoptotic stimuli. Science 2000; 288:874–877.

63. Li F, Ambrosini G, Chu EY, et al. Control of apoptosis and mitotic spindle checkpoint by survivin. Nature 1998; 396:580–584.

64. Roy N, Deveraux QL, Takahashi R, et al. The c-IAP-1 and c-IAP-2 proteins are direct inhibitors of specific caspases. EMBO J 1997; 16:6914–6925.

65. Deveraux QL, Roy N, Stennicke HR, et al. IAPs block apoptotic events induced by caspase-8 and cytochrome c by direct inhibition of distinct caspases. EMBO J 1998; 17:2215–2223.

66. Wang CY, Mayo MW, Korneluk RG, et al. NF-kappaB antiapoptosis: induction of TRAF1 and TRAF2 and c-IAP1 and c-IAP2 to suppress caspase-8 activation. Science 1998; 281:1680–1683.

67. Li X, Yang Y, Ashwell JD. TNF-RII and c-IAP1 mediate ubiquitination and degradation of TRAF2. Nature 2002; 416:345–349.

68. McEleny KR, Watson RW, Coffey RN, et al. Inhibitors of apoptosis proteins in prostate cancer cell lines. Prostate 2002; 51:133–140.

69. Metkar SS, Anand M, Manna PP, et al. Ceramide-induced apoptosis in fas-resistant Hodgkin's disease cell lines is caspase independent. Exp Cell Res 2000; 255:18–29.

70. Bratton DL, Fadok VA, Richter DA, et al. Polyamine regulation of plasma membrane phospholipid flip-flop during apoptosis. J Biol Chem 1999; 274:28113–28120.

71. Blankenberg FG, Katsikis PD, Tait JF, et al. In vivo detection and imaging of phosphatidylserine expression during programmed cell death. Proc Natl Acad Sci USA 1998; 95:6349–6354.

72. Span LF, Pennings AH, Vierwinden G, et al. The dynamic process of apoptosis analyzed by flow cytometry using Annexin-V/propidium iodide and a modified in situ end labeling technique. Cytometry 2002; 47:24–31.

73. Bratton DL. Release of platelet activation factor from activated neutrophils. Transglutaminase-dependent enhancement of transbilayer movement across the plasma membrane. J Biol Chem 1993; 268:3364–3373.

74. Martin SJ, Finucane DM, Amarante-Mendes GP, et al. Phosphatidylserine externalization during CD95-induced apoptosis of cells and cytoplasts requires ICE/CED-3 protease activity. J Biol Chem 1996; 271:28753–28756.

75. Bassé F, Stout JG, Sims PJ, Wiedmer T. Isolation of an erythrocyte membrane protein that mediates Ca^{2+}-dependent transbilayer movement of phospholipid. J Biol Chem 1996; 271:17205–17210.

76. Bratton DL, Fadok VA, Richter DA, et al. Appearance of phosphatidylserine on apoptotic cells requires calcium-mediated nonspecific flip-flop and is enhanced by loss of the aminophospholipid translocase. J Biol Chem 1997; 272:26159–26165.

77. Zhao J, Zhou Q, Wiedmer T, Sims PJ. Level of expression of phospholipid scramblase regulates induced movement of phosphatidylserine to the cell surface. J Biol Chem 1998; 273:6603–6606.

78. Martin SJ, Reutelingsperger CP, McGahon AJ, et al. Early redistribution of plasma membrane phosphatidylserine is a general feature of apoptosis regardless of the initiating stimulus: inhibition by overexpression of Bcl-2 and Abl. J Exp Med 1995; 182:1545–1556.

79. Cornelissen M, Philippe J, De Sitter S, De Ridder L. Annexin V expression in apoptotic peripheral blood lymphocytes: an electron microscopic evaluation. Apoptosis 2002; 7:41–47.

80. Schmeiser K, Grand RJ. The fate of E- and P-cadherin during the early stages of apoptosis. Cell Death Differ 1999; 6:377–386.

81. Caulin C, Salvesen GS, Oshima RG. Caspase cleavage of keratin 18 and reorganization of intermediate filaments during epithelial cell apoptosis. J Cell Biol 1997; 138:1379–1394.

82. Wen LP, Fahrni JA, Sergiu T, et al. Cleavage of focal adhesion kinase by caspases during apoptosis. J Biol Chem 1997; 272:26056–26061.

83. Kothakota S, Azuma T, Reinhard C, et al. Caspase-3 generated fragment of gelsolin: effector of morphological change in apoptosis. Science 1997; 278:294–298.

84. Vallorosi CJ, Day KC, Zhao X, et al. Truncation of the beta-catenin binding domain of E-cadherin precedes epithelial apoptosis during prostate and mammary involution. J Biol Chem 2000; 275:3328–3334.

85. Muntzing J. Androgen and collagen as growth regulators of the rat ventral prostate. Prostate 1980; 1:71–78.

86. Tenniswood M, Guenette RS, Lakins J, et al. Active cell death in hormone-dependent tissues. Cancer Metastasis Rev 1992; 11:197–220.

87. Kyprianou N, English HF, Isaacs JT. Activation of a Ca^{2+}-Mg^{2+}-dependent endonuclease as an early event in castration-induced prostatic cell death. Prostate 1988; 13:103–117.

88. Mukae N, Enari M, Sakahira H, et al. Molecular cloning and characterization of human caspase-activated DNase. Proc Natl Acad Sci USA 1998; 95:9123–9128.

89. Samejima K, Tone S, Earnshaw WC. CAD/DFF40 nuclease is dispensable for high molecular weight DNA cleavage and stage 1 chromatin condensation in apoptosis. J Biol Chem 2001; 276:45427–45432.

90. Lechardeur D, Drzymala L, Sharma M, et al. Determinants of the nuclear localization of the heterodimeric DNA fragmentation factor (ICAD/CAD). J Cell Biol 2000; 150:321–334.

91. Torriglia A, Perani P, Brossas JY, et al. A caspase-independent cell clearance program: the LEI/L-DNase II pathway. Ann N Y Acad Sci 2000; 926:192–203.

92. Ly L, Luo X, Wang X. Endonuclease G is an apoptotic DNase when released from mitochondria. Nature 2001; 412:95–99.

93. Van Loo G, Schotte P, Van Gurp M, et al. Endonuclease G: a mitochondrial protein released in apoptosis and involved in caspase-independent DNA degradation. Cell Death Differ 2001; 8:1136–1142.

94. Furr BJA. The development of Casodex™ (bicalutamide): preclinical studies. Eur Urol 1996; 29:83–95.

95. Waller AS, Sharrard RM, Berthon P, Maitland NJ. Androgen receptor localisation and turnover in human prostate epithelium treated with the antiandrogen, casodex. J Mol Endocrinol 2000; 24:339–351.

96. Guenette RS, Tenniswood M. The role of growth factors in the suppression of active cell death in the prostate: an hypothesis. Biochem Cell Biol 1994; 72:553–559.

97. Nickerson T, Pollack M. Bicalutamide (Casodex)-induced prostate regression involves increased expression of genes encoding insulin-like growth factor binding proteins. Urology 1999; 54:1120–1125.

98. Rajah R, Valentinis B, Cohen P. Insulin-like growth factor (IGF)-binding protein-3 induces apoptosis and

mediates the effects of transforming growth factor-b1 on programmed cell death through a p53 and IGF-independent mechanism. J Biol Chem 1997; 272:12181–12188.

99. Miyake H, Nelson C, Rennie PS, Gleave ME. Overexpression of insulin-like growth factor binding protein-5 helps accelerate progression to androgen-independence in the human prostate LNCaP tumor model through activation of phosphatidylinositol 3′-kinase pathway. Endocrinology 2000; 141:2257–2265.

100. Wen Y, Hu MC, Makino K, et al. HER-2/neu promotes androgen-independent survival and growth of prostate cancer cells through the Akt pathway. Cancer Res 2000; 60:6841–6845.

101. Murillo H, Huang H, Schmidt LJ, et al. Role of PI3K signaling in survival and progression of LNCaP prostate cancer cells to the androgen refractory state. Endocrinology 2001; 142:4795–4805.

102. Bubendorf L, Sauter G, Moch H, et al. Prognostic significance of Bcl-2 in clinically localized prostate cancer. Am J Pathol 1996; 148:1557–1565.

103. Gibbons NB, Watson RW, Coffey RN, et al. Heat-shock proteins inhibit induction of prostate cancer cell apoptosis. Prostate 2000; 45:58–65.

104. Kirschenbaum A, Liu X, Yao S, Levine AC. The role of cyclooxygenase-2 in prostate cancer. Urology 2001; 58:127–131.

105. Polek TC, Weigel NL. Vitamin D and prostate cancer. J Androl 2002; 23(1):9–17.

106. Katiyar SK, Mukhtar H. Tea in the chemoprevention of cancer: epidemiologic and experimental studies [Review]. Int J Oncol 1996; 8:221–238.

107. Paschka AG, Butler R, Young CY. Induction of apoptosis in prostate cancer cell lines by the green tea component, (–)-epigallocatechin-3-gallate. Cancer Lett 1998; 130(1–2):1–7.

108. Gupta S, Ahmad N, Nieminen AL, Mukhtar H. Growth inhibition, cell-cycle dysregulation, and induction of apoptosis by green tea constituent (–)-epigallocatechin-3-gallate in androgen-sensitive and androgen-insensitive human prostate carcinoma cells. Toxicol Appl Pharmacol 2000; 164(1):82–90.

109. Liao S, Umekita Y, Guo J, et al. Growth inhibition and regression of human prostate and breast tumors in athymic mice by tea epigallocatechin gallate. Cancer Lett 1995; 96(2):239–243.

110. Gupta S, Hastak K, Ahmad N, et al. Inhibition of prostate carcinogenesis in TRAMP mice by oral infusion of green tea polyphenols. Proc Natl Acad Sci USA 2001; 98:10350–10355.

111. Pylkkanen L, Makela S, Santti R. Animal models for the preneoplastic lesions of the prostate. Eur Urol 1996; 30:243–248.

112. Mentor-Marcel R, Lamartiniere CA, Eltoum IE, et al. Genistein in the diet reduces the incidence of poorly differentiated prostatic adenocarcinoma in transgenic mice (TRAMP). Cancer Res 2001; 61:6777–6782.

113. Fritz WA, Wang J, Eltoum IE, Lamartiniere CA. Dietary genistein down-regulates androgen and estrogen receptor expression in the rat prostate. Mol Cell Endocrinol 2002; 186:89–99.

114. Rosenberg Zand RS, Jenkins DJ, Brown TJ, Diamandis EP. Flavonoids can block PSA production by breast and prostate cell lines. Clin Chim Acta 2002; 317:17–26.

8

Laparoscopic radical prostatectomy
Xavier Cathelineau and Guy Vallancien

History

Théodore Billroth, in Vienna, performed the first transperineal radical prostatectomy in 1867. In 1900, Hugh Hampton Young, assisted by his colleague, Halstead, standardized this transperineal technique and, in 1904, published his preliminary results based on a series of 40 patients.

In 1949, Thomas Millin, from Dublin, developed the retropubic approach to the prostate and, in 1980, Patrick Walsh, from Baltimore, described the nerve preservation technique by dissecting the fascia flush with the prostate, in order to preserve both the blood supply and the innervation necessary for preservation of erections.

Laparoscopic surgery, which was developed in gynecology during the 1940s, and then in gastrointestinal surgery from 1986 onwards, especially following development of the technique by Philippe Mouret, in Lyon, and François Dubois, in Paris, was not immediately extended to the field of urology The first laparoscopic nephrectomy was performed in 1990 by Ralph Clayman, in St Louis, but the urological community remained reticent for a long time about the value of these time-consuming techniques, which had only limited indications. From 1995 onwards, the development of intracorporeal suture, allowing repair of anomalies of the ureteropelvic junction and nephrectomies for cancer, led to a renewed interest in laparoscopy.

In 1992, the first attempt to perform laparoscopic prostatectomy in two cases was published by Schuessler et al in an abstract presented to the American Urology Association Congress. In 1997, the same team[1] published nine cases of laparoscopic radical prostatectomy and reached the conclusion that this technique did not provide any advantages over open surgery, due to the duration and difficulty of the operation, especially when performing the vesicourethral anastomosis.

In the same year, Raboy et al[2] published a case of extraperitoneal radical prostatectomy. In December 1997, Richard Gaston (Bordeaux, France), in a personal communication, indicated that he had performed a transperitoneal radical prostatectomy in less than 6 hours. Six weeks later, Bertrand Guillonneau and Guy Vallancien[3,4] started to perform their first radical prostatectomies. Five months later, Claude Abbou and colleagues,[5] in Créteil, also started to perform this new surgical technique.

The essential driving force that encouraged French surgeons to develop this surgery was the experience acquired by their gastrointestinal surgery colleagues. They hoped to reduce operative bleeding and postoperative pain, shorten the convalescence time and improve the quality of the vesicourethral suture as a result of endoscopic vision and the use of long needle holders. They also hoped to be gradually able to ensure preservation of neurovascular bundles, without increasing the oncological risks of this type of surgery.

The step from open surgery to laparoscopic surgery constitutes a completely new experience for the surgeon, who must learn a new endoscopic anatomy and new operative procedures and must work with new instruments. It therefore represents a profound change, which explains the difficulties encountered when trying to develop this surgery in places not adequately equipped. Laparoscopy requires appropriate instruments, an intellectual investment (long training) and a physical investment (this surgery is more tiresome than open surgery). Most importantly, surgeons must be assisted by motivated teams, composed of instrument nurses, scrub nurses, anesthetists and the hospital administration. It would be impossible to perform laparoscopic surgery without such an environment.

Indications and contraindications

Indications

The indications for laparoscopic radical prostatectomy are exactly the same as for open radical prostatectomy. The development of the laparoscopic procedure has not changed the indications or the selection of patients for surgical treatment.

The best indication is probably the young patient, who has a prostate specific antigen (PSA) of less than 15 ng/ml, with less than 50% of positive biopsies and Gleason score less than 8.

Laparoscopic radical prostatectomy is feasible for some T3N0M0 graded tumors, with the condition that the neurovascular bundles are taken.

Salvage laparoscopic radical prostatectomy is also feasible after radiotherapy or brachytherapy, but the patient must be informed of the risk of temporary colostomy.

Contraindications

Anesthetic contraindications

There are no specific anesthetic contraindications for laparoscopic radical prostatectomy. Contraindications for this procedure are the same as those for all laparoscopic procedures.

The main absolute contraindication for a laparoscopic approach is high intracranial pressure whatever its origin (primary or secondary to intracranial process).

The relative anesthetic contraindications are severe emphysema, severe cardiac injury, chronic respiratory disease and glaucoma.

Anatomic contraindications

There are no anatomic contraindications for laparoscopic radical prostatectomy. High body mass index (BMI) is not a contraindication but the very obese patient (e.g. over 120 kg) is probably not a good indication, exactly the same as in open surgery.

Obviously, some cases are more difficult, and, especially at the beginning of the experience, the surgeon has to be aware of these difficulties.

Difficult cases

Different factors can increase the difficulty of the procedure, especially:

- previous hormone therapy
- previous transuretheral resection of prostate (TURP) or prostatectomy
- prostatitis.

All these factors can alter the prostatic and periprostatic tissues and make the surgery considerably more difficult. Moreover, a very small (less than 20 g) or a very large (more than 100 g) prostate can increase the difficulty of the dissection.

According to previous experience, the surgeon should probably avoid these cases at the beginning of the learning curve. In any case, conversion is not a sign of shame but a sign of wisdom.

Operative technique

Transperitoneal approach: the Montsouris technique[6]

Medical preparation

Prophylactic antibiotics are not given to the patient. They do not decrease the risk of infection but can induce selection of bacteria, especially enterococci.

Thromboembolic complications are prevented by injection of low molecular weight heparin on the day before the operation, which is continued for at least 7 days postoperatively, associated with wearing of varicose veins stockings during hospitalization.

No gastrointestinal or skin preparation is required.

Preoperative preparation of the patient

- The operation is performed under general anesthesia.
- The patient is placed in the dorsal supine position, with the lower limbs in abduction allowing intraoperative access to the rectum.
- An exaggerated Trendelenburg position is essential, at least for the initial posterior phase of the operation.
- The upper limbs are positioned alongside the body to avoid the risk of stretch injuries to the brachial plexus.
- An adhesive elastic bandage is placed in cross fashion over the thorax, which ensures better comfort for the patient than shoulder rests.
- The surgeon stands to the left of the patient and the assistant stands to the right. The camera is attached to a voice-controlled robotic arm.

Material

There are no specific instruments for laparoscopic radical prostatectomy. As for all the other laparoscopic procedures, adapted material is primordial. All the instruments must be checked before the procedure, especially bipolar forceps and scissors, in order to detect any leak which could induce a burning of an intra-abdominal organ.

Main steps of the operation

Insufflation is performed with a Veress needle in the umbilicus or left hypochondrium.

The 10 mm trocar for the scope is placed in the umbilicus. Four other trocars are used for the surgeon and the assistant, arranged according to the surgeon's usual practice: either in a triangular pattern (the operator uses a left pararectal trocar and a right pararectal trocar, and the assistant uses a trocar in the right iliac fossa and an inter-umbilicopubic trocar) or in a parallel pattern (the operator uses a trocar in the left iliac fossa and a left pararectal trocar, and the assistant uses two symmetrical trocars on the right side).

Pelvic lymph node dissection with frozen section examination is performed according to the preoperative findings.

The operation comprises seven successive steps:

- *Posterior phase*: The posterior peritoneum is incised over the vasa deferentia, which are sectioned, and the seminal vesicles are completely dissected. The median part of Denonvilliers' fascia is incised.
- *Anterior phase*: The anterior parietal peritoneum is incised from one umbilical artery to the other providing access to the retropubic space after section of the urachus. The pelvic fascia is incised as far as the puboprostatic ligaments, which are sectioned. The prostatic apex is completely dissected. Santorini's venous plexus and the preprostatic venous drainage are then ligated with 2-0 Vicryl (this stitch can also be placed after the dissection of the prostatic vascular pedicles, just before cutting the urethra).
- *Vesicoprostatic dissection*: Vesicoprostatic dissection is performed by preserving, as far as possible, the fibers of the bladder neck. Dissection of the posterior surface of the bladder neck provides access to the plane of the seminal vesicles and vasa deferentia.
- *Dissection of prostatic pedicles and neurovascular bundles*: The prostatic vascular pedicles are selectively coagulated with bipolar forceps. Neurovascular bundles are preserved depending on anatomic and oncologic conditions.

- *Section of the urethra*: The urethra is sectioned away from the prostatic apex. The recto-urethralis muscle is also sectioned and the prostate is then completely released (a bougie in the rectum can be useful to identify the rectum in the case of difficult posterior dissection).
- *Vesicourethral anastomosis*: This is performed by interrupted 3-0 Vicryl sutures. An 18 F Foley catheter is inserted. The absence of anastomotic leak is verified intraoperatively.
- *Extraction of the operative specimen*: The prostate is placed in a laparoscopic bag and removed by enlarging the umbilical incision.

At closure, a Redon drain is inserted in the retropubic space or the pouch of Douglas. The 5 mm trocar orifices are closed in one layer and the 10 mm trocar orifices are closed in two layers.

Postoperative management

The bladder catheter is left in place for 3–7 days depending on the quality of the suture (cystography is not performed).

Analgesia is limited to paracetamol (8 g by i.v. injection) during the first 24 hours, followed, on day 1, by oral paracetamol/dextropropoxyphene prn. Major analgesics are not administered routinely, but are prescribed prn. The i.v. infusion is stopped on day 1.

Oral fluids are started on day 1 and a normal diet can generally be resumed on day 2.

Variants of the transperitoneal approach

Transperitoneal approach with initial anterior approach

Rassweiler and colleagues[7] reported their experience with a modified version of the Montsouris technique. An initial anterior approach is performed, providing access to the retropubic space. The pelvic fascia is incised, the puboprostatic ligaments are sectioned and Santorini's venous plexus is ligated. The urethra is then sectioned and, when the neurovascular bundles are preserved, they are dissected in an ascending direction. The vesicoprostatic dissection is then performed, prior to dissection of the seminal vesicles and section of the vasa deferentia. The anastomosis is performed with interrupted sutures.

Overall, this technical modification is designed to reproduce the various steps of retropubic prostatectomy.

Number of trocars

Most teams[6,8,9] performing laparoscopic radical prostatectomy use five trocars, which may be arranged in different ways according to the surgeon's usual practice. Rassweiler[7] adds a sixth 5 mm trocar at McBurney's point, which is designed to improve exposure, especially during seminal vesicle dissection.

Use of an arm for the scope

The use of an arm for the scope provides valuable assistance when performing a laparoscopic procedure such as radical prostatectomy, as it ensures a fixed image and frees one of the assistant's hands, allowing more active participation in the operative procedure.

Many teams[6-9] use a voice-controlled robotic arm (automated endoscope system for optimal positioning, AESOP), but other types of arm are also available, including less expensive, manually guided, compressed air arms.

Modalities of dissection of neurovascular bundles

Preservation of the neurovascular bundles precludes the use of mechanical staplers for section of the superior prostatic pedicles. Control and section of these pedicles and preservation of neurovascular bundles require precise dissection, ideally performed by selective bipolar coagulation[6,8,10] or even the use of clips.[9] The choice between these two approaches is a matter of personal preference, as neither technique has been shown to be superior to the other.

Technical modalities of vesicourethral anastomosis

The vesicourethral anastomosis can be performed with interrupted sutures or a running suture. Whatever the choice, the rules are the same and in particular the necessity of using both hands with forehand and backhand.

The running suture has the advantage of being less time consuming, but it requires constant good quality traction to ensure a perfectly leak-proof suture. In every case, the operator's experience and that of the team appear to be essential for both the rapidity and the quality of the procedure.

Extraperitoneal approach

In 1997, Raboy et al[2] described, for the first time, their experience of extraperitoneal laparoscopic radical prostatectomy. In 2001, Bollens and colleagues[11] reported their experience of 46 cases performed according to this technique.

The scope is introduced via a 10 mm trocar placed at the inferior margin of the umbilicus. Four trocars are used: two 10 mm trocars placed in the left iliac fossa and right iliac fossa; a 5 mm trocar is introduced about 5 cm above the pubic symphysis; and the last 5 mm trocar is placed in the right flank.

The first phase of the procedure consists of creation of a prevesical working space. Bladder neck dissection is performed prior to seminal vesicle dissection. The pelvic fascia is then incised and Santorini's venous plexus is ligated, following which the neurovascular bundles are dissected before coagulation and section of the superior prostatic pedicles. Denonvilliers' fascia is then incised, releasing the posterior surface of the prostate. Next, the apex is dissected and the urethra is sectioned. The anastomosis is performed by interrupted sutures.

Overall, the advantages of the extraperitoneal approach, according to its supporters, would be a reduction of the risk of damage to intraperitoneal organs and a similar surgical approach to that of open retropubic prostatectomy. Its disadvantages would be a limited working space, and the difficulty of the anastomosis due to the more limited mobilization of the bladder.

Perioperative complications (Tables 8.1 and 8.2)

Improvement of the surgical technique has allowed a reduction of the morbidity of radical prostatectomy.

Comparative studies of the complications according to the surgical technique are often difficult and must always take into account not only the operator's level of experience with the technique, but also the patient characteristics and finally the modalities of evaluation of complications, especially functional complications.

Morbidity is related not only to the technique itself, but also to the patient's comorbidities, particularly the ASA3 score[12] and blood loss.

The mortality rate is currently close to 0%, regardless of the technique used (retropubic, perineal or laparoscopic).[13-16]

Table 8.1 Complications of radical prostatectomy

	Dillioglugil et al[17]	Lerner et al[20]	Heinzer et al[35]	Lepor et al[37]	Catalona et al[13]	*Guillonneau et al[16]	*Rassweiler et al[10]
Number of patients	472	1000	150	1000	1870	567	180
Rectal injury	3/0.6	6/0.6	3/2	5/0.5	1/0.05	8/1.4	1.1
Ileocolic injury	nc	nc	nc	nc	nc	4/0.7	nc
Ileus	15/3.2	nc	nc	4/0.4	nc	6/1.1	2.8
Bladder injury	nc	nc	nc	nc	nc	9/1.6	nc
Ureteral injury	1/0.3	nc	7/4.7	1/0.1	1/0.05	3/0.5	0
Deep venous thrombosis	6/1.3	13/1.3	4/2.7	2/0.2	39/2	2/0.4	0
Pulmonary embolism	5/1	7/0.7	nc	4/0.4	nc	0	0
Anastomotic leakage	3/0.6	nc	15/10	2/0.2	nc	46/8.1	2.2
Lymphocele	12/2.5	1/0.1	3/2	1/0.1	11/0.6	1/0.2	0
Hydronephrosis	1/0.3	nc	nc	nc	nc	nc	2.8
Acute renal failure	2/0.4	nc	2/1.3	nc	nc	1/0.2	nc
Pelvic hematomas	nc	1/0.1	nc	nc	nc	5/0.9	8.9
Wound	13/2.7	/0.9	nc	9/0.9	15/0.8	7/1.2	0.6
Nerve injury	7/1.5	nc	nc	1	5/0.3	3/0.5	0
Myocardial infarction	2/0.4	7/0.7	0	5/0.5	2/0.1	0	nc
Cerebral vascular accident	1/0.3	nc	nc	nc	0	0	nc
Death	2/0.4	nc	1/0.7	1/0.1	0	0	nc
Anastomotic stricture	nc	nc	nc	10/1	71/3.8	nc	2.8
Total complications	73/16	35/3.5			143/8	95/16.7	nc

* Laparoscopic approach. nc, no cases.

Table 8.2 Evolution of the complication rate with experience in laparoscopy (Montsouris experience)

	Patients 1–200	Patients 200–400	Patients 400–567
Lymphadenectomy (%)	25	19	14
Mean operative time (min)	234	190	180
Mean estimated blood loss (ml)	372	398	350
Transfusions (%)	7.5	5	3.8
Conversions (%)	3.5	0	0
Rectal injuries (No.)	3	1	4
Reinterventions (%)	6	7	9

Considering the different phases of the laparoscopic procedure, complications can be divided according each step:

1. Patient positioning
2. Insufflation and placement of trocars
3. Dissection
4. Extraction of surgical specimen and removal of trocars
5. Early postoperative phase
6. Late postoperative phase.

Complications of patient positioning

The main complications at this step are compartment syndrome, peripheral neuropathy and scapular pain.

The risk is related to protections used for the positioning and also, obviously, to the length of time of the procedure. Therefore, the surgeon should always check the protection of the patients and to be aware of the length of time of the operation (conversion is sometimes the best solution).

These complications are exceptional (less than 0.1%) and their risk decreases significantly with experience of the surgeon and the team.

Complications of insufflation and trocar placement

The main risk is vascular or bowel injury with the first trocar. There is no rule on whether to use an open or a laparoscopic procedure and the choice depends on which is more useful and the experience of each team.

Small vessel injury can also occur during the placement of other trocars, especially to the epigastric artery (0.3%).

Intraoperative complications

Blood loss

Median intraoperative bleeding reported by experienced teams performing retropubic prostatectomy varies between 1000 and 1500 ml.[13,17] Dillioglugil et al[17] reported a transfusion rate of 29% for all the series and 15% for the last 135 patients among a total of 472. For Catalona et al,[13] using the technique of hemodilution, most of the patients received autologous transfusion during or after surgery and 9% also needed heterologous postoperative transfusion. In the same series, the rate of hematoma was 0.05%.

The median blood loss during laparoscopic prostatectomy varies from 370 ml[18] to 1230 ml[10] for patient series with a comparable experience.[10,18] The transfusion rates for these two series were 7% and 30%, respectively, at the beginning of their experience.

Guillonneau et al[16] reported, for their last 100 patients, a mean estimated blood loss of 290 ml and a transfusion rate of 3.5%. The rate of hematoma in this series was 1%.

Digestive injuries

Digestive injuries are rare and directly related to the operator's experience and to the patient's history (especially previous radiotherapy).

The rate of rectal injuries is similar regardless of the technique (retropubic or laparoscopic), ranging from 0.5 to 2%.[10,17,18]

In laparoscopic procedures, using a rectal bougie can help to identify the rectal wall but cannot ensure risk-free surgery.

Ureteric injuries

Ureteric injuries are also rare, occurring in 0.05–0.3% of cases, regardless of technique.

Complications of specimen extraction and trocar removal

The complications which can occur are bleeding from the orifice of the 10 mm trocar, and ileum injury (with the endobag or during the opening for extraction of the specimen). These complications are exceptional.

Early postoperative complications

Thromboembolic complications

These constitute the main cause of postoperative mortality in open procedures.[19,20] Dillioglugil et al[17] reported 2% thromboembolic accidents, while Rassweiler et al[10] and Guillonneau et al[16] reported a thromboembolic accident rate of less than 0.5%. Prophylactic anticoagulation and early mobilization (especially after laparoscopic procedure) decrease the frequency of these complications.

Anastomotic leaks

Anastomotic leaks are often missed when minimal and correctly drained and their incidence is therefore often underestimated. The length time that the bladder catheter has to be retained is directly related to the quality of the anastomosis.

Lymphoceles

These are now less frequent, whatever the procedure (laparoscopic or open), due to better selection of patients requiring pelvic lymph node dissection.

Late postoperative complications

Urinary incontinence and impotence are the two most frequent and most disabling functional sequelae. Stenosis of the vesicourethral anastomosis is observed more rarely.

Urinary incontinence (Table 8.3)

The quality of continence after radical prostatectomy is difficult to assess, as reflected by the marked variability of incontinence rates reported in the literature. This variability is related to three main factors: definition of incontinence, modalities of evaluation and follow up.

- *The definition of incontinence* varies considerably from one study to another: total absence of protection or use of a maximum of one protection. Geary et al[21] reported that 80.1% of patients did not require any protection, while Eastham et al,[22]

Table 8.3 Continence

Study	No. of patients	Follow-up months	Evaluation	Mean age	= 1 pad/day (%)
Catalona et al[13]	1325	50	Physician	63 (38–79)	8
Geary et al[21]	458	>18	Physician	64.1 ± 0.3	19.9
Leandri et al[29]	620	12	Physician	68 (46–84)	5
Steiner[31]	593	12	Physician	? (34–76)	5.5
Turk et al[8] *	125	9	Physician	60 (37–72)	8
Bollens et al[11] *	50	6	Physician	63 (47–71)	15
Igel et al[19]	692	–	Physician	–	21
Rassweiler et al[7] *	100	6	Questionnaire	68 (55–74)	22
Fontaine et al[27]	116	51.6	Patient quest.	65.2 (48–76)	19.8
McCammon et al[23]	203	40.3	Patient quest.	63.7 (43–73)	23.7
Jonler et al[26]	86	22.5	Patient quest.	64 (49–75)	47
Bates et al[30]	83	22	Patient quest.	65 (49–73)	24
Walsh et al[14]	64	18	Patient quest.	57 (36–67)	7
Wei & Montie[24]	145	12	Patient quest.	62.3 (40–80)	13
Talcott et al[33]	94	12	Patient quest.	61.5	39
Guillonneau et al[16]*	567	12	Patient quest.	63 (49–77)	21
Abbou[9]*	29	12	Patient quest.	64.8 (47–77)	13.8

* Laparoscopic approach. Patient quest., patient questionnaire.

considering patients who required a maximum of one protection to be continent, reported that 91% of patients were continent. No consensus has therefore been reached concerning the definition of incontinence. In Table 8.3 continence is defined as complete absence of either occasional or permanent protection.

- *The modalities of evaluation* also vary from one author to another: clinical interview by the surgeon, clinical interview by another doctor, self-administered questionnaire. The method of data collection is essential to obtain completely objective information. Development of a validated questionnaire, based on a standardized definition, would facilitate comparison of the various results reported in the literature.[23,24]

- *The follow up* also frequently differs from one series to another. Although about one half of patients are 'dry' between 1 and 3 months, and most are dry at 1 year, some patients can still recover for up to 2 years. A follow up of at least 12 months is therefore essential.[21,22,25,26]

Furthermore, the main predisposing factor for postoperative incontinence appears to be age greater than 70 years.[13,15,22,28,29] The respective roles of preoperative continence, stage of the disease, and development of anastomotic stenosis are also discussed.[13,14,21,22,30]

Finally, some authors consider that certain technical modifications appear to facilitate preservation of continence: quality of apical dissection,[14] neurovascular bundle preservation,[31] preservation of the bladder neck, and preservation of puboprostatic ligaments.

In any case, the experience of the surgeon is an essential factor to improve the recovery of continence.

Impotence (Table 8.4)

As for continence, objective evaluation of sexual potency encounters a number of difficulties: absence of a consensual definition of sexual potency, various methods of evaluation and variable follow up.

Table 8.4 Potency

Study	No. of patients	Mean age	Follow-up months	Evaluation	Impotence (%)	Definition
Leandri et al[29]	620	68	12	Physician	29	Intercourse
Igel et al[19]	692			Physician	97.5	Erection
Turk et al[8] * bilateral unilateral	44 5 39	60	?	Physician	41 nc nc	Intercourse with sildenafil
Rassweiler et al[10] * unilateral	100 10	68	?	Physician	 6/10	Intercourse Intercourse with sildenafil or PGE1
Geary et al[21] bilateral unilateral	459 69 203	64,1	18	Questionnaire	44.4 68.1 86.7	Intercourse
Catalona et al[13] bilateral unilateral	858 798 60	63	18	Questionnaire	33.5 32 53	Intercourse
Fowler et al[34]	739	?	24	Patient quest. + questionnaire	79	Erection
Walsh et al[14]	64	57	18	Patient quest.	14	Intercourse; one-third with sildenafil
Stanford et al[28] bilateral unilateral	1291	62,9	18	Patient quest. + questionnaire	59 44 46.6	Intercourse
No preservation					34.4	
Talcott et al[33] bilateral	94 19	61,5	12	Patient quest.	 4/19	Incomplete erection
Bollens et al[11] * bilateral	50 6	63	6	Patient quest.	 1/6	Intercourse with sildenafil or PGE1
Abbou[9]*	25	64.8	12	Patient quest.	11/25	Erection (intercourse ?)

* Laparoscopic approach. nc, no cases; Patient quest., patient questionnaire.

- *The definition of sexual potency* varies according to the criteria adopted: erection with or without sexual intercourse, erection allowing sexual intercourse.
- *The methods of evaluation* of sexual potency are also very heterogeneous, as shown in Table 8.4: clinical interview by the surgeon, clinical interview by another doctor, self-administered questionnaire. The possible use of a treatment for erectile dysfunction, not systematically reported, also makes it difficult to compare various series.
- *Follow up* also constitutes an important parameter in this evaluation. While a large number of series have demonstrated the possibility of late recovery, most studies are limited to a relatively short follow up. The assessment of recovery of sexual function requires a follow up of at least 18 months.[14,32]

Other elements must also be taken into account, such as quality of erections before surgery, patient's age, and type of surgery (preservation of one or two neurovascular bundles). Moreover, the surgeon's experience is essential for preserving the neurovascular bundles.

Finally, the selection of patients eligible for preservation of neurovascular bundles is an important factor, rarely mentioned in the literature.[13]

Anastomotic stenosis
Stenosis of the vesicourethral anastomosis occurs in 0.5–4% of cases.[13]

Oncologic results

The aim of the laparoscopic procedure, which is to increase the quality of the dissection and to reduce morbidity, is only acceptable if oncologic efficacy is demonstrated.

For patients with organ-confined disease, at 3 years, Catalona et al[13] had a recurrence-free survival of 93%. Similar results are observed by the Johns Hopkins group where their 5-year recurrence-free rate was 97% for organ-confined cancer. In series using a retropubic approach, the rate of positive margins ranges between 15 and 40% depending on the experience of the team and the preservation or not of the neurovascular bundles.

In their experience of laparoscopy, after 3 years, Guillonneau et al[38] observed that 92% of the pT2a and pT2b patients had a PSA < 0.1 ng/ml. Among the patients with a PSA < 10 ng/ml and a Gleason score less than 7, 95.5% had a PSA < 0.2 ng/ml. The overall rate of positive margin was 17%. No port seeding was observed.

Remote-controlled assisted radical prostatectomy

Laparoscopy is probably a transitional technique between open surgery and remote-controlled surgery. As it is no longer necessary to open the abdomen to operate and almost all of the necessary instruments can be introduced via trocars, it is only logical to develop remote-controlled surgery because the laparoscopy position is not very ergonomic. The surgeon stands to the side of the patient and has to operate by crossing his hands over the midline, especially for sutures. This position can cause scapular pain. The vesicourethral suture at the bottom of the lesser pelvis is also a difficult procedure, requiring an experienced operator to ensure a good quality anastomosis.

Many articles have been written on experimental remote-controlled surgery in animals, but very few have yet been published in man. A first series of 10 cases of remote-controlled assisted radical prostatectomy has been published.[39] The operating time was 9 hours. It should be noted that this team started to perform remote-controlled assisted radical prostatectomy without any previous experience of laparoscopic surgery.

Claude Abbou and colleagues[40] published one case and, more recently, Guglielmo et al[41] and Pasticier et al[42] also published their cases. In the United States, Mani Menon's team[43] in Detroit, after 1 year of training in pelvic laparoscopy, has acquired a certain experience with remote-controlled laparoscopic surgery (70 cases).

The Institut Montsouris experience, based on 30 cases, together with the cases operated on in Detroit, illustrates the following advantages of remote-controlled surgery:

- Good ergonomy for the surgeon, whose forearms are supported to allow precise manipulation of the joysticks.
- A possible reduction of the amplitude of displacement of the remote-controlled robotic arms and especially 6 degrees of freedom, allowing rotation of the remote-controlled needle holders in all directions, makes suturing much easier.
- The 3-dimensional vision provided by a dual scope is extremely precise, but is not specific to remote-controlled surgery.

The disadvantages of remote-controlled surgery, at the present time, are the absence of practical bipolar coagulation to ensure reliable hemostasis and a slight increase in intraoperative bleeding compared to laparoscopy. As good quality bipolar coagulation is essential to ensure an optimal laparoscopic procedure, engineers are currently working to rapidly develop this instrument.

The future of surgery is clearly remote-controlled surgery, as it is less tiring for the surgeon and ensures more precise sutures.

Teaching could be ensured by virtual reconstitution of prostatectomies from operative videos. The trainee surgeon would be able to practice on the operating console in the same position as when performing remote-controlled laparoscopic surgery.

Finally, a senior surgeon would be able to control two or three operating rooms, each equipped with a remote-controlled system and console operated by a junior surgeon. The senior surgeon would be in a separate room, supervising the external and endoscopic screens of each room under his direction. His console could be connected in a fraction of a second to the other operating consoles in the event of difficulties. Such 'industrialization of surgery' will probably considerably change our everyday practice. Performing surgery at distant sites would appear to be more difficult: a surgeon would still need to be present on site to insert the trocars and to treat any complications. The transmitted image could be used to help another surgeon seeking advice, but there is no future for remote-controlled surgery of the entire procedure.

In conclusion, remote-controlled surgery does not currently provide any significant benefit for the patient. Bleeding is higher than with laparoscopic surgery, but the development of a hemostasis system, such as good quality bipolar forceps, should reduce bleeding. Suture is easier, but a surgeon experienced in laparoscopy can achieve similar results. For the operator, the operation is less tiring and the various procedures are facilitated. Virtual teaching systems must be developed to allow trainee operators to learn the basic techniques of remote-controlled surgery.

References

1. Schuessler WW, Schulam PG, Clayman RV, Kavoussi LR. Laparoscopic radical prostatectomy: initial short-term experience. Urology 1997; 50(6):854–857.
2. Raboy A, Ferzli G, Albert P. Initial experience with extraperitoneal endoscopic radical retropubic prostatectomy. Urology 1997; 50(6):849–853.
3. Guillonneau B, Cathelineau X, Barret E, et al. Laparoscopic radical prostatectomy: technical and early oncological assessment of 40 operations. Eur Urol 1999; 36:14–20.
4. Guillonneau B, Vallancien G. Laparoscopic radical prostatectomy: the Montsouris experience. J Urol 2000; 163:418.
5. Abbou CC, Salomon L, Hoznek A, et al. Laparoscopic radical prostatectomy: preliminary results. Urology 2000; 55(5):630–634
6. Guillonneau B, Vallancien G. Laparoscopic radical prostatectomy: the Montsouris technique. J Urol 2000; 163:1643–1649.
7. Rassweiler J, Sentker L, Seemann O, et al. Heilbronn laparoscopic radical prostatectomy. Technique and results after 100 cases. Eur Urol 2001; 40:54–64.
8. Turk I, Deger S, Winkelmann B, et al. Laparoscopic radical prostatectomy. Technical aspects and experience with 125 cases. Eur Urol 2001; 40(1):46–52; discussion 53.
9. Hoznek A, Salomon L, Olsson LE, et al. Laparoscopic radical prostatectomy. The Creteil experience. Eur Urol 2001; 40(1):38–45.
10. Rassweiler J, Sentker L, Seemann O, et al. Laparoscopic radical prostatectomy with the Heilbronn technique: an analysis of the first 180 cases. J Urol 2001; 166(6):2101–2108.
11. Bollens R, Vanden Bossche M, Roumeguere T, et al. Extraperitoneal laparoscopic radical prostatectomy. Results after 50 cases. Eur Urol 2001; 40(1):65–69.
12. Koch MO, Smith JA Jr. Clinical outcomes associated with the implementation of a cost-efficient programme for radical retropubic prostatectomy. Br J Urol 1995; 76(1):28–33.
13. Catalona WJ, Carvalhal GF, Mager DE, Smith DS. Potency, continence and complication rates in 1,870 consecutive radical retropubic prostatectomies. J Urol 1999; 162(2):433–438.
14. Walsh PC, Marschke P, Ricker D, Burnett AL. Patient-reported urinary continence and sexual function after anatomic radical prostatectomy. Urology 2000; 55:58–61.
15. Zincke H, Bergstralh EJ, Blute ML, et al. Radical prostatectomy for clinically localized prostate cancer: long-term results of 1,143 patients from a single institution. J Clin Oncol 1994; 12(11):2254–2263.
16. Guillonneau B, Rozet F, Cathelineau X, et al. Perioperative complications of laparoscopic radical prostatectomy: the Montsouris 3-year experience. J Urol 2002; 167(1):51–56.
17. Dillioglugil O, Leibman BD, Leibman NS, et al. Risk factors for complications and morbidity after radical retropubic prostatectomy [Review]. J Urol 1997; 157(5):1760–1767.
18. Guillonneau B, Rozet F, Barret E, et al. Laparoscopic radical prostatectomy: assessment after 240 procedures. Urol Clin North Am 2001; 28(1):189–202.
19. Igel TC, Barrett DM, Segura JW, et al. Perioperative and postoperative complications from bilateral pelvic lymphadenectomy and radical retropubic prostatectomy. J Urol 1987; 137(6):1189–1191.
20. Lerner SE, Blute ML, Lieber MM, Zincke H. Morbidity of contemporary radical retropubic prostatectomy for localized prostate cancer. Oncology (Huntingt) 1995; 9(5):379–382; discussion 382, 385–386, 389.
21. Geary ES, Dendinger TE, Freiha FS, Stamey TA. Incontinence and vesical neck strictures following radical retropubic prostatectomy [Review]. Urology 1995; 45(6):1000–1006.
22. Eastham JA, Kattan MW, Rogers E, et al. Risk factors for urinary incontinence after radical prostatectomy [Review]. J Urol 1996; 156(5):1707–1713.
23. McCammon KA, Kolm P, Main B, Schellhammer PF. Comparative quality-of-life analysis after radical prostatectomy or external beam radiation for localized prostate cancer. Urology 1999; 54(3):509–516.
24. Wei JT, Montie JE. Comparison of patients' and physicians' rating of urinary incontinence following radical prostatectomy. Semin Urol Oncol 2000; 18(1):76–80.
25. Donnellan SM, Duncan HJ, MacGregor RJ, Russell JM. Prospective assessment of incontinence after radical retropubic prostatectomy: objective and subjective analysis. Urology 1997; 49(2):225–230.
26. Jonler M, Madsen FA, Rhodes PR, et al. A prospective study of quantification of urinary incontinence and quality of life in patients undergoing radical retropubic prostatectomy. Urology 1996; 48(3):433–440.
27. Fontaine E, Izadifar V, Barthelemy Y, et al. Urinary continence following radical prostatectomy assessed by a self-administered questionnaire. Eur Urol 2000; 37(2):223–227.
28. Stanford JL, Feng Z, Hamilton AS, et al. Urinary and sexual function after radical prostatectomy for clinically localized prostate cancer: the Prostate Cancer Outcomes Study. JAMA 2000; 283(3):354–360.
29. Leandri P, Rossignol G, Gautier JR, Ramon J. Radical retropubic prostatectomy: morbidity and quality of life. Experience with 620 consecutive cases. J Urol 1992; 147(3 Pt 2):883–887.

30. Bates TS, Wright MP, Gillatt DA. Prevalence and impact of incontinence and impotence following total prostatectomy assessed anonymously by the ICS-male questionnaire. Eur Urol 1998; 33(2):165–169.

31. Steiner MS. Continence-preserving anatomic radical retropubic prostatectomy. Urology 2000; 55: 427–435.

32. Kim ED, Nath R, Slawin KM, et al. Bilateral nerve grafting during radical retropubic prostatectomy: extended follow-up. Urology 2001; 58(6):983–987.

33. Talcott JA, Rieker P, Propert KJ, et al. Patient-reported impotence and incontinence after nerve-sparing radical prostatectomy. J Natl Cancer Inst 1997; 89(15):1117–1123.

34. Fowler FJ Jr, Barry MJ, Lu-Yao G, et al. Patient-reported complications and follow-up treatment after radical prostatectomy. The National Medicare Experience: 1988–1990 (updated June 1993). Urology 1993; 42(6):622–629.

35. Heinzer H, Graefen M, Noldus J, et al. Early complication of anatomical radical retropubic prostatectomy: lessons from a single-center experience. Urol Int 1997; 59(1):30–33.

36. Hoznek A, Salomon L, Olsson LE, et al. Laparoscopic radical prostatectomy. The Creteil experience. Eur Urol 2001; 40(1):38–45.

37. Lepor H, Nieder A, Ferrandino M. Intraoperative and postoperative complications of radical retropubic prostatectomy in a consecutive series of 1000 cases. J Urol 2001; 166:1729–1733.

38. Guillonneau B, Gerard C, El Fettouh H, et al. Mid-term oncological follow-up of laparoscopic radical prostatectomy: mono-institutional experience based on 800 consecutive patients. 97th Annual Meeting, AUA, Orlando, May 2002.

39. Binder J, Kramer W. Robotically assisted laparoscopic radical prostatectomy. BJU Int 2001; 87:408–410.

40. Abbou CC, Hoznek A, Salomon L, et al. Laparoscopic radical prostatectomy with a remote controlled robot. J Urol 2001; 165:1964–1966.

41. Guglielmo B, Nakada SY, Rassweiler JJ. Future developments and perspectives in laparoscopy. Eur Urol 2001; 40:84–91.

42. Pasticier G, Rietbergen JBW, Guillonneau B, et al. Robotically assisted laparoscopic radical prostatectomy: feasibility study in men. Eur Urol 2001; 40:70–74.

43. Menon M, Tewari A, Baize B, Guillonneau B, Vallancien G. Prospective comparison of radical retropubic prostatectomy and robot-assisted anatomic prostatectomy: the Vattikuti Urology Institute experience. Urology 2002; 60:864–868.

9

Robotic surgery and nanotechnology

Jyoti Shah and Ara Darzi

Introduction

Big incisions are the anathema of surgery. Minimally invasive surgery or laparoscopy has changed this drastically by making these incisions smaller and cosmetically acceptable. Although the introduction of laparoscopy in urology has been slow compared to general surgery, it is now the operation of choice for many procedures. Now, just as we are getting used to smaller incisions, even these are coming under scrutiny. Technological advances have put this very mark of surgery under attack. The incision is shrinking, perhaps even disappearing altogether.

This chapter describes the advances in robotic surgery and their impact in urology, and speculates on the role of nanotechnology in the future of urology.

Robotic surgery

The principle of robots was described even before the term was coined. Aristotle developed the concept of automation and had unwittingly described the industrial revolution centuries before it had happened.[1] In 1921 Karl Capek's play, *Rossum's Universal Robots* opened in which he first coined the term 'robot' and it is perhaps from this plot that the misconception of robots as evil beings has stemmed. The subsequent rise of the robot industry was predicted by Isaac Asimov, a scientist and writer, who in 1941 proposed three laws of robotics.[2,3] Since this time, robots have been used widely in industrial manufacturing, space exploration and sea operations. They are now making their way into surgery.

Open surgery requires precise movements that are made by the surgeon. Laparoscopic surgery requires even smaller and more precise movements, although the difficulty is that they are made within a confined space. This tends to make laparoscopic procedures time consuming and the surgeon easily tires.[4] The use of long laparoscopic instruments amplifies the surgeon's normal tremor and the trocar through which the instruments are passed provides a fulcrum effect. There is a mapping error as the hand of the surgeon and the tip of the instrument move in opposite directions and the use of flat screen monitors leads to reduced depth perception. Perhaps the greatest problem, however, is the reduction in the range of motion to only 4 degrees of freedom (DOF).[5]

The term 'degree of freedom' refers to the number of possible movements that can be made at a joint and is used to describe the robot's dexterity. Complete freedom of movement requires 6 DOF. Hence in open surgery there is complete freedom of movement, but in laparoscopic surgery there are only 4 DOF. Thus laparoscopic instruments limit the surgeon's abilities and great skill and training is required. One study has shown that when comparing surgical performance using systems with 4 and 6 DOF, the time required to complete the task and the error rate were significantly less when surgeons used a system with 6 DOF.[6] It is problems such as these that have led to the development of robots in surgery.

What are robots?

Robots are mechanical systems that are controlled by a computer system with sensors and motors. They produce fast, precise movements that are repeatable without fatigue. They can also work in environments that may be uncomfortable for humans.

Humans can control the computer in two ways; off-line robots perform preprogrammed tasks with only human supervision. Clearly this is inappropriate for surgery.[7] In contrast, on-line robot control makes use of human judgment to dictate movements. In surgery there is synergy between the forces that the surgeon experiences upon tissue contact and the visual feedback obtained. This haptic feedback is obtained in real time and is the basis of many new systems that have been designed.[8]

A master–slave system such as the *da Vinci* system is an example of an on-line robotic control. The surgeon sits at a console that is at a remote site (Figs 9.1 and 9.2). The operating field is displayed up to 10 times the actual size with a choice between a 2-dimensional or 3-dimensional display. In the latter the surgeon restores binocular cues to the visual system. The surgeon's hands are placed in a device called a data glove. This is the master. Any movements the surgeon makes in the

data glove are translated by the computer to movements at the robot arms within the patient in real time (Fig. 9.3). This is the slave.[9] The system can scale down the surgeon's movements by 100-fold and reduce any tremor. The greatest advantage is they restore complete freedom of movement with 6 DOF at the slave.

In spite of these advantages, there are shortcomings with currently available systems. For example many of the instruments are suboptimal and limited in their variability (Fig. 9.4). Many countries have only recently established training mechanisms for laparoscopic surgery; considerable experience and training is required for robotic surgery. This is different from that required for laparoscopic surgery. We have yet to establish which of the operations in the urological armamentarium will actually benefit from robotic surgery. Another major hurdle is the cost of the system and the

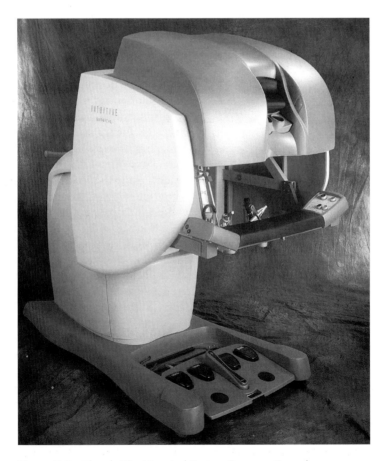

Figure 9.1 The *da Vinci* Surgical System Surgeon Console.

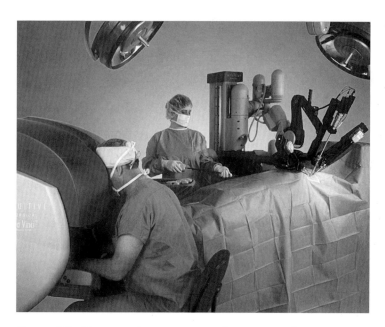

Figure 9.2 The operating room set-up for a master–slave system.

instruments.[10] Perhaps the greatest hurdle is acceptance by the urological community and the public in general, many of whom are still skeptical about laparoscopy!

Current robotic systems

Neurosurgery and orthopedics pioneered the use of robots in surgery. Neurosurgery requires great precision. There are fixed anatomical landmarks for robotic registration and positional accuracy can be achieved to ~2 mm.[11] Presently there are neuronavigators, stereotactic localizers and robotic assistants.

In the field of orthopedics, surgeons are using the RoboDoc system (Integrated Surgical Systems, Inc., Sacramento, CA, USA) to prepare the femoral canal for prosthetic implants. The system produces fewer gaps and cavities can be obtained with 10 times greater accuracy than by manual reaming.[12] One study found radiographic evidence in 900 patients of better position of the implant and elimination of the intraoperative femoral fracture rate.[13]

Obstetrics and gynecology are using the Zeus robotic system, another master–slave system (Computer Motion Inc., Goleta, CA, USA) to perform tubal ligation reversal. The pregnancy rate

at 12 months is 50% compared to 80% after standard laparoscopic tubal reversal.[14]

Many cardiac centers in Europe have successfully performed coronary artery bypass procedures on a beating heart using the *da Vinci* system. This has enabled intracardiac procedures to be carried out with incisions that are less than 1 cm in size, thereby reducing the morbidity associated with cardiac surgery.[15] The same system has also been used to perform mitral valve repairs and replacements, with results comparable to those of existing minimally invasive mitral valve procedures.[16,17]

The scaling down of movements with robotic systems is ideal for surgical specialties such as gynecology, cardiac surgery and microsurgery where small but precise movements are essential. The robotic-assisted microsurgery system (RAMS) is a device that consists of a laptop computer, a joystick, a mouse and a slave robot arm with 6 DOF. The system has been used for procedures of the eye, face and hand with results suggesting that when RAMS is used, the procedures are faster and more precise than when the surgeon operates alone.[18]

General surgical procedures such as Heller's myotomy, rectopexy, sigmoid colectomy and many others have been performed at our institution with postoperative results comparable to open surgery,

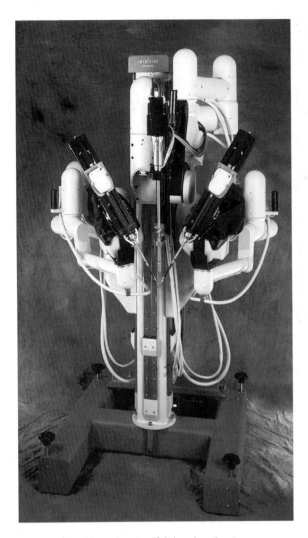

Figure 9.3 The robot itself ('the slave').

albeit with less morbidity and earlier return to normal levels of activity.

Robots in urology

Eliminating human assistance

An important aspect of operating laparoscopically is the assistance that is received. This involves retracting of instruments and positioning the endoscope. Hence control of the surgeon's operating field is in the hands of another individual. Human assistance is costly, an unskilled assistant can in fact impair the procedure leading to increased stress levels in the operating theater, and the assistant can easily tire. As a result, systems

have been developed that hold and position a laparoscopic instrument, thereby eliminating the problems of the human assistant. The AESOP (Automated Endoscope System for Optimal Positioning, Computer Motion) was the first robot to receive Food and Drug Administration approval in the USA and attaches to the operating table while holding the laparoscope. It has hand or foot control and a recent upgrade allows it to be driven by voice control.[19] Kavoussi et al[20] have used it extensively for robot-assisted laparoscopic procedures such as nephrectomy, pyeloplasty, ureterolysis and retroperitoneal lymph node dissection with more accurate and effective positioning when compared to humans. Hence the use of a robotic assistant may be more effective and economical than human assistants for laparoscopic surgery.

Benign prostatic hyperplasia

Although medical therapy for benign prostatic hyperplasia is now increasingly used as first line treatment, transurethral resection of the prostate (TURP) is still a commonly used procedure. In 1989 a robot was developed at Imperial College, London (PROBOT) using a six-axis Puma robot, a Wickham Endoscope Liquidizer and Aspirator and a potato to model the prostate and saline irrigation.[21] Trials carried out in patients showed the model to produce results that are comparable to the standard TURP, although the technology is inaccurate in determining prostate dimensions using transrectal ultrasound (TRUS).[22] These problems are currently being addressed.

Prostate biopsy

Another system that is still at the research stage is a prostate biopsy model that draws parallels with the robotic system for biopsy of mammary lesions. Developed in Italy, this model obtains biopsies from the prostate with an accuracy of 1–2 mm in animal models once the surgeon has selected biopsy sites. Initial studies have shown the device to be more reliable as it maintains position without any drift and the procedure is quicker when using the robot.[23]

Percutaneous renal access

The Imperial College group has also investigated the use of a robotic system for percutaneous renal access. This is a challenging procedure requiring

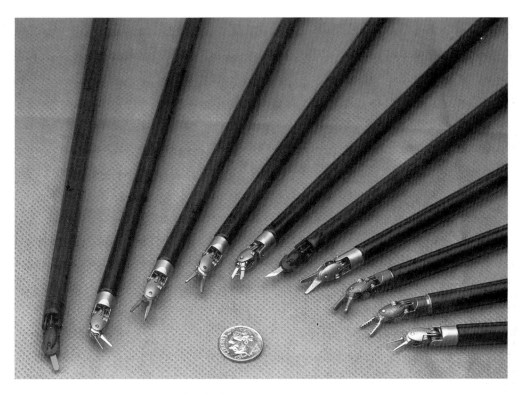

Figure 9.4 The instruments used with the *da Vinci* system.

precision in needle location in a 3-dimensional calyx with images that are 2-dimensional. The system that was developed was a passive robot with 5 DOF and an access needle on a C-arm with positional sensors. Initial experiments have shown that the system can target a calyx within 1.5 mm.[24] More recently, a group at John Hopkins University has developed an active robot to obtain percutaneous renal access. The Percutaneous Access of the Kidney (PAKY) positions and advances the needle using a radiolucent needle driver with an active translational mechanism. Experiments in porcine kidneys have shown that the robot locates the desired calyx 83% of the time with an in vitro positioning accuracy of 0.43 nm.[25,26]

da Vinci and Zeus master–slave systems
The *da Vinci* and Zeus master–slave systems have effectively given the surgeon an extra hand with which to operate. The surgeon can now control the laparoscope eliminating the inherent problems of the human assistant and also have two free hands. The first case of laparoscopic radical prostatectomy was reported in 1992, and since that time

the procedure has gained popularity[27] (See Chapter 8). Nowadays, the *da Vinci* system is being used at select centers around the world to perform this operation. After initial feasibility studies, the procedure was combined with the Walsh retrograde and Campbell antegrade procedures.[28] Early studies indicate that the mean hospital stay after a robotic radical prostatectomy is 36 hours, with 63% of these patients discharged home within 23 hours. The mean duration of postoperative catheterization in this group is 11 days. Additionally the postoperative complications and margin rates are comparable to patients who undergo conventional radical retropubic prostatectomy.[29] The Zeus system has also been used to perform robot-assisted laparoscopic pyeloplasty in pig models. Initial studies demonstrated feasibility and five out of six robotic anastomoses were watertight compared to three of four conventional laparoscopic pyeloplasties.[30]

At our institution, the *da Vinci* system has been used successfully for robot-assisted laparoscopic adrenalectomy demonstrating a more widespread indication for use of the robot system in urology.

Telepresence

All these procedures carried out with master–slave systems involve the surgeon sitting at a console several feet away from the actual operating theater. Why then can the surgeon not be further away, perhaps even in another country? This is telepresence and is the next step for robots in urology. Telepresence uses a computer interface to transmit the surgeon's actions from a primary workstation to a remote operative site with real-time visualization. In 1998 the first remote open urological procedure was carried out, although retraction, suctioning and suture cutting was carried out by an assistant at the site of the actual operation.[31] Using a similar technique a clinical laparoscopic adrenalectomy in Innsbruck, Austria was telementored successfully from Baltimore, USA.[32] For this system of operating to work clinically, signal transmission needs to be instantaneous. It has been shown that delays of greater than 0.3 seconds can significantly limit the ability to perform telesurgery.[33] Audio communication is also of great importance as it gives the surgeon data that are not visually available at a remote site. Today, advances in telecommunications allow excellent motion images using only 3 ISDN telephone lines.

Technology is moving fast. Robotic devices can now help the urologist perform safer, quicker and more accurate procedures. These advantages are combined with an economic incentive. Moreover, remote surgeons who may be the best in the world for that procedure can operate on patients from another country – this could become routine surgical practice very soon. The potential for telepresence also extends to a very real application for mentoring and surgical education.

Nanotechnology

Urology has moved from large incisions to small incisions in a very short space of time. Clearly the next step is no incisions. Robots are already being miniaturized with applications such as navigating through the gastrointestinal tract. An 18 mm robot that can propel itself through the colon has been developed.[34] At the Massachusetts Institute of Technology (MIT), a one-inch machine with the sensory functions of touch and light, the motor function of bilateral grippers, a computer with 256 bytes of RAM and 2000 bytes of memory and

three self-contained batteries has been developed.[35] It is therefore only a matter of time before one is available for urological procedures. Taking this miniaturization a step further will involve machines no bigger than the size of a red blood cell. This is the world of nanotechnology.

Yet again, Isaac Asimov's name appears. In 1966 he wrote a science fiction classic called *Fantastic Voyage* about a technology called miniaturization. By shrinking the atoms of objects, he eloquently described the voyage of a five-man medical crew who use a submarine to destroy a life-threatening blood clot in the brain of a man with intellectual capital. The technology was unbelievable at the time, but Asimov had again underestimated his prescience. We are far closer to this technology than many realize.

Nanotechnology is the science of creating machines that manipulate matter in the same way that it is created – one atom at a time.[36] The word originates from 'nanometer' – one billionth of a meter.[37] This technology requires a new way of thinking, often called nanothink, which was first suggested by Nobel Prize winner Richard Feynman, a physicist. In 1959 he said: 'The principles of physics, as far as I can see, do not speak against the possibility of maneuvering things atom by atom'.[38] This has since become a classical milestone.

In medicine, nanotechnology will mimic the life process. It is really already in existence. Consider the nanoscale molecular machinery that is within the living cell, converting fuel, making energy, proteins and enzymes as directed by the cell's DNA. At our institution, atomic force microscopy is being used on red blood cells to measure and manipulate on a nanoscale (Fig. 9.5a–c). The goal of nanomedicine will be to create nanorobots (or nonobots) that can carry out vital engineering works or medical preprogrammed tasks at the molecular level without the need for any incisions. They will effectively be the workhorses of nanotechnology.[39]

The anatomy of a nanobot

The typical nanobot will probably be a robot that is 0.5–3 microns in diameter. The upper limit of 3 microns is due to the maximum size for capillary passage. The bulk of the nanobot will comprise of carbon in the form of diamond due to its strength and inertness. This form of carbon is 1000 times

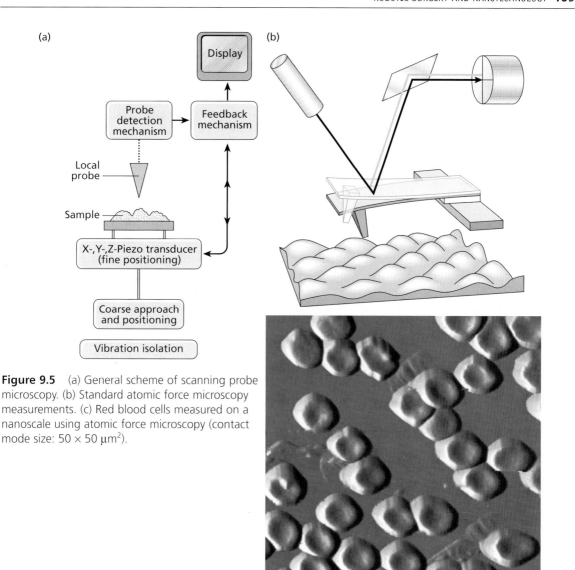

(a)

(b)

Figure 9.5 (a) General scheme of scanning probe microscopy. (b) Standard atomic force microscopy measurements. (c) Red blood cells measured on a nanoscale using atomic force microscopy (contact mode size: $50 \times 50 \ \mu m^2$).

as strong as steel but 50 000 times as thin as human hair.[39] Initial studies have shown that the smoother and more flawless the diamond surface, the less immune activity stimulation there is. This equates with less leukocyte activity, less fibrinogen adsorption, a strong hydrophobicity and minimal opsonization.[40] The interior will need to be a highly controlled environment so that external fluids cannot intrude, and therefore it is likely to be both airtight and watertight.

The nanobot could be introduced into the body via the femoral artery and be propelled around the body by a number of means:

- An electric motor that would fit within a cube that is 1/64 of an inch in diameter
- Vibrating cilia
- Body temperature ceramic superconductors
- The nanobot could crawl along the surface of the circulatory system by the use of appendages, which would grip the walls without causing any damage to them.[41]

Drexler originally proposed that nanobots could be powered by metabolizing glucose and oxygen, similar to human cells.[42] Another power source suggested by Freitas is acoustic power.[40] In vivo nanobots could be sent new commands while at work by supervising physicians, which would be picked up by acoustic sensors on the nanobot. The messages could then be computed and implemented appropriately. IBM has described the ability to impregnate various proteins onto a silicon finger. This is effectively an antigen receptor relationship and when the two bind, the silicon finger bends releasing energy. This energy can then be used as an alternative power source for the nanobot, or to open the gate for delivery of a drug.[43]

Some nanobots can be excreted from the body in the usual manner, whilst others could be designed such that they need to be removed by medical personnel in an apheresis-like process. They will not need to replicate within the human body.

What could a nanobot do?

The nanobot could be effective in removing unwanted tissues such as arteriosclerotic plaques by means of physical separation from the wall by the nanobot. They could deliver potent chemotherapeutic agents to the actual cancer site, thereby eliminating the majority of side effects. Nanobots could be preprogrammed to seek out and destroy viruses or bacteria. The enhanced precision would allow them to avoid damage to other healthy tissues.[44] In this manner when a nanobot detects a molecule that does not fit the profile of a healthy cell, the nanobot would grasp the 'abnormal' molecule. Depending upon the program of the nanobot, it could either repair this molecule or destroy it.[45] Such nanobots could also monitor the levels of different compounds and store information in an internal memory, with specific data about time and location. They could be filtered out of the body and analyzed.

A specific example of a spherical nanobot is the respirocyte.[46] This measures 1 micron in diameter and floats in the bloodstream. It is made of 18 billion atoms that are mostly carbon. It works as a tiny pressure tank that has up to 9 billion oxygen and carbon dioxide molecules. These are released in a controlled manner by a rotor system.[47] When the nanobot is in the lung where the partial pressure of oxygen is high and that of carbon dioxide is low, the computer in the nanobot tells the delivery system to load up with oxygen and dump the carbon dioxide. This process is then reversed in tissues where there is low oxygen. In essence the respirocyte mimics the actions of a red blood cell, but is able to deliver 236 times more oxygen per unit volume than a human red blood cell.[48] The physician, using an ultrasound-like transmitter, can modify and control behavior of the respirocyte once within the body. Respirocytes could be controlled to stop working and lie dormant, for example, and once the therapeutic purpose has been achieved they could be extracted from the circulation.

Another example of a nanobot in action is in providing oxygen to tissues already suffering from ischemic injury, such that they can no longer properly metabolize oxygen. In this situation, the direct release of ATP with selective absorption of critical metabolites would function as artificial mitochondria. They could be released into the circulation and work autonomously for hours. This discovery with ATPase motors was cited as one of the most promising new technologies of 1999.[49]

Recently there have been several breakthroughs for nanotechnology. A company in Dublin (Nanomat) has established a method of binding nanocrystals of various drugs with a substance that can seek out tissue in specific organs of the human body. This system will avoid the side effects associated with current drug delivery systems. Zyvex (a company in Texas) is building the first assembler that is able to pick up individual atoms and move them around. Meanwhile in The Netherlands, a scientist has created the first single molecule transistor.[50]

Conclusion

Clearly this technology has unlimited potential in every sphere of medicine. How long will it be before these systems are actually being used? Computing technology is growing exponentially, and the foundations and principles of nanotechnology have already been laid. So significant is the support for nanomedicine that President Clinton said on January 21, 2000:

> My 2001 budget supports a major new National Nanotechnology Initiative, worth $500 million ... the ability to manipulate matter at the atomic and molecular level. Imagine the

possibilities: ... detecting cancerous tumors when they are only a few cells in size. Some of our research goals may take 20 or more years to achieve, but that is precisely why there is an important role for the federal government.[51]

Surgical tools started off as crude and large; so were the incisions. Recently the way we treat has moved to a smaller incision and smaller instruments. At the cellular level, however, even a fine scalpel causes injury that is only permissible as cells have the ability to regenerate. The nanotechnology agenda shows a way into the future that will allow us to build nanobots, computer-controlled machines even smaller than the size of the cell, enabling intervention at the molecular level, without any incision. This sophisticated technology will not be like Karl Capek's robot, but instead controlled at every stage of their 'fantastic voyage'. Today we have the artificial heart, but within the next 20–30 years nanotechnologists predict that we will have the artificial mitochondrion.

References

1. Malone R. The robot book. New York: Push Pin Press, 1978.
2. Clarke R. Asimov's laws for robotics: implications for information technology. Computer (Parts 1 and 2) 1993; Dec:53–61; 1994; Jan:57–65.
3. Shah J, Mackay S, Rockall T, et al. 'Urobotics': robots in urology. BJUI 2001; 88:313–320.
4. Rosser JC, Rosser LE, Salvagi RS. Skill acquisition and assessment for laparoscopic surgery. Arch Surg 1997; 132:200–204.
5. Schurr MO, Breitwieser H, Meizer A, et al. Experimental telemanipulation in endoscopic surgery. Surg Laparosc Endosc 1996; 6:167–175.
6. Falk V, McLoughlin J, Guthart G, et al. Dexterity enhancement in endoscopic surgery by a computer-controlled mechanical wrist. Min Inv Therapy Allied Tech 1999; 8:235–241.
7. Caddedu JA, Stoianovici D, Kavoussi LR. The use of robotics in urological surgery. Urol Int 1997; 4:11–14.
8. Hurmuzlu Y, Ephanov A, Stoianovici D. Effect of a pneumatically driven haptic interface on the perceptional capabilities of human operators. Presence 1998; 7(3):290–307.
9. Furukawa T, Wakabayash G, Ozawa S, et al. Surgery using master–slave manipulators and telementoring. Nippon Geka Gakkai Zasshi 2000; 101(3):293–298.
10. Buckingham RA, Buckingham RO. Robots in operating theatres. BMJ 1995; 311:1479–1482.
11. Tseng CS, Chung CW, Chen HH, et al. Development of a robotic navigation system for neurosurgery. Stud Health Technol Inform 1999; 68(4):358–359.
12. Paul HA, Bargar WL, Mittlestadt B, et al. Development of a surgical robot for cementless total hip arthoplasty. Clin Orthop 1992; 285:57–66.
13. Bargar WL, Bauer A, Börner M. Primary and revision total hip replacement using the RoboDoc system. Clin Orthop 1998; 354:82–91.
14. Yoon TK, Sung HR, Kang HG, et al. Laparoscopic tubal anastomosis: fertility outcome in 202 cases. Fertil Steril 1999; 72(6):1121–1126.
15. Loulmet D, Carpentier A, d'Attellis N, et al. Endoscopic coronary artery bypass grafting with the aid of robotic assisted instruments. J Thorac Cardiovasc Surg 1999; 118:4–10.
16. Falk V, Autschbach R, Walther T, et al. Computer enhanced mitral valve surgery – towards a total endoscopic procedure. Semin Thorac Surg 1999; 11:244–249.
17. Mishra YK, Malhotra R, Mehta Y, et al. Minimally invasive mitral valve surgery through an anterolateral minithoracotomy. Ann Thorac Surg 1999; 68(4):1520–1524.
18. Siemionow M, Ozer K, Siemionow W, et al. Robotic assistance in microsurgery. J Reconstr Microsurg 2000; 16(8):643–649.
19. Sackier JM, Wang Y. Robotically assisted laparoscopic surgery: from concept to development. Surg Endosc 1994; 8:63–66.
20. Kavoussi LR, Moore RG, Partin AW, et al. Telerobotic assisted laparoscopic surgery: initial laboratory and clinical experience. Urology 1994; 44(1):15–21.
21. Nathan MS, Davies BL, Hibberd B, et al. Devices for automated resection of the prostate. Proceedings of the First International Symposium on Medical Robotics and Computer Assisted Surgery, Pittsburgh, Pennsylvania. 1994:342–344.
22. Davies BL, Hibberd RD, Ng WS, et al. The development of a surgeon robot for prostatectomies. Proc Inst Mech Eng [H] 1991; 205:35–38.
23. Rovetta A, Sala R, Wen Z, et al. Sensorization of a surgeon robot for prostate biopsy operation. Proceedings of the First International Symposium on Medical Robotics and Computer Assisted Surgery, Pittsburgh, Pennsylvania. 1994:345.
24. Potamianos P, Davies BL, Hibberd B. Intra-operative registration for percutaneous surgery. Proceedings of the Second International Symposium on Medical Robotics and Computer Assisted Surgery, Baltimore. 1995:156.
25. Bzostek A, Schreiner S, Barnes A, et al. An automated system for precise percutaneous access of the renal collecting system. Proceedings of the First Joint Conference Computer Vision, Virtual Reality and Robotics in Medicine and Medical Robotics and Computer-Assisted Surgery, Grenoble, France. 1997:779.
26. Caddedu JA, Bzostek A, Screiner S, et al. A robotic system for percutaneous renal access. J Urol 1997; 158(4):1589–1593.
27. Schuessler WW, Kavoussi LR, Clayman RV, et al. Laparoscopic radical prostatectomy: initial case report. J Urol 1992; 147:246A.
28. Abbou CC, Saloman L, Hoznek A, et al. Laparoscopic radical prostatectomy: preliminary results. Urology 2000; 55(5):630–634.
29. Menon M, Tewari A, Baize B, et al. Prospective comparsion of radical retropubic prostatectomy and

robot-assisted anatomic prostatectomy: the Vattikuti Urology Institute experience. Urology 2002; 60(5):864–868.

30. Sung TS, Gill IS, Hsu TH. Robotic-assisted laparoscopic pyeloplasty: a pilot study. Urology 1999; 53:1099–1103.

31. Bowersox JC, Cornum RL. Remote operative urology using a surgical telemanipulator system: preliminary observations. Urology 1998; 52:17.

32. Janetschek G, Bartsch G, Kavoussi LR. Transcontinental interactive laparoscopic telesurgery between the United States and Europe. J Urol 1998; 160:1413.

33. Funda J, Lindsay TS, Paul RP. Teleprogramming: toward delay-invariant remote manipulation. Presence 1992; 1:29–44.

34. Carrozza MC, Lencioni L, Magnani B, et al. The development of a microrobotic system for colonoscopy. Proceedings of the First Joint Conference Computer Vision, Virtual Reality and Robotics in Medicine and Medical Robotics and Computer-Assisted Surgery, Grenoble, France. 1997:779.

35. Lehr H, Ehrfeld W, Hagemann B, et al. Development of micro- and millimotors. MITAT 1997; 6:191.

36. Freitas RA Jr. Nanomedicine. www.foresight.org/ Nanomedicine

37. Crandall BC, ed. Molecular engineering. In: Nanotechnology: molecular speculations on global abundance. Cambridge, MA: MIT Press; 1996:2–6.

38. Feynman RP. There's plenty of room at the bottom. Engineering & Science 1960; 23:22. Reprinted in Gilbert HD, ed. Miniaturization. New York: Reinhold, 1961.

39. Lemonick MD. Will tiny robots build diamonds one atom at a time? Time 2000; June 19:94–98.

40. Freitas RA Jr. Nanomedicine FAQ. www.foresight.org/ Nanomedicine/NanoMedFAQ.html

41. Rubenstien L. A practical nanorobot for treatment of various medical problems. Eighth Foresight Conference on Molecular Nanotechnology, July 2001.

42. Drexler KE. Engines of creation: the coming era of nanotechnology. New York: Archer Press/Doubleday; 1986:Ch. 7.

43. Gunther B. Basics of nanotechnology. MITAT 1995; 4:331.

44. Ralph C Merkle. Nanotechnology and medicine. www.zyvex.com/nanotech/nanotech/AndMedicine.html

45. Drexler KE, Peterson C, Pergamit G. Unbounding the future: the nanotechnology revolution. New York: Simon & Schuster; 1992:Ch. 10.

46. Freitas RA Jr. Respirocytes: high performance artificial nanotechnology red blood cells. Nanotechnology Magazine 1996; 2:8–13.

47. Drexler KE. Nanosystems: molecular machinery, manufacturing and computation. New York: Wiley; 1992.

48. Freitas RA Jr. Exploratory design in medical nanotechnology: a mechanical artificial red cell. Artificial Cells 1998; 26:411–430.

49. Fantastic voyage: tiny pharmacies propelled through the body could result from Cornell breakthrough in molecular motors. News Release, 1999.

50. Voss D. Nanomedicine nears the clinic. Jan/Feb 2000. http://www.technologyreview.com/articles

51. The National Nanotechnology Initiative. Washington DC: Office of the President. January 2000.

10

Marginally worse? Positive resection limits after radical prostatectomy

Simon RJ Bott

Positive resection limits after radical prostatectomy

Over the last two decades we have seen a progressive downstaging of prostate cancer at diagnosis. As public awareness has increased and with advent of prostate specific antigen (PSA) in the late 1980s, a growing number of men are presenting with potentially curable localized disease. Coupled to this are the improvements in operative techniques, which have resulted in acceptable continence and potency rates and more latterly, with the introduction of laparoscopic prostatectomy, a shorter hospital stay.

Yet, even with the most sophisticated preoperative staging techniques, an average of 28% of those undergoing radical prostatectomy are found to have positive surgical margins, although later series have a lower margin positive rate.[1] Furthermore, once positive margins have been established, the optimum treatment remains controversial.

Defining positive surgical margins

Before a radical prostatectomy specimen is step sectioned, each half of the whole gland is painted with two different colored inks. This enables orientation of the section taken for histological examination and assessment of the margin status. The prostate is then sectioned, stained and mounted. A positive surgical margin is defined as the presence of tumor at the inked surface of the resected specimen[2–5] and implies incomplete excision of malignant tissue.

Several sites are designated with margin status, including the apex – the urethral limit, the base (which includes the bladder neck margin), vasal and circumferential – anterior, lateral, rectal or posterior surface.

Stamey subdivided positive surgical margins into two groups.[4] In the first group the cancer is cut through when it is outside the prostate boundaries into the fat, having penetrated the capsule – a positive extraprostatic limit (Fig. 10.1a). In the second group the cancer is cut through inside the glandular area of the prostate due to inadvertent surgical excision of the periprostatic fascia and prostate capsule, which are missing from histological specimen – a positive intraprostatic limit (Fig. 10.1b). The first group may be further subdivided into focal (where limited tumor reaches the inked limit in one or two sites) or extensive (where multiple positive margins were present at different sites in the prostate).[6,7] Epstein et al[7] demonstrated significantly different progression rates between those with negative (Fig. 10.1c) compared with equivocal (intraprostatic positive margin), focal and extensive extraprostatic surgical margins. However, the subclassification of positive margins has not been standardized.[8]

Positive margins and PSA relapse

The identification of a positive extraprostatic margin suggests inadequate cancer clearance and most investigators consider the presence of positive surgical margins an independent predictor of disease recurrence after radical prostatectomy. Patients are at significant risk of biochemical relapse (50–60% at 5 years) and subsequent clinical relapse, although by no means every patient will suffer eventual disease recurrence.[2,7,9–11] Epstein et al,[9] from Johns Hopkins Hospital, reported 79% of men with negative margins were progression free over a 10-year period compared with 55% of those with positive margins (p < 0.00001). The Johns Hopkins group subsequently demonstrated the effect of Gleason grade on outcome in men with positive margins. They reported that positive surgical margins had no impact on 10-year probability of biochemical recurrence in men with Gleason score less than 7. However, men who had

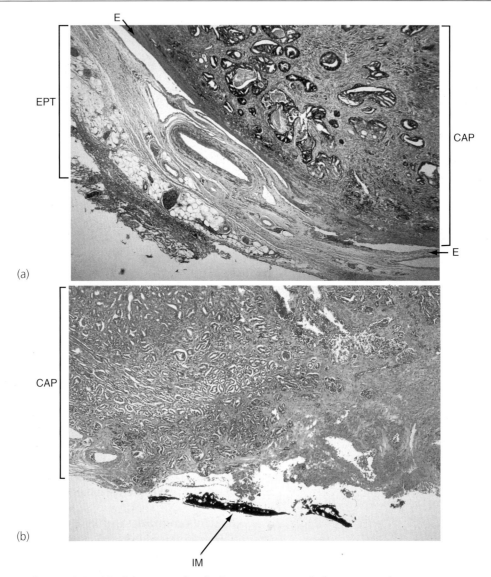

Figure 10.1　(a) High power of radical prostatectomy wholemount section demonstrating organ confined prostate cancer. (b) High power of radical prostatectomy wholemount section demonstrating an intraprostatic positive surgical margin.

a Gleason score of 7 and positive surgical margins did significantly worse than those with extra-capsular extension and negative margins.[12]

Grossfeld and colleagues[13] calculated that, after adjusting for PSA, pathologic tumor stage and Gleason grade, patients with positive margins were 2.6 times more likely to have disease recurrence than those with negative margins. Furthermore patients with positive margins were significantly more likely to receive adjuvant or non-adjuvant secondary treatment (p = 0.0001). Stamey et al[14] contested these findings however, stating that

margin status is not an independent predictor of failure after radical prostatectomy when adjusting for the percentage of Gleason 4 and 5 cancers, tumor volume and lymph node status.

Cheng and co-workers examined the correlation between margin status and PSA relapse in a series of 377 patients from the Mayo Clinic.[11] Their overall margin positivity rate was 29%; 19% of patients had positive margins without extracapsu-lar disease (intraprostatic), 14% had extracapsular extension with negative margins and 10% had both extracapsular extension and positive margins. Men

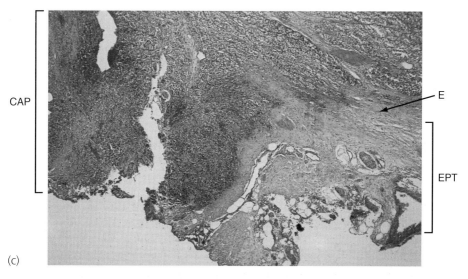

(c)

Figure 10.1 (c) High power of radical prostatectomy wholemount section demonstrating extraprostatic carcinoma with a positive surgical margin. CAP, prostate cancer; E, edge of prostate; EPT, extraprostatic tissue; IM, inked margin.

with organ-confined disease and negative margins had a 90% 5-year progression-free survival. In the cohort with positive margins the 5-year progression-free survival was 78% for those without extracapsular extension and 55% for those with extracapsular extension.

Other authors have shown that intraprostatic positive margins have little or no effect on outcome, at least in the medium term.[2,6] Ohori et al[2] reported 100% of men with intraprostatic positive margins were free from tumor recurrence after 5 years compared with 42% with positive margins and extracapsular extension. Barocas et al[15] compared 91 cases who had isolated intraprostatic margins with three groups matched for age, Gleason grade, preoperative PSA and clinical stage, at Johns Hopkins. Their follow up was on average only 31 months, but they were able to show a 4.3% recurrence rate for men with organ-confined prostate cancer, 9.8% for specimen-confined, margin negative cases, 10.9% for men with a positive intraprostatic surgical margin, but otherwise organ-confined disease, and a 25% relapse rate for men with extracapsular disease and positive surgical margins. They concluded, from this small series, that inadvertent capsular incision, resulting in a positive intraprostatic limit, gave similar PSA outcomes to specimen-confined disease.

Factors predisposing to cancer relapse

Features such as the location, extent and number of positive margins may have an impact on disease recurrence.[16,17] Blute et al[16] reported that the site of positive margins was a significant predictor of progression. Patients with pT2N0 disease who had a single margin at either the apex/urethra (the most common) or anterior/posterior prostate or multiple positive margins in these sites had only slightly decreased PSA free rates compared with patients with negative margins at 5 years (79%, 78%, 82% compared with 86% with negative margins). However, patients in whom the prostate base limit was positive had significantly lower clinical or PSA failure-free rates – 56% at 5 years. The risk of PSA progression was 1.68 times higher in men with positive margins after matching for Gleason score, preoperative PSA and DNA ploidy in this series.

From Miami, Öbek and colleagues reported similar findings from their series of 495 men with clinical T1–T3 disease who underwent radical prostatectomy.[17] After a mean follow up of 25.3 months their recurrence rate was significantly higher in men with positive compared with negative surgical margins, 27.8% versus 6.9% respectively, despite a quarter of margin positive cases receiving adjuvant androgen deprivation. The recurrence rate for various margin positive sites was 29% at the apex, 30% posterior, 33% anterior, 36% lateral; 48% posterolateral and 57% bladder neck. These were not isolated margins and patients with other adverse pathologic features, for example seminal vesicle and lymph node involvement were not excluded. However, they concluded that time to recurrence was shorter in patients older than 70, with a Gleason score of 7 or more, seminal vesicle invasion, multiple positive margins and a positive margin at the bladder neck or on the posterolateral surface of the prostate. Of men with multiple positive margins, 43% developed disease recurrence, compared with 24% of men with a single positive margin.

Several authors have cited a bladder neck positive margin as having a particularly poor progression-free outcome. They are usually associated with other adverse pathologic features:

- they occur as solitary positive margins in only 0–5% of specimens
- they are more frequently associated with Gleason score 7 or greater disease or preoperative PSA values exceeding 20 ng/ml, large volume tumors and seminal vesicle invasion.

Positive vas deferens margins are also associated with a poor prognosis. In a series of 105 men undergoing radical prostatectomy, seven (6.7%) cases had vasal involvement; in these patients there was a significant correlation with seminal vesicle involvement, extracapsular extension, extensive carcinoma, Gleason score 7–10 and positive bladder neck margins. All five men with follow up developed disease recurrence.[71]

Several groups have highlighted the prognostic difference between a focal compared with an extensive positive margin.[1,9] They reported that focal margins were associated with recurrence in 40% and extensive margins had a 65% risk of progression after 5-years' follow up. Therefore the site, number and extent of positive surgical margins all provide valuable prognostic information.

Positive margins without cancer relapse

Several explanations are given for why a positive margin is not always associated with tumor recurrence. The surgery results in ischemia and fibrosis, both of which may destroy small areas of residual carcinoma as the malignant tissue is unable to survive in its new environment. Alternatively, it may be a result of the desmoplastic response. This is where the extraprostatic prostate cancer cells are more adherent to the prostate than the surrounding adipose tissue. When the prostate is lifted away from the surrounding tissue the malignant cells adhere to the specimen. Finally the process required to prepare the specimen for histological examination may result in inadvertent damage leading to the false impression of positive surgical margins.

The histological method used to assess radical prostatectomy specimens varies and this may account, in part, for the variation in reported margin status. Coronal sections are taken serially at 2–6 mm. Hall et al[18] demonstrated that sections taken at 4–6 mm intervals missed 12% of positive margins compared with 2–3 mm sections.

The apex may be examined by two different techniques. The distal 1.5 cm of the prostate is amputated and tissue is sectioned in a sagittal plane, with the urethra at the centre – the cone technique (Fig. 10.2). Alternatively a 'thin shave' transverse section is taken of the apex around the urethra. This tissue block is sectioned from its inferior aspect and examined (Fig. 10.3). The cone technique allows examination of the prostate at its most distal limit, although only 5 μm for every 3–5 mm section of the distal margin are examined histologically. The shave technique on the other hand is simpler and less time consuming to perform and the entire surface area of the distal margin is examined. However, with the latter technique there is at least a theoretical risk of overdiagnosing positive apical margins as the inked surface is firstly 'roughed down' and so the section taken for microscopic examination is several microns within the prostate.

The definition of a positive apical margin is variable. Epstein and co-workers,[7] using the shave technique, classified an apical margin as positive if it:

1. showed skeletal muscle without benign prostate glands and contained tumor
2. contained benign glands and any amount of tumor of high grade, or
3. benign glands and extensive tumor of any grade.

Where there are benign glands and a small focus of low-grade tumor the margin is classified as equivocal and margins are designated negative where no tumor is seen. Stamey et al[4] describe apical margins in the same way as margins elsewhere in

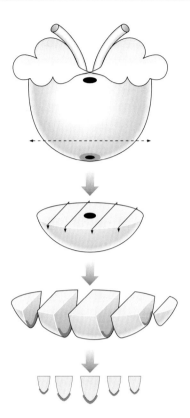

Figure 10.2 The cone technique for assessing margin status at the apex of the prostate.

the prostate: margin negative, margin positive with (CP+) or without (CP–) capsular penetration. Van den Ouden et al[10] defined an apical limit as positive if tumor is in the distal 5 mm of the prostate. Comparative data are not yet established on PSA relapse in patients with isolated positive apical margins when these differing definitions and techniques are employed.

Avoiding positive margins

Undoubtedly the best way to minimize the risk of positive surgical margins is by careful and appropriate patient selection aided by meticulous surgical technique.

Case selection

Case selection involves correctly identifying those patients most likely to benefit from the treatment. This is of paramount importance in men considered for radical prostatectomy, particularly in

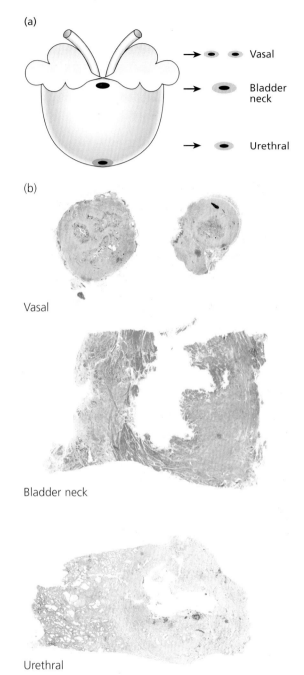

Figure 10.3 (a) The shave technique for assessing margin status at the vasal, bladder neck and apical surgical limits. (b) Low power of the vasal, bladder neck and apical shave limits.

terms of reducing the incidence of positive surgical margins. Although there is no absolute means of identifying those individuals with pre-existing microscopic invasion of extraprostatic tissue, methods are now available to establish those at highest risk. The most useful of these are the three components incorporated in the tables devised, and subsequently updated, by Partin et al,[19,20] namely the clinical stage, the PSA and the Gleason score from the preoperative prostate biopsy. High clinical stage, high preoperative PSA, high Gleason grade as well as large tumor volume and multiple positive biopsies all increase the risk of positive surgical margins.[3,21,22]

While clinical staging using digital rectal examination (DRE) is inaccurate at assessing pathologic stage it is a useful predictor of positive margins. In a recent review positive surgical margin rates were: 5% for T1a, 22% for T1b, 23% for T1c, 17% for T2a, 36% for T2b, 27% for T2c and 40% for T3a clinical stage.[1]

Depending on the tumor site, clinical stage indirectly reflects tumor volume. Gomez et al[23] showed patients with negative margins had a mean tumor volume of 4.8 ml compared with 12.3 ml in those with positive margins. As tumor size is difficult to assess preoperatively, attempts have been made to compare tumor volume with the preoperative prostate biopsy findings. Ackerman and colleagues demonstrated the presence of two or more positive biopsy cores as the most significant risk factor for positive margin status.[3] Hammerer et al[24] showed that men in whom margins were positive had a mean 3.79 positive cores compared with 1.89 in those with negative margins.

PSA is also a useful predictor of the risk of positive margins. As the PSA rises the risk increases; the mean PSA for a patient with positive margins is 16.8–29.0 ng/ml, whereas for men with negative margins it is 9.27–16.6 ng/ml.[3,10]

Watson et al[5] compared Gleason sum at biopsy with margin status; they found that of men who had a Gleason score of 7 or greater, 43% had positive margins compared with 30% of men with a Gleason score of less than 7. Although a higher Gleason score increases the risk of positive margins, Ohori et al[25] emphasized the need to combine the Gleason score with the PSA and DRE. This combination identified 60% of poorly differentiated tumors of which 81% were organ confined.

Newer techniques are evolving in an attempt to augment or improve on the 'classical three' preoperative predictors (biopsy Gleason grade, clinical stage and preoperative PSA score). DNA ploidy has been reported as an independent predictor of outcome after radical prostatectomy,[11] although it has not been adequately assessed for use in predicting margin status.

Race is an independent predictor of positive surgical margins and disease-free survival in patients with positive surgical margins.[26] In patients matched for pathologic stage, Gleason grade and tumor volume, African–American men were found to have a higher incidence of positive margins compared with white Americans (48% vs 33% respectively, p = 0.001). Furthermore, African–American men had a higher incidence of positive margins at the bladder base; however in this study, the location of the positive margin did not have an effect on the disease-free survival.[26]

Preoperative imaging

The ability of imaging modalities to correctly stage prostate cancer remains limited, even in the best hands using state-of-the-art equipment. Extracapsular extension is often microscopic and current techniques are not of sufficient resolution to detect small breaches in the capsule. The apex of the prostate is the most frequent site for a positive margin but as the capsule is ill defined in this region,[27] it is difficult to distinguish extracapsular from organ-confined tumor. Clearly intraprostatic positive margins are not visualized preoperatively.

Where macroscopic tumor extension is present, endorectal magnetic resonance imaging (eMRI) is the most sensitive and specific technique available; nevertheless there is still a high rate of false positives as well as considerable interobserver variability. Cornud et al[28] reported eMRI to have a sensitivity of 33% and a specificity of 100% at detecting extracapsular disease, excluding intraprostatic margins. They concluded that eMRI is only accurate in a minority of highly selected high risk hypervascular tumors. D'Amico et al[21] suggested eMRI should be used in cases where there is intermediate risk of extraprostatic disease. They defined intermediate as those who have a PSA of less than 4 ng/ml and a Gleason biopsy score of 7, a PSA 4–10 ng/ml and Gleason score 5–7 or a PSA 10–20 ng/ml and a Gleason sum of 2–7. Using this algorithm eMRI correctly detected all prostate cancers with extra-prostatic extension. More recently D'Amico et al[29] assessed the role of eMRI in predicting biochem-ical outcome after radical prostatectomy. While eMRI failed to add any useful clinical information in 81% of over a thousand cases, it was clinically and statistically relevant in the 5-year PSA outcomes in the remaining 191 patients in the intermediate risk group.

Other modalities including transrectal ultra-sound (TRUS), pelvic CT, and body coil MRI are not sufficiently accurate to detect extracapsular extension. TRUS is no better than DRE in predicting extracapsular extension in prospective multicenter studies.[30] CT has a reported sensitivity of between 55 and 75% and body coil MRI between 20 and 70% at detecting extracapsular disease.[31] Positron emission tomography (PET), a non-invasive imaging modality, has been investigated for its use in staging prostate cancer. It relies on the increased uptake in tumors of a radiolabelled choline analog. This technique is still under evaluation; however it is likely only to be of benefit in the staging of prostate cancer that has meta-stasized as the false positive rate for extracapsular disease is unacceptably high.[32] In practice radio-logic evidence of extracapsular disease is usually sought only in those men with a high risk – those with a PSA > 20 ng/ml or with a Gleason score of 8 or more.

Surgical technique

There are three approaches to radical prostatec-tomy: retropubic, perineal and laparoscopic. The incidence of positive surgical margins is very similar for each technique but the location of the margins is dependent upon the approach. The apex is the most common site for positive margins in the retropubic and laparoscopic approaches, whilst the anterior prostate is the most common site for the perineal approach.[1,5,15,16,33] Table 10.1 shows the incidence and site of positive margins.

The majority of radical prostatectomy proce-dures are performed via the retropubic approach in the 'anatomic' manner originally described and subsequently adapted by Walsh. Others have made further modifications such as preserving the bladder neck; proponents argue this maneuver results in an earlier restoration of continence and a lower risk of bladder neck stricture. Unfortunately the scope for making the operation more 'radical' is not very great, as important structures (e.g. the distal sphincter) limit the dissection. However, there are a number of ways in which the chance of positive surgical margins can be minimized without compromising the important aim of maintaining urinary continence.

The apex of the prostate

As stated, the most common location of a positive surgical margin is at the apex of the prostate.[5,16] This is because there is only scant periprostatic tissue at this point and the fibromuscular 'capsule' found elsewhere is absent at the apex. What is more, as prostate cancer has a tendency to invade perineural spaces the short inferior neurovascular pedicle at the apex renders extraprostatic extension more common.[4] Particular care is required not to excise excess 'normal' tissue in this region because of the proximity of the sphincter mechanism and

Table 10.1 Location of non-iatrogenic solitary positive surgical margins after radical prostatectomy

Author	Stage	No. of margins	% site of solitary positive surgical margin						
			Apical	Anterior	Posterior	Lateral	Posterolateral	Bladder neck	Other
Radical retropubic prostatectomy									
Epstein et al[34]	T1c	29	31 shave	24	10	7	24	–	3
Watson et al[5]	T1c	17	59 shave	6	18	–	18	–	
Van Poppel et al[35]	T3	19	37 cone	–	–	–	53	–	10
Kirby (unpublished data)	T1c–T3	131	79 shave				16	2	2
Radical perineal prostatectomy									
Weldon et al[36] cone	T1–2	88	7	25	–	–	16	7	45
Laparoscopic radical prostatectomy									
Abbou et al[37]	T2–3	4	50	–	–	–	–	50	–

the neurovascular bundles. Potency or continence may occasionally have to be sacrificed in order to obtain the primary objective of cancer cure.

In order to limit positive apical margins while preserving the neurovascular bundle and sphincter mechanism, it is firstly important to mobilize a sufficient length of membranous urethra to enable visualization of the most distal anterior part of the prostate. This is best achieved by ensuring adequate division of the puboprostatic ligaments and the fibromuscular bands anterior to the urethra and tethered to the apex of the prostate.[38]

Usually the urethra enters the prostate slightly anterior and proximal to the apex in the 'prostatic notch'. The more distal apex is hidden by the urethra in the retropubic approach. When the urethra is divided in this notch, proximal to the apex, there is a risk of incising into the concealed posterior prostate tissue when dividing the posterior urethra. To prevent this the urethra should be transected at a point distal to the anterior apical tissue. Once this has been accomplished the rectourethralis muscle needs to be divided completely without damaging the rectum. Failure to do this risks violation of the prostate capsule posteriorly. Once the rectourethralis has been divided, the prostate may be bluntly dissected away from the rectum, ensuring Denonvillier's fascia remains intact. If retrograde dissection proves difficult or the capsule is breached, an antegrade approach should be considered.

The neurovascular bundles

A decision has to be made, based upon the preoperative investigations and pre-existing erectile function, whether or not to spare either or both neurovascular bundles in an attempt to preserve potency. The neurovascular bundles lie outside the capsule and fascia of the prostate; cancer control is therefore not compromised by preserving the bundles, provided the tumor is organ confined. Pound et al[39] reported on the series of 1623 men who underwent radical prostatectomy at Johns Hopkins Hospital. They compared the actuarial recurrence-free probabilities according to tumor stage and margin status in men potent and impotent postoperatively. The groups were similar for age, Gleason grade and stage. With all stages there was no difference in actuarial recurrence-free probability between the potent and impotent men.

The commonest site of capsular penetration is in the region of the neurovascular bundles, posterolateral to the prostate. Moreover, Catalona and Bigg[40] reported that all men who had extracapsular extension in the region of the neurovascular bundles also had positive surgical margins. This has led some to excise the neurovascular bundle on the side of the prostate with the palpable nodule or positive biopsies. This may not suffice as 80% of men with a palpable nodule have bilateral tumor involvement. However, the contralateral tumor burden is usually, but not invariably, less, and in appropriately selected patients nerve sparing can be performed without compromising margin status.[10,25] A patient should generally fulfill certain criteria before a nerve-sparing technique is utilized:

1. The prostate biopsies should be positive on one side only and ideally only one or two out of six cores should contain tumor. Daniels et al[41] demonstrated that bilateral positive cores correlate with large tumors and an increased probability of capsular penetration and positive surgical margins.
2. The patient should have T1, T2a or T2b clinical stage. T1a and T1b are the most suitable for nerve-sparing surgery as they rarely invade the neurovascular bundles.[42] In T1c prostate cancer Wieder and Soloway[1] recommend excising the neurovascular bundle on the side of the positive biopsies. Daniels and colleagues reported that men with T2a and T2b prostate cancer, in whom the contralateral biopsies were cancer free, had low-volume, localized disease and had a low risk of positive surgical margins with contralateral nerve-sparing.[41]
3. The patient should have normal erectile function before surgery and should express a wish to stay potent postoperatively.

Other factors to take into consideration before embarking on nerve-sparing radical prostatectomy include the preoperative PSA, the Gleason score and the site of the tumor. The PSA and Gleason are independent predictors of margin status as outlined above. Tumors situated in the apex are more likely to spread into the perineural spaces as a result of the short length of the inferior pedicle.[4] Preserving the neurovascular bundles in men with apical tumors may increase the risk of positive margins. Consequently, Stamey et al[4] suggested wide excision of all tissues proximal to the membranous urethra to the levator muscles, including the neurovascular bundles and periprostatic fascia, in men with apical lesions.

Several studies have shown no statistically significant difference between nerve-sparing and non-nerve-sparing in terms of margins in appropriately selected patients. Overall, nerve-sparing procedures are associated with a 7–46% positive margin rate compared with 13–46% for the non-nerve sparing technique.[4,10,40] However, in men with induration in or around the lateral pedicle, wide excision of the neurovascular bundle on that side does seem to improve the chances of negative surgical margins and decrease the risk of disease recurrence; however using this criteria 30% of patients will have their neurovascular bundles excised unnecessarily as the cancer is organ confined.[43] There is no significant effect on potency in men under 50 years of age when one neurovascular bundle is excised; however with advancing age sexual function is better in men in whom both bundles are preserved. In general, decisions about whether or not to spare the neurovascular bundles on each side should be made on the basis of the criteria listed above, rather than on the basis of more subjective operative findings.

The bladder neck

To avoid positive surgical margins a third point of surgical technique is the method of dissection of the prostate away from the bladder neck. Bladder neck sparing was developed in an attempt to reduce the risk of anastomotic stricture and accelerate the return of urinary continence, while maintaining the surgical objective of cancer clearance.[44] Positive margins at the location of the bladder neck are reported in up to 25% of cases when all bladder neck dissection techniques are included. Bladder neck positive margins may be iatrogenic; where there is extracapsular disease and a positive surgical margin there are, almost invariably, positive margins elsewhere. In fact solitary positive bladder neck margins were found in only 1% of specimens in one study.[44] These authors concluded bladder neck preservation did not compromise surgical outcome and that more extensive resection at the bladder neck would not have been curative. This is consistent with other reports that

correlate genuine positive bladder neck margins with poorer prognosis disease as outlined earlier. As positive bladder neck margins when associated with extracapsular disease coexist with poor prognosis disease it is unlikely the bladder neck margin affects the overall outcome. What is more, several authors have demonstrated an earlier return to urinary continence and reduced incidence of bladder neck contracture.[44,45] Other authors have confirmed there is no negative impact on margin status following bladder neck preserving surgery but they have failed to show any significant improvement on return of urinary continence[45] or bladder neck contracture.[46]

Neoadjuvant androgen deprivation

Neoadjuvant androgen deprivation has been shown to reduce the incidence of positive surgical margins and extracapsular disease in a number of studies.[47–49] This may be because the whole prostate shrinks allowing wider resection margins, downstaging of the tumor itself or because of difficulties with accurate pathologic assessment after hormonal treatment.[1] Either way, there is no evidence from long-term prospective randomized trials that neoadjuvant androgen deprivation has any effect on biochemical relapse or survival.[49] Furthermore, difficulties may arise giving the prostate specimen a Gleason grade as androgen withdrawal affects the glandular architecture, so important prognostic information may be lost. Given the current data the routine use of neoadjuvant androgen deprivation before radical prostatectomy is unjustified.[49]

Adjuvant treatment options for patients with positive surgical margins

The aim of adjuvant therapy after radical prostatectomy in patients with positive surgical margins is to prevent or delay PSA and subsequent clinical relapse and to prolong survival. However, there is currently no consensus on what, if any, and when such treatment should be offered to these patients. Treatment options have included adjuvant external beam radiotherapy (EBRT), adjuvant androgen deprivation and surveillance with delayed EBRT or androgen ablation at the time of recurrence.[1] Adjuvant radiotherapy is used in an attempt to delay local recurrence or cure residual local disease;

adjuvant androgen ablation is primarily used to delay progression of systemic disease. As there is no standard regime, trials set up to elucidate the effects of adjuvant therapy are difficult to compare or to subject to meta-analysis. Furthermore, the effect of the lead-time bias complicates survival comparisons between those treated with adjuvant versus salvage EBRT. Despite these difficulties in interpreting the data, freedom from biochemical recurrence after adjuvant or salvage EBRT is quoted as 30–65%.[49]

Adjuvant radiotherapy

Potential indications for adjuvant radiotherapy include detectable postoperative PSA,[51] high Gleason score or extracapsular disease, seminal vesicle invasion,[39,51] lymph node involvement[22,39,51] and positive surgical margins.[6,39] Of these, positive surgical margins are usually associated with the smallest amount of residual disease and potentially the highest chance of success following adjuvant radiotherapy.[52]

There are no data yet available from randomized controlled trials to compare the efficacy of adjuvant EBRT for patients with positive surgical margins. Several non-randomized, retrospective studies have suggested improved local control and prolonged PSA progression-free periods, but no overall survival benefit.[52–54]

Leibovich et al[53] retrospectively matched two groups of patients with pT2 disease and a positive margin at a single site. They found 88% of men who had adjuvant radiotherapy after radical prostatectomy were free of biochemical and clinical relapse over 5 years compared with 59% of those who had surgery but no adjuvant therapy. Their conclusion was that adjuvant radiotherapy improved clinical disease-free survival. However, this and other trials failed to show enhanced metastasis-free rates or an overall survival benefit over the period of the study.[53,55,56]

Salvage radiotherapy

By definition, giving adjuvant treatment to all cases of positive surgical margins will result in some patients receiving radiotherapy, with its potential inherent complications, unnecessarily. Some investigators have therefore opted to delay treatment until there is evidence of disease recurrence, either by a detectable or rising PSA or a biopsy-proven local recurrence. This begs the question at what PSA threshold should salvage radiotherapy be given if equivalent results to adjuvant therapy are to be achieved?

The American Society for Therapeutic Radiology and Oncology Consensus Panel examined the use of salvage EBRT in patients with PSA relapse after radical prostatectomy. They recommended a dose of at least 64 Gy given when the PSA level is less than 1.5 ng/ml.[57] Nudell and colleagues reported a cohort of 105 men treated with either adjuvant or salvage EBRT.[58] They defined disease free as the achievement and maintenance of a PSA of < 0.2 ng/ml, giving a 5-year overall disease-free survival of 43%. Outcomes were equivalent for the adjuvant and salvage EBRT groups where therapeutic irradiation was administered when the serum PSA was low (< 1.0 ng/ml).

Patients who receive radiotherapy after surgery fare better if the PSA falls to an undetectable level than those with a persistently detectable PSA (66% at 40 months compared with 20% at 12 months, respectively).[51] What is more, men in whom the PSA rises more than 1 year after surgery and patients who have a low to moderate grade tumor have a better response to salvage EBRT.[51,59] Peschel et al,[54] reporting on a series of 52 men who had either adjuvant or salvage EBRT, found the preoperative PSA level and seminal vesicle involvement were significant risk factors for biochemical recurrence following postoperative radiotherapy. However, the risk of recurrence was most significant for a preradiotherapy PSA of 0.3 ng/ml, suggesting a PSA threshold of 0.3 ng/ml.

Not all patients with positive margins coupled with other adverse prognostic indicators after radical prostatectomy should be considered for radiotherapy. At 2 years after salvage radiation treatment Cadeddu et al[60] found no patients with Gleason score 9 or more, seminal vesicle invasion or lymph node metastases were PSA free. Data are not yet available; however these patients may gain some disease-free advantage by receiving either adjuvant hormonal monotherapy or adjuvant hormonal therapy with EBRT.

Early reports indicated a significant incidence of postradiotherapy complications: chronic radiation proctitis and/or cystitis in 27% of patients and 5% of men requiring a colostomy and 5% a urinary diversion.[56] However, with newer conformal and intensity modulated radiotherapy techniques the incidence of such complications is far lower.[57] Importantly there is no significant effect on urinary continence[61] or potency[62] following the administration of 45–54 Gy of adjuvant radiotherapy.

Adjuvant androgen deprivation

In another hormone sensitive cancer, breast cancer, adjuvant therapy has had a highly significant effect on both tumor recurrence and cancer-related mortality. This approach provides a rationale for the use of adjuvant androgen ablation therapy in patients following radical prostatectomy with positive surgical margins or in whom the serum PSA does not become undetectable. Various adjuvant hormonal treatment options are available, including luteinizing hormone releasing hormone (LHRH) analog monotherapy, maximum androgen blockade, androgen antagonists, 5-alpha reductase inhibitors and bilateral orchidectomy. To date no survival benefit has been shown from hormonal deprivation for men with positive margins without lymph node metastases.[42,63] Furthermore, initiating hormone therapy may result in short- and long-term side effects including gynecomastia, breast pain and osteoporosis.

Results from several trials have shown a significant improvement in disease-free survival using hormonal deprivation as adjunctive treatment after radical prostatectomy. In a prospective randomized study Prayer-Galetti et al[64] observed a 25% improvement in disease-free survival after radical prostatectomy in patients with 'C stage' prostate cancer who received the LHRH analog goserelin compared with the no adjuvant treatment control group. Messing et al[63] reported improved overall survival and reduced risk of recurrence in node-positive patients treated with goserelin/orchidectomy rather than observation after radical prostatectomy.

The bicalutamide early prostate cancer program is currently underway to assess the effect of bicalutamide either as immediate or as adjunctive hormonal therapy in men who have undergone radical prostatectomy or EBRT with curative intent. Following a median follow-up period of 2.6 years the risk of disease progression was 13.9% in the placebo arm and 7.3% in the treated group.[65] The results from the subgroup of patients with positive margins have not yet been published. Moreover the survival data will not be available for some time as the median actuarial time after surgery from PSA elevation to the development of metastases is 8 years and to death a further 5 years.[66]

Combined androgen deprivation and adjuvant radiotherapy

The European Organization of Research and Treatment of Cancer (EORTC) and Radiation Therapy Oncology Group (RTOG) randomized prospective trials both demonstrated improved overall survival, freedom from local recurrence and freedom from distant metastases for patients with high grade or clinically advanced disease treated with androgen deprivation and primary radiotherapy.[67,68] Yet data on the use of combination therapy in patients with suspected or proven residual disease after radical prostatectomy are scant.

Eulau et al[69] examined men who received androgen ablation 2 months before, and continuing for a mean of 6 months during and after 60–70 Gy of adjuvant radiotherapy compared to those receiving adjuvant EBRT alone. The mean follow-up time was 3.1 years for those who had androgen suppression and 4.6 years for those who received radiotherapy alone. Of the study group, 56% had no biochemical recurrence compared with 27% in the control group and 100% versus 70% had no evidence of clinical recurrence, respectively. Positive margins were not a significant risk factor for biochemical recurrence after adjuvant treatment in either group. The follow-up period in this study was short and the duration of androgen withdrawal not standardized.

Several authors have postulated that adjuvant radiotherapy alone may fail to provide a survival benefit because of undetectable micrometastases present at the time of radiotherapy.[56,70] Anti-androgens induce apoptosis in hormone sensitive prostate cancer cells irrespective of their location. It is not surprising therefore that the risk of biochemical relapse is reduced at least in the short term with androgen deprivation. Whether there is any survival advantage, as seen when androgen ablation is used with primary radiotherapy in poor prognosis disease, remains to be seen from ongoing randomized trials.

Conclusions

A positive surgical margin is associated with increased risk of disease progression and decreased disease-specific survival. Appropriate patient selection is essential to reduce the risk of positive surgical margins, utilizing the preoperative PSA, biopsy Gleason score and findings on DRE together with, in selected cases, endorectal MRI.

African–American men with clinically localized prostate cancer have a higher incidence of positive surgical margins and poorer disease-free survival than their white compatriots.

While intraprostatic positive margins may not lead to biochemical or clinical recurrence in the medium term, the patient may develop recurrence in the long term, as remaining benign tissue is capable of malignant transformation, and the patient has the anxiety associated with a detectable PSA after radical prostatectomy.

The use of neoadjuvant androgen deprivation does reduce the incidence of positive margins, but to date has not been shown to affect disease-free survival.

Surgical measures to reduce postoperative complications including nerve sparing and bladder neck preservation do not appear to increase the incidence of positive margins if employed in appropriate cases.

It is inevitable that, with the inadequacies of current staging techniques, positive surgical margins will occur, although as men are presenting sooner in their disease course the rate of positive margins is also falling.

It appears from retrospective data that adjuvant radiotherapy is of benefit, at least in terms of local disease control, to patients with positive margins in the absence of seminal vesicle or lymph node involvement. However, in men whose postoperative PSA becomes undetectable it is probably safe to watch and irradiate if the PSA starts to climb, provided the PSA is below 1.5 ng/ml. Large trials, currently underway in Europe and North America, are expected to shed more light on the role of androgen deprivation in patients with positive surgical margins. Chemotherapeutic agents are also undergoing trials and these may play a role in the future either as adjuvant therapy or at the time of progression in men with positive surgical margins.

References

1. Wieder JA, Soloway MS. Incidence, etiology, location, prevention and treatment of positive surgical margins after radical prostatectomy for prostate cancer. J Urol 1998; 160(2):299–315.
2. Ohori M, Wheeler TM, Kattan MW, et al. Prognostic significance of positive surgical margins in radical prostatectomy specimens. J Urol 1995; 154(5):1818–1824.
3. Ackerman DA, Barry JM, Wicklund RA, et al. Analysis of risk factors associated with prostate cancer extension to the surgical margin and pelvic node metastasis at radical prostatectomy. J Urol 1993; 150(6):1845–1850.
4. Stamey TA, Villers AA, McNeal JE, et al. Positive surgical margins at radical prostatectomy: importance of the apical dissection. J Urol 1990; 143(6):1166–1172.
5. Watson RB, Civantos F, Soloway MS. Positive surgical margins with radical prostatectomy: detailed pathological analysis and prognosis. Urology 1996; 48(1):80–90.
6. Blute ML, Bostwick DG, Seay TM, et al. Pathologic classification of prostate carcinoma: the impact of margin status. Cancer 1998; 82(5):902–908.
7. Epstein JI, Pizov G, Walsh PC. Correlation of pathologic findings with progression after radical retropubic prostatectomy. Cancer 1993; 71(11):3582–3593.
8. Sakr WA, Wheeler TM, Blute M, et al. Staging and reporting of prostate cancer – sampling of the radical prostatectomy specimen. Cancer 1996; 78(2):366–368.
9. Epstein JI, Partin AW, Sauvageot J, Walsh PC. Prediction of progression following radical prostatectomy. A multivariate analysis of 721 men with long-term follow-up. Am J Surg Pathol 1996; 20(3):286–292.
10. van den Ouden D, Bentvelsen FM, Boeve ER, Schroder FH. Positive margins after radical prostatectomy: correlation with local recurrence and distant progression. Br J Urol 1993; 72(4):489–494.
11. Cheng L, Darson MF, Bergstralh EJ, et al. Correlation of margin status and extraprostatic extension with progression of prostate carcinoma. Cancer 1999; 86(9):1775–1782.
12. Epstein JI, Pound CR, Partin AW, Walsh PC. Disease progression following radical prostatectomy in men with Gleason score 7 tumor. J Urol 1998; 160(1):97–100.
13. Grossfeld GD, Chang JJ, Broering JM, et al. Impact of positive surgical margins on prostate cancer recurrence and the use of secondary cancer treatment: data from the CaPSURE database. J Urol 2000; 163(4):1171–1177.
14. Stamey TA, McNeal JE, Yemoto CM, et al. Biological determinants of cancer progression in men with prostate cancer. JAMA 1999; 281(15):1395–1400.
15. Barocas DA, Han M, Epstein JI, et al. Does capsular incision at radical retropubic prostatectomy affect disease-free survival in otherwise organ-confined prostate cancer? Urology 2001; 58(5):746–751.
16. Blute ML, Bostwick DG, Bergstralh EJ, et al. Anatomic site-specific positive margins in organ-confined prostate cancer and its impact on outcome after radical prostatectomy. Urology 1997; 50(5):733–739.
17. Öbek C, Sadek S, Lai S, et al. Positive surgical margins with radical retropubic prostatectomy: anatomic site-specific pathologic analysis and impact on prognosis. Urology 1999; 54(4):682–688.

18. Hall GS, Kramer CE, Epstein JI. Evaluation of radical prostatectomy specimens. A comparative analysis of sampling methods. Am J Surg Pathol 1992; 16(4):315–324.

19. Partin AW, Kattan MW, Subong EN, et al. Combination of prostate-specific antigen, clinical stage, and Gleason score to predict pathological stage of localized prostate cancer. A multi-institutional update. JAMA 1997; 277(18):1445–1451.

20. Partin AW, Mangold LA, Lamm DM, et al. Contemporary update of prostate cancer staging nomograms (Partin Tables) for the new millennium. Urology 2001; 58(6):843–848.

21. D'Amico AV, Whittington R, Malkowicz SB, et al. Critical analysis of the ability of the endorectal coil magnetic resonance imaging scan to predict pathologic stage, margin status, and postoperative prostate-specific antigen failure in patients with clinically organ-confined prostate cancer. J Clin Oncol 1996; 14(6):1770–1777.

22. Zincke H, Oesterling JE, Blute ML, et al. Long-term (15 years) results after radical prostatectomy for clinically localized (stage T2c or lower) prostate cancer. J Urol 1994; 152(5 Pt 2):1850–1857.

23. Gomez CA, Soloway MS, Civantos F, Hachiya T. Bladder neck preservation and its impact on positive surgical margins during radical prostatectomy. Urology 1993; 42(6):689–693.

24. Hammerer P, Henke P, Meyer-Moldenhauer W, Huland H. Preoperative evaluation of tumour aggressiveness in patients with localised prostate carcinoma. J Urol 1995; 153(428(A)).

25. Ohori M, Goad JR, Wheeler TM, et al. Can radical prostatectomy alter the progression of poorly differentiated prostate cancer? J Urol 1994; 152(5 Pt 2):1843–1849.

26. Shekarriz B, Tiguert R, Upadhyay J, et al. Impact of location and multifocality of positive surgical margins on disease-free survival following radical prostatectomy: a comparison between African–American and white men. Urology 2000; 55(6):899–903.

27. Ayala AG, Ro JY, Babaian R,. The prostatic capsule: does it exist? Its importance in the staging and treatment of prostatic carcinoma. Am J Surg Pathol 1989; 13(1):21–27.

28. Cornud F, Hamida K, Flam T, et al. Endorectal color doppler sonography and endorectal MR imaging features of nonpalpable prostate cancer: correlation with radical prostatectomy findings. AJR Am J Roentgenol 2000; 175(4):1161–1168.

29. D'Amico AV, Whittington R, Malkowicz B, et al. Endorectal magnetic resonance imaging as a predictor of biochemical outcome after radical prostatectomy in men with clinically localized prostate cancer. J Urol 2000; 164(3 Pt 1):759–763.

30. Yu KK, Hricak H. Imaging prostate cancer. Radiol Clin North Am 2000; 38(1):59–85, viii.

31. Manyak MJ, Javitt MC. The role of computerized tomography, magnetic resonance imaging, bone scan, and monoclonal antibody nuclear scan for prognosis prediction in prostate cancer. Semin Urol Oncol 1998; 16(3):145–152.

32. DeGrado TR, Coleman RE, Wang S, et al. Synthesis and evaluation of 18F-labeled choline as an oncologic tracer for positron emission tomography: initial findings in prostate cancer. Cancer Res 2001; 61(1):110–117.

33. Guillonneau B, Vallancien G. Laparoscopic radical prostatectomy: the Montsouris technique. J Urol 2000; 163(6):1643–1649.

34. Epstein JI, Walsh PC, Brendler CB. Radical prostatectomy for impalpable prostate cancer: the Johns Hopkins experience with tumors found on transurethral resection (stages T1A and T1B) and on needle biopsy (stage T1C). J Urol 1994; 152(5 Pt 2):1721–1729.

35. Van Poppel H, De Ridder D, Elgamal AA, et al. Neoadjuvant hormonal therapy before radical prostatectomy decreases the number of positive surgical margins in stage T2 prostate cancer: interim results of a prospective randomized trial. The Belgian Uro-Oncological Study Group. J Urol 1995; 154(2 Pt 1):429–434.

36. Weldon VE, Tavel FR, Neuwirth H, Cohen R. Patterns of positive specimen margins and detectable prostate specific antigen after radical perineal prostatectomy. J Urol 1995; 153(5):1565–1569.

37. Abbou CC, Salomon L, Hoznek A, et al. Laparoscopic radical prostatectomy: preliminary results. Urology 2000; 55(5):630–634.

38. Walsh PC, ed. Radical retropubic prostatectomy. In: Cambell's urology, 6th edn. Philadelphia: WB Saunders; 1992:2865–2886.

39. Pound CR, Partin AW, Epstein JI, Walsh PC. Prostate-specific antigen after anatomic radical retropubic prostatectomy. Patterns of recurrence and cancer control. Urol Clin North Am 1997; 24(2):395–406.

40. Catalona WJ, Bigg SW. Nerve-sparing radical prostatectomy: evaluation of results after 250 patients. J Urol 1990; 143(3):538–543.

41. Daniels GF Jr, McNeal JE, Stamey TA. Predictive value of contralateral biopsies in unilaterally palpable prostate cancer. J Urol 1992; 147(3 Pt 2):870–874.

42. Zincke H, Utz DC, Taylor WF. Bilateral pelvic lymphadenectomy and radical prostatectomy for clinical stage C prostatic cancer: role of adjuvant treatment for residual cancer and in disease progression. J Urol 1986; 135(6):1199–1205.

43. Graefen M, Hammerer P, Michl U, et al. Incidence of positive surgical margins after biopsy-selected nerve-sparing radical prostatectomy. Urology 1998; 51(3):437–442.

44. Soloway MS, Neulander E. Bladder-neck preservation during radical retropubic prostatectomy. Semin Urol Oncol 2000; 18(1):51–56.

45. Licht MR, Klein EA, Tuason L, Levin H. Impact of bladder neck preservation during radical prostatectomy on continence and cancer control. Urology 1994; 44(6):883–887.

46. Poon M, Ruckle H, Bamshad BR, et al. Radical retropubic prostatectomy: bladder neck preservation versus reconstruction. J Urol 2000; 163(1):194–198.

47. Montironi R, Diamanti L, Santinelli A, et al. Effect of total androgen ablation on pathologic stage and resection limit status of prostate cancer. Initial results of the Italian PROSIT study. Pathol Res Pract 1999; 195(4):201–208.

48. Soloway MS, Sharifi R, Wajsman Z, et al. Randomized prospective study comparing radical prostatectomy alone versus radical prostatectomy preceded by androgen

blockade in clinical stage B2 (T2bNxM0) prostate cancer. The Lupron Depot Neoadjuvant Prostate Cancer Study Group. J Urol 1995; 154(2 Pt 1):424–428.

49. Lee HH, Warde P, Jewett MA. Neoadjuvant hormonal therapy in carcinoma of the prostate. BJU Int 1999; 83(4):438–448.

50. Meng M, Carroll P. Local therapy for prostate-specific antigen recurrence after definitive treatment. Prostate Cancer Prostatic Dis 2001; 4:1–8.

51. Coetzee LJ, Hars V, Paulson DF. Postoperative prostate-specific antigen as a prognostic indicator in patients with margin-positive prostate cancer, undergoing adjuvant radiotherapy after radical prostatectomy. Urology 1996; 47(2):232–235.

52. Anscher MS, Robertson CN, Prosnitz R. Adjuvant radiotherapy for pathologic stage T3/4 adenocarcinoma of the prostate: ten-year update. Int J Radiat Oncol Biol Phys 1995; 33(1):37–43.

53. Leibovich BC, Engen DE, Patterson DE, et al. Benefit of adjuvant radiation therapy for localized prostate cancer with a positive surgical margin. J Urol 2000; 163(4):1178–1182.

54. Peschel RE, Robnett TJ, Hesse D, et al. PSA based review of adjuvant and salvage radiation therapy vs. observation in postoperative prostate cancer patients. Int J Cancer 2000; 90(1):29–36.

55. Jacobson GM, Smith JA, Jr, Stewart JR. Postoperative radiation therapy for pathologic stage C prostate cancer. Int J Radiat Oncol Biol Phys 1987; 13(7):1021–1024.

56. Gibbons RP, Cole BS, Richardson RG, et al. Adjuvant radiotherapy following radical prostatectomy: results and complications. J Urol 1986; 135(1):65–68.

57. Cox JD, Gallagher MJ, Hammond EH, et al. Consensus statements on radiation therapy of prostate cancer: guidelines for prostate re-biopsy after radiation and for radiation therapy with rising prostate-specific antigen levels after radical prostatectomy. American Society for Therapeutic Radiology and Oncology Consensus Panel. J Clin Oncol 1999; 17(4):1155.

58. Nudell DM, Grossfeld GD, Weinberg VK, et al. Radiotherapy after radical prostatectomy: treatment outcomes and failure patterns. Urology 1999; 54(6):1049–1057.

59. Grossfeld GD, Tigrani VS, Nudell D, et al. Management of a positive surgical margin after radical prostatectomy: decision analysis. J Urol 2000; 164(1):93–99.

60. Cadeddu JA, Partin AW, DeWeese TL, Walsh PC. Long-term results of radiation therapy for prostate cancer recurrence following radical prostatectomy. J Urol 1998; 159(1):173–177.

61. Petrovich Z, Lieskovsky G, Langholz B, et al. Comparison of outcomes of radical prostatectomy with and without adjuvant pelvic irradiation in patients with pathologic stage C (T3N0) adenocarcinoma of the prostate. Am J Clin Oncol 1999; 22(4):323–331.

62. Formenti SC, Lieskovsky G, Skinner D, et al. Update on impact of moderate dose of adjuvant radiation on urinary continence and sexual potency in prostate cancer patients treated with nerve-sparing prostatectomy. Urology 2000; 56(3):453–458.

63. Messing EM, Manola J, Sarosdy M, et al. Immediate hormonal therapy compared with observation after radical prostatectomy and pelvic lymphadenectomy in men with node-positive prostate cancer. N Engl J Med 1999; 341(24):1781–1788.

64. Prayer-Galetti T, Zattoni F, Capizzi A, et al. Disease free survival in patients with pathological "C Stage" prostate cancer at radical prostatectomy submitted to adjuvant hormonal treatment. Eur Urol 2000; 38:504 [abstract 48].

65. Wirth M, Tyrrell C, Wallace M, et al. Bicalutamide (Casodex) 150 mg as immediate therapy in patients with localized or locally advanced prostate cancer significantly reduces the risk of disease progression. Urology 2001; 58(2):146–151.

66. Pound CR, Partin AW, Eisenberger MA, Chan DW, Pearson JD, Walsh PC. Natural history of progression after PSA elevation following radical prostatectomy. JAMA 1999; 281(17):1591–1597.

67. Bolla M, Gonzalez D, Warde P, et al. Improved survival in patients with locally advanced prostate cancer treated with radiotherapy and goserelin. N Engl J Med 1997; 337(5):295–300.

68. Lawton CA, Winter K, Murray K, et al. Updated results of the phase III Radiation Therapy Oncology Group (RTOG) trial 85–31 evaluating the potential benefit of androgen suppression following standard radiation therapy for unfavorable prognosis carcinoma of the prostate. Int J Radiat Oncol Biol Phys 2001; 49(4):937–946.

69. Eulau SM, Tate DJ, Stamey TA, et al. Effect of combined transient androgen deprivation and irradiation following radical prostatectomy for prostatic cancer. Int J Radiat Oncol Biol Phys 1998; 41(4):735–740.

70. Anscher MS, Prosnitz LR. Multivariate analysis of factors predicting local relapse after radical prostatectomy – possible indications for postoperative radiotherapy. Int J Radiat Oncol Biol Phys 1991; 21(4):941–947.

71. Billis A, Freitas LL, Magna LA. Vas deferens involvement in radical prostatectomy. Prevalence and significance. United States and Canadian Academy of Pathology (USCAP) Annual Meeting. Feb 2002. Abstract 647.

11

Adjuvant therapy for prostate cancer

*Manfred P Wirth, Michael Froehner
and Oliver W Hakenberg*

Introduction

Today, prostate cancer is the most commonly diagnosed malignancy and the second leading cause of cancer death in males in the United States[1] and many other countries in the Western world. Growing public awareness and the widespread testing of prostate specific antigen (PSA) have led to an increased detection of localized and potentially curable tumor stages.[2] Whereas radical prostatectomy results in disease-specific 10-year survival rates of approximately 90% in organ-confined disease,[3] the survival rates are unsatisfactory when the disease has spread outside the prostate gland. In a multicenter trial with 298 stage cT3 patients treated by pelvic lymphadenectomy with or without radical prostatectomy, the disease-specific 10-year survival was only 57%.[4] Considering the tumor differentiation, there is an analog situation. In tumors with a Gleason score of 2–6, radical prostatectomy offers excellent long-term cure rates, whereas disease-specific 15-year survival is clearly less favorable in the subset of Gleason score 7–10 tumors.[5] In the especially problematic subgroup of patients with Gleason score 8–10 disease, tumor-specific 15-year survival after radical prostatectomy is under 50%.[5] Similarly unfavorable results were observed after radiotherapy alone for locally advanced prostate cancer[6] and after radiotherapy for tumors with unfavorable Gleason scores of 7–10, respectively,[5] Overall, with clinically localized disease, biochemical relapse after radical prostatectomy is observed in about 35% of patients within 10 years.[7] In clinically locally advanced tumors or even lymph node positive cancers, the vast majority of patients will experience biochemical failure within 10 years after radical prostatectomy alone.[4,8] Considerable interest has therefore focused on the development of adjuvant hormonal or (after radical prostatectomy) radiotherapeutic interventions to improve the cure rates after curatively intended treatment of prostate cancer and to delay symptomatic progression as much as possible. In addition, efforts have been undertaken to decrease the side effects and costs of hormonal therapy. This chapter will discuss the current status and ongoing studies in the field of adjuvant treatment for prostate cancer.

Rationale for adjuvant hormonal treatment in prostate cancer – pros and cons

Adjuvant treatment after the resection or destruction of all macroscopic tumor tissue is intended to prevent progression of suspected microscopic residual cancer. In early breast cancer, which may be considered an analogous hormone-sensitive malignancy, adjuvant tamoxifen treatment has led to significantly improved tumor control and survival rates compared to local measures alone.[9] It has therefore been hypothesized that – given a similar biology of both tumors – immediate hormonal treatment might also be beneficial in prostate cancer.[10]

An appropriate adjuvant therapy requires the availability of effective drugs without severe and irreversible side effects and the ability to identify patients who are at high risk of tumor progression.

The traditional forms of hormonal manipulation in prostate cancer, i.e. orchiectomy and estrogen treatment, suffer from considerable disadvantages limiting their suitability in the adjuvant setting. The application of estrogens has been shown to be accompanied by severe cardiovascular side effects.[11] Orchiectomy, on the other hand, is an irreversible measure followed by impotence and – in the long run – by osteoporosis and the associated risk of pathologic fractures.[12] Furthermore, the classical form of treatment for prostate cancer, castration, first described 60 years ago,[13] is not appropriate for the increasing number of sexually and physically active men confronted with the diagnosis of prostate cancer. Many of these cancers are detected due to screening, and castration would have a negative impact on the quality of life, especially on libido and sexual potency.[14] During the last decades, other forms of hormonal deprivation – for example luteinizing hormone releasing hormone (LHRH) analogs, antiandrogens – have been developed which allow reversible treatment with fewer side effects and have opened new perspectives in the adjuvant treatment of prostate cancer.

Non-steroidal antiandrogens such as bicalutamide, flutamide or nilutamide competitively inhibit the activity of androgens at the androgen receptor site thus maintaining or even increasing the serum testosterone level. Currently, bicalutamide is the best-tolerated available substance in this group.[14] In two combined randomized trials with a total of 480 patients with locally advanced prostate cancer (stage T3–T4), bicalutamide monotherapy (150 mg daily) was as effective as castration considering overall survival and time to progression after a median follow up of 6.3 years.[15] Significant benefits were observed in the bicalutamide monotherapy group concerning sexual interest (p = 0.029) and physical capacity (p = 0.046).[15] In a randomized study with 220 stage C or D prostate cancer patients comparing bicalutamide monotherapy (150 mg daily) to combined androgen blockade with either flutamide or nilutamide as antiandrogens, no significant differences concerning progression-free and overall survival were observed.[16] In another randomized trial with a total of 1453 patients enrolled, Tyrrell et al[17] compared bicalutamide 150 mg daily with castration as palliative treatment for M1 or T3–T4M0 prostate cancer. Bicalutamide was as effective as castration in M0 patients whereas there was a small survival advantage for castration among M1 patients, with however, a better tolerability profile and quality of life in the bicalutamide arm. Altogether, bicalutamide monotherapy is a valuable option especially for younger and sexually active patients with locally advanced prostate cancer. Current evidence suggests that it is as effective as castration in men with a limited tumor burden (with a PSA level up to 400 ng/ml).[14] The properties of bicalutamide – effective and reversible androgen withdrawal with an acceptable side effect profile – make it appear a suitable candidate for application in the adjuvant setting.

Two further types of hormonal treatment should be discussed briefly: complete and intermittent androgen blockade. Conclusive evidence for the superiority of complete androgen blockade (i.e. the combination of an antiandrogen such as bicalutamide with surgical or medical castration) as primary treatment for metastatic prostate cancer is still lacking despite a large number of randomized trials available[18] and the results obtained in patients with metastatic disease should not be simply extrapolated to non-metastatic disease.[19] Therefore, in the setting of locally advanced non-metastatic prostate cancer, the application of complete androgen blockade should still be restricted to randomized trials. Even less evidence supports the use of intermittent androgen deprivation (i.e. temporary androgen withdrawal, for instance by a LHRH analog). To date, only a few studies with small numbers of patients, heterogeneous inclusion criteria and short follow up are available.[20] Therefore, it is still only possible to speculate on the role of adjuvant intermittent hormonal therapy which should be considered as a highly experimental treatment approach.

Whereas androgen deprivation may delay prostate cancer progression and resolve tumor-associated symptoms, it is not known whether it is capable of eradicating microscopic residual disease. Even in the presence of unresectable prostate cancer, the optimal time to start treatment remains unknown. Since long-term androgen deprivation is accompanied by considerable side effects and costs, an immediate start of hormonal treatment in patients with advanced prostate cancer is still discussed controversially.

In a randomized study with 938 patients with locally advanced or asymptomatic metastatic prostate cancer,[21] there was a significant survival advantage for those who were treated with immediate hormonal therapy. However, this study has been criticized because some patients in the delayed arm died without receiving hormonal therapy thus diminishing the reliability of the data. Nevertheless, there were some important results in this trial supporting the use of immediate therapy.

Some severe complications attributed to progressive disease occurred significantly less often in the immediate treatment arm (spinal cord compression, ureteral obstruction, extraskeletal metastases). A re-evaluation after a longer follow up confirmed the protective impact of early hormonal treatment on progression-related complications. The influence on survival was, however, not as high as seen earlier in the study.[22]

Altogether, at present, there is no conclusive evidence that every patient with advanced prostate cancer needs immediate treatment. Although an increasing amount of data support early hormonal deprivation in this situation, especially considering the prevention of progression-related complications, further randomized trials are needed to prove the value of this treatment and to identify subgroups of patients who are most likely to benefit from early hormonal manipulation. The findings from studies with advanced prostate cancer may not be applied uncritically to the adjuvant situation. Currently, only a paucity of data are available in favor of immediate hormonal therapy after curative treatment of early prostate cancer. Furthermore, adjuvant hormonal treatment after contemporary therapies for localized prostate cancer (i.e. radical prostatectomy, external beam radiotherapy, and brachytherapy) is associated with a measurable decrease in quality of life due to the side effects of androgen deprivation.[23]

Which endpoints are suitable for clinical trials on adjuvant treatment for prostate cancer?

Overall and disease-specific survival are accepted endpoints in adjuvant prostate cancer trials. After radical prostatectomy treatment for clinically non-metastatic prostate cancer, the disease-specific 10-year survival exceeds 50% even in the prognostically unfavorable subgroups with a high Gleason score.[5] That and the fact that probably only a small survival benefit of immediate treatment exists, mean large multicenter trials with long-term follow up are required to detect possible survival differences. The considerable proportion of intercurrent deaths complicate the detection of possible advantages of adjuvant treatment after radical prostatectomy. It may be expected that, at a follow up of 10 years after radical prostatectomy, more

than 50% of registered deaths will not be attributable to prostate cancer.[5]

Trials with locally advanced tumors treated by radiotherapy, on the other hand, include an unknown but presumably significant proportion of patients with undetected lymph node involvement and micrometastatic disease. Differences may thus be expected to be detected earlier. In a population of 405 radiotherapy patients followed by Barry et al,[5] only approximately one in three deaths during up to 10 years of follow up has not been attributed to prostate cancer. It is therefore not surprising that the majority of currently available data supporting adjuvant hormonal treatment is derived from trials in the setting of radiotherapy for locally advanced disease.

Survival without objective clinical progression (i.e. without local failure, bony or visceral metastases) is another possible endpoint of adjuvant studies and results may be expected much earlier than survival data. The use of clinical progression as a study endpoint however, raises controversies about the degree of the real benefit. Until a possible survival advantage of immediate treatment is proven, it remains unclear whether side effects and costs do or do not outweigh possible benefits. Monitoring quality of life is of great interest in this situation. PSA progression may be used as an endpoint in studies with adjuvant local radiotherapy after radical prostatectomy. This endpoint is, however, problematic in the setting of adjuvant endocrine treatment. Since androgen withdrawal nearly always results in a PSA decline in previously non-hormonally treated prostate cancer, PSA should not lead to wrong conclusions in trials with adjuvant endocrine treatment for prostate cancer.

Prognostic factors in early prostate cancer

Not all patients can be expected to benefit from adjuvant treatment. Particularly in patients with organ-confined disease, the general application of adjuvant therapy would expose the large majority of patients to unnecessary side effects and considerably increase treatment costs. It is essential to identify subgroups of patients with unfavorable tumor characteristics who are at a high risk of failure after treatment with curative intent. Excluding patients with lymph node or seminal vesical involvement who are known to be at a very high risk of progression after radical prostatectomy, Epstein et al[24] identified 721 patients with clinically organ-confined prostate cancer. Gleason score, in the extent of capsular penetration, and the status of the surgical margins were all independent prognostic factors. In addition to these parameters, Kupelian et al[25] demonstrated that the preoperative PSA value is the most reliable clinical predictor of biochemical failure after radical prostatectomy. While in patients with a preoperative PSA value of less than 4 ng/ml the 10-year progression risk was only 13%, it was 72% in patients with a PSA value of more than 20 ng/ml.[25]

Patients with a Gleason score of 6 or less who underwent radical prostatectomy have a prostate cancer-specific 10-year survival of more than 90%.[5] Adjuvant treatment is likely to be of little benefit in this population. Nevertheless, further research is needed in the field of prognostic markers in early prostate cancer, since the estimation of the risk of progression is still not adequate for individual patients.[26] After resolving this prognostic uncertainty, future studies in early prostate cancer might need fewer patients and shorter follow-up periods to assess the efficacy of adjuvant treatment.

Adjuvant hormonal treatment after radiotherapy

Reliable data derived from prospective randomized trials on adjuvant hormonal treatment of prostate cancer are available in the external beam radiotherapy setting (Table 11.1). The first randomized trials started in the 1960s; however, a survival benefit of hormonal therapy was not demonstrated until the 1990s. Bolla et al[27] randomized 415 patients with T1–T4N0–x prostate cancer either to receive radiotherapy alone (n = 208) or radiotherapy plus goserelin starting at the first day of irradiation and continued for 3 years (n = 207). The majority of patients had locally advanced T3–T4 disease. Patients who survived for 5 years had a significantly increased probability of being free of disease recurrence in the adjuvant treatment arm (85% vs 48%, p < 0.001).[27]

Adjuvant therapy with LHRH analogs starting at the beginning of radiotherapy significantly improved the overall survival rate at 5 years (79% vs 62%, p = 0.001). However, concern has been expressed about the uncommonly poor survival in the arm treated with radiotherapy alone, which was even less favorable than had been observed in a comparable population of stage D patients treated with hormonal therapy alone.[34] In another prospective randomized trial (n = 91, median follow up 9.3 years), Granfors et al[30] observed a significantly better clinical progression-free (p = 0.005) and overall survival (p = 0.02) and a trend towards improved disease-specific survival (p = 0.06) in patients with tumor stages T1–4N0–1 treated by orchiectomy and subsequent radiotherapy compared to those treated by radiotherapy alone. There was, however, mainly a benefit for patients with

Table 11.1 Effect of adjuvant hormonal treatment after radiotherapy in selected studies

Adjuvant study (authors)	Inclusion criteria	Progression-free survival	Survival
Bolla et al[27] *	T1–T4N0–x	Advantage for adjuvant treatment	Advantage for adjuvant treatment
Pilepich et al[28] * Lawton et al[29] *	Stage C or D1	Advantage for adjuvant treatment	Advantage for adjuvant treatment in subgroup with Gleason score 8–10
Granfors et al[30] *	T1–T4N0–1	Advantage for adjuvant treatment	Advantage for adjuvant treatment in N1 subgroup
Arcangeli et al[31]	Tumors confined to the pelvis	No advantage for adjuvant treatment	Disadvantage for adjuvant treatment
Hanks et al[32] *	T2b–T4, PSA < 150 ng/ml	Advantage for adjuvant treatment	Advantage for adjuvant treatment in subgroups with unfavorable tumors (cT3–T4 or cT2 with Gleason score 8–10 and all patients with Gleason score 8–10 together, respectively)
Wirth et al[33] *	T1b–T4N0–1M0	Advantage for adjuvant treatment	Not available

* Prospective randomized trials.

lymph node metastases. No significant difference was seen in patients without lymph node involvement, possibly due to the small sample size.

In another prospective randomized trial on adjuvant hormonal treatment in the radiotherapy setting with 945 analyzable patients with tumor stage C or D1 published by Pilepich et al,[28] the 5-year disease control rate was significantly improved (local failure: 84% vs 71%, p < 0.0001, systemic failure: 83% vs 70%, p < 0.001, disease-free survival: 60% vs 44%, p < 0.0001) in patients treated by adjuvant LHRH analogs. There were, however, no differences concerning overall survival with the exception of a subgroup of patients with Gleason score 8–10. A recent update confirmed the favorable impact of adjuvant hormonal treatment on both overall (p = 0.036) and disease-specific survival (p = 0.019), on local (p < 0.0001) and distant disease control (p < 0.0001) and disease-free survival (p < 0.0001) after external beam radiotherapy in the Gleason score 8–10 subset.[29]

Locally advanced cancers are very likely to harbor micrometastatic disease, and adjuvant hormonal treatment is certainly a reasonable approach in this situation.[29,35] In a prospective randomized study in patients with locally advanced prostate cancer (T2b–T4, PSA < 150 ng/ml), Hanks et al[32] compared goserelin and flutamide treatment for 2 months prior to and during radiotherapy and continuing for 24 months after radiotherapy to no further endocrine treatment after completion of local therapy. 1520 patients were eligible; the median follow up was 4.8 years. The group with continued treatment experienced a significantly improved disease-free survival, biochemical, local and distant control. Subsets with unfavorable tumors (cT3–T4 or cT2 with Gleason score 8–10 and all patients with Gleason score 8–10 together, respectively) showed a significantly better disease-specific survival at 5 years. Overall 5-year survival was significantly improved in the subgroup of all patients with Gleason score 8–10 (90% vs 78%, p = 0.007). In the whole study group however, there was only a trend favoring adjuvant treatment concerning disease-specific 5-year survival (92% vs 87%, p = 0.07) and no difference concerning overall 5-year survival (78% vs 79%).[32]

Conflicting data also exist. In a retrospective series with 264 patients and a median follow up of 100 months, Arcangeli et al[31] compared supplementary immediate endocrine treatment started up to 9 months prior to radiotherapy and continued for 2 or more years or until tumor progression occurred versus deferred hormonal therapy at relapse. Patients with tumors confined to the pelvis were included. After a median follow up of 100 months, there was no advantage for immediate treatment concerning the incidence of local and distant failure and disease-specific mortality. Due to a decreased number of deaths due to intercurrent disease, overall survival at 10 years was even higher in the group with radiotherapy only (p = 0.03).

In summary, there seems to be an advantage for adjuvant hormonal treatment after radiotherapy with curative intent for high risk patients with stage C or D1 prostate cancer.[27–30,32,34–36] It remains unknown however, whether the observed survival advantage can be attributed to hormonal therapy alone, since mainly poor-risk patients (with locally advanced disease and/or high Gleason scores) benefit from adjuvant androgen deprivation, whereas in earlier stages the differences tend to diminish. It is possible that adjuvant hormonal treatment suppresses unnoticed micrometastatic disease which – if left untreated – might result in rapid and life-threatening tumor progression.[34] An important problem in this setting is that studies comparing adjuvant hormonal therapy after radiotherapy with hormonal treatment alone are lacking to date.

Adjuvant hormonal treatment after radical prostatectomy

Compared with the body of knowledge supporting adjuvant endocrine treatment after radiotherapy for prostate cancer, fewer and more conflicting data are reported in the radical prostatectomy setting (Table 11.2). The first randomized trials comparing radical prostatectomy plus placebo with radical prostatectomy plus adjuvant hormonal treatment (5 mg diethylstilbestrol) had already been undertaken by the Veterans Administration Cooperative Urological Research Group (VACURG) in the 1960s.[11] No advantage for the adjuvant treatment had been demonstrated. More disappointingly, the application of 5 mg diethylstilbestrol had been associated with a significant excess of cardiovascular mortality, a fact which finally became the best-known result of the VACURG

Table 11.2   Effect of adjuvant hormonal treatment after radical prostatectomy in selected studies

Adjuvant study (authors)	Inclusion criteria	Progression-free survival	Survival
Zincke et al[8]	pN+	Advantage for adjuvant treatment	Advantage for adjuvant treatment in diploid subgroup
Seay et al[37]	pN+	Advantage for adjuvant treatment	Advantage for adjuvant treatment in diploid subgroup after 10 years
Messing et al[38] *	pN+	Advantage for adjuvant treatment	Advantage for adjuvant treatment
Wirth et al[39] *	Stage C	Advantage for adjuvant treatment	Not available
Prayer-Galetti et al[40] *	Stage C	Advantage for adjuvant treatment	Not available
Wirth et al[33] *	T1b–T4N0–1M0	Advantage for adjuvant treatment	Not available
Zincke et al[41]	Seminal vesicle involvement	Advantage for adjuvant treatment	Advantage for adjuvant treatment

* Prospective randomized trials.

studies.[11] Thus, estrogens currently play only a marginal role in the adjuvant treatment of prostate cancer.

Several retrospective studies showed advantages for immediate androgen deprivation after radical prostatectomy in men with lymph node metastases.[41] In a series of 370 patients with stage D1 (lymph node positive) tumors, Zincke et al[8] found that immediate hormonal treatment significantly delayed the time to progression after radical prostatectomy regardless of the ploidy pattern. A survival advantage, however, was only observed in patients with diploid tumors (p = 0.02). In the latter prognostically favorable subgroup, however, only seven of 138 patients eventually died of prostate cancer. The authors concluded that deferred treatment in stage D1 prostate cancer patients is only acceptable for non-diploid tumors, whereas patients with diploid tumors should receive immediate treatment.[8] A later series from the same institution again revealed no disease-specific survival advantage in non-diploid tumors.[37] In diploid tumors, there was a trend towards improved disease-specific survival in the adjuvant treatment group after 15 years of follow up (83% vs 49%, p = 0.1014). Thus, the authors claimed a survival advantage for adjuvant treatment in the diploid group after 10 years (p < 0.002), with, however, only a few patients followed for such a long period and with remarkable imbalance in the distribution of events between both arms. Whereas almost all deaths in the adjuvant group occurred earlier than 10 years of follow up (and only one

event has been observed later), there is a surprising contrary situation in the group without immediate treatment: only one event was observed prior to a follow up of about 9 years and all other events occurred very late in follow up. In both groups the patients with diploid and those with non-diploid tumors, adjuvant treatment was associated with a lower probability of disease progression.[37] Recently, more support for adjuvant hormonal therapy for stage D1 disease came from a randomized trial (n = 98, median follow up 7.1 years).[38] In this trial immediate hormonal therapy was compared with observation alone in prostate cancer patients with minimal lymph node disease treated by radical prostatectomy and pelvic lymph node dissection. The risk of tumor recurrence and death due to prostate cancer in the arm treated immediately was significantly reduced.[38] Other studies, however, have yielded conflicting results. An ongoing European Organization of Research and Treatment of Cancer (EORTC) study with 302 stage D1 patients who did not undergo radical prostatectomy showed no advantage for immediate treatment concerning cancer-specific survival after a median follow up of 6 years.[42] The above quoted series by Seay et al[37] demonstrated a (marginal) disease-specific survival advantage only for diploid tumors and only after a follow up of more than 10 years.

These conflicting results raise questions concerning possible biases which possibly influenced the results of the trial by Messing et al.[38] Specifically, concern has been expressed about the small size of the study (the study was closed long before the intended number of patients was enrolled because of the significantly better outcome in the intervention arm) and the absence of a correlation between histologic grade and survival. These factors could have created imbalances that would account for the surprisingly large difference in survival within a relatively short period of time.[42]

When studies in patients with lymph node metastases are excluded, no conclusive evidence for the efficacy of adjuvant endocrine treatment after radical prostatectomy is presently available.[26,41,43] Only a limited amount of data on adjuvant treatment in stage pT3 have been published. In a retrospective study, Zincke et al[41] compared 157 men with seminal vesicle involvement (stage pT3bN0M0) who received adjuvant orchiectomy or oral hormones with 550 who did not. Adjuvantly treated patients had a significantly better 10-year outcome concerning biochemical progression-free survival (67% vs 23%, p < 0.001), systemic progression-free survival (90% vs 78%, p < 0.001) and disease-specific survival (95% vs 87%, p = 0.046). Among tumor stage pT3, cancers with seminal vesicle involvement are a subset with a particularly unfavorable prognosis (73% progression within 10 years[24]), and results obtained in this setting may not be transferred to the whole stage pT3 population.

We conducted a controlled randomized multi-center study in which 356 patients with stage C disease were randomized into two groups: group 1 received flutamide as adjuvant treatment, group 2 received no further treatment. In a preliminary analysis, tumor progression (a PSA value > 5 ng/ml, two PSA values > 2 ng/ml more than 3 months apart with increasing tendency or three PSA values > 1 ng/ml more than 3 months apart with increasing tendency, or clinical progression) was significantly delayed by adjuvant treatment with flutamide. However, when clinical recurrence only was considered, there was no detectable difference, possibly due to the small number of events up to the last follow up (flutamide group: 4/139, control group: 5/144, Table 11.1).[39,44] At present, a re-evaluation of the study is ongoing. The side effects of flutamide such as gynecomastia and nausea are considerable disadvantages, limiting its suitability as an adjuvant treatment. In our study, approximately every fifth patient discontinued flutamide due to side effects.[39,44]

Preliminary results from another prospective randomized trial with 201 stage C patients enrolled have been reported by Prayer-Galetti et al.[40] The authors reported a 25.2% progression advantage for adjuvant goserelin acetate treatment at a median follow up of 5 years. However, PSA relapse and objective progression were not distinguished. It may be supposed that this difference is mainly attributable to the authors' definition of recurrence (one PSA greater than 0.5 ng/ml) which is certainly not a generally accepted cut-off in the setting of a randomized trial comparing adjuvant LHRH analog treatment with expectant management. Furthermore, the application of long-term LHRH analogs in the relatively low risk population of (nodal negative) stage C prostate cancer in patients with a long life expectancy (selected for radical prostatectomy) raises questions about the side effects of treatment concerning impotence, loss of libido and osteoporosis.

The Bicalutamide Early Prostate Cancer Program

In the largest currently ongoing trials on adjuvant treatment of prostate cancer, the Bicalutamide Early Prostate Cancer Program with 8115 patients enrolled, the non-steroidal antiandrogen bicalutamide is being assessed as adjuvant therapy after primary treatment with curative intent or as an immediate and only treatment in patients with early prostate cancer (T1b–T4N0–1M0). The program comprises three double-blind, parallel-group trials (one in North America, one in Scandinavia and one in a number of countries worldwide), all of which enrolled and randomized patients on a 1:1 basis to either bicalutamide 150 mg once daily or placebo.[10] In North America, more than 80% of the patients enrolled had previously undergone radical prostatectomy, compared to about 60% in Europe and less than 20% in Scandinavia. In North America, more than 70% of patients entered had a tumor stage of less than T3, compared with approximately 60% in Europe and Scandinavia.[10]

Recruitment to the program, which began in 1995, was completed in 1998, and first results are now available.[10,33,45] A total of 3603 patients were enrolled in Europe, South Africa, Australia and Mexico (trial 24) of the Bicalutamide Early Prostate Cancer Program. After a median follow up of 2.6 years, a significant delay in the time to PSA doubling and a significant reduction in the risk of objective progression (confirmed by biopsy, bone scan, computed tomography, ultrasound or magnetic resonance imaging) were observed in the bicalutamide group (p < 0.001).[33] The difference was more apparent in men with locally advanced disease.[45] For survival analysis, however, further maturation of data is required.[33] The overall withdrawal rate was similar in both treatment arms, while the withdrawal rate due to side effects was higher in the bicalutamide than in the placebo group (24.5% vs 7.7%). Mild to moderate gynecomastia and breast pain were the major side effects of bicalutamide treatment and the main reason for side-effect associated withdrawal of treatment. Prophylactic low-dose breast gland irradiation may prevent this complication (Table 11.3).[33]

Adjuvant radiotherapy after radical prostatectomy

Currently, no prospective randomized studies have been published regarding adjuvant radiotherapy after radical prostatectomy. However, it has been shown by retrospective analyses that local recurrence can effectively be prevented by adjuvant radiotherapy.[46] In a matched-pair analysis, Valicenti and Gomella[47] found that the application of adjuvant radiotherapy to patients with adverse prognostic criteria after radical prostatectomy

(high Gleason score, PSA > 10 ng/ml, seminal vesicle involvement) resulted in a significantly improved biochemical disease-free 5-year survival (89% vs 55%, p = 0.002). Improved disease control was observed above a level of 61.2 Gy.[47]

Grossfeld et al[48] developed a decision model for the application of adjuvant radiotherapy versus expectant management in patients with a margin-positive disease after radical prostatectomy. The authors recommended adjuvant radiotherapy in cases with low to intermediate grade cancer without seminal vesicle involvement and multiple positive margins that are considered to be at a high risk of local rather than systemic failure.[48] Leibovich et al[49] performed a retrospective analysis of 76 men with stage pT2N0 disease and a single positive margin who underwent adjuvant radiation therapy within 3 months of radical prostatectomy, matched 1:1 with 76 controls who were managed expectantly. Patients who underwent adjuvant irradiation had an improved outcome after 5 years concerning biochemical disease-free survival (88% vs 59%, p = 0.005) and local or distant recurrence-free survival (16% vs 0%, p = 0.015).

Non-randomized clinical trials available to date do not show that adjuvant radiotherapy improves overall survival. There are however, prospective trials being undertaken at present which can be expected to answer this question.[50] In the meantime, adjuvant radiotherapy after radical prostatectomy cannot be considered a standard treatment. It remains to be seen whether delayed secondary radiotherapy, if and when local recurrence occurs, is not equally effective. This approach would spare patients with positive surgical margins (who might develop metastases rather than local recurrence) the potential complications of local radiotherapy. Although adjuvant radiotherapy is capable of reducing the risk of local progression, positive margins after radical prostatectomy alone should not uncritically be treated by adjuvant local radiotherapy. About 50% of patients with positive margins will not experience recurrence within 10 years[24] and would unnecessarily be exposed to the side effects of adjuvant radiotherapy. Furthermore, if positive margins are accompanied by high Gleason score and locally advanced disease, adjuvant local radiotherapy will be unlikely to prevent recurrence since these patients are at a high risk of systemic failure.

Table 11.3 Most frequent side effects in the bicalutamide and placebo arm of the Europe, South Africa, Australia, and Mexico trial of the Bicalutamide Early Prostate Cancer Program[33]

Side effect	Bicalutamide 150 mg (n = 1798) (%)	Placebo (n = 1805) (%)
Gynecomastia alone	17.4	5.3
Breast pain alone	17.6	3.1
Gynecomastia and breast pain	47.5	2.1
Hot flushes	9.3	4.6
Flu syndrome	8.6	9.5
Back pain	8.2	10.9
Impotence	8.0	5.3

PSA-based onset of delayed radiotherapy is another possible option in the management of patients who are at an increased risk of local failure. PSA relapse precedes clinical recurrence by years.[7] If the histopathologic parameters and PSA kinetics support local rather than systemic failure (PSA relapse-free interval > 2 years after radical prostatectomy, PSA doubling time > 12 months, PSA velocity ≥ 0.75 ng/ml per year, histopathologic stage pT3a or R1, Gleason score ≤ 7),[51] prostate bed radiotherapy will be an acceptable approach. Local radiotherapy for PSA failure should be applied with PSA levels of not more than 1.5 ng/ml in standard fractionation with a dosage of 64 Gy.[52] Patients with PSA relapse who fail the criteria which suggest local recurrence are thus rather candidates for systemic (hormonal) treatment, since local measures like radiotherapy are unlikely to be able to control the disease in these cases.

Summary

To date, cure of prostate cancer is not possible with hormonal treatment alone. However, modern types of hormonal therapy such as antiandrogen monotherapy allow palliative treatment of locally advanced prostate cancer with tolerable side effects as effectively as castration.

Despite considerable research efforts in the field of adjuvant treatment of prostate cancer, many questions remain unanswered. At present, studies demonstrating an advantage for adjuvant treatment have mainly shown this advantage for patients with lymph node metastases or for those with a high probability of micrometastatic disease and early systemic progression. These patients probably really need immediate treatment. However, there is a different situation in early (pT2–T4pN0M0) prostate cancer, where no randomized studies have so far been completed regarding survival data. A delay of objective and PSA progression has been demonstrated; however, to date it remains unclear whether this delay will translate into a true survival advantage. The maturation of data of ongoing trials are awaited to answer this question. However, it is also necessary to identify risk groups by application of conventional and the development of new prognostic markers. Furthermore, the appropriate duration of adjuvant treatment is still unknown. Currently available evidence supports adjuvant hormonal treatment after treatment with curative intent for prostate cancer only in those patients with a considerable risk of early distant progression. In subsets with a lower risk, adjuvant hormonal manipulation should be restricted to new and ongoing randomized trials which should not only focus on progression- and survival-associated endpoints but also on quality of life and costs.

Finally, it should be emphasized that the decision on any type of adjuvant treatment after radical prostatectomy or radiotherapy should be made individually after counseling of the patient on all available treatment options (including watchful waiting) concerning the potential benefits and side effects of each management strategy.

References

1. Jemal A, Thomas A, Murray T, Thun M. Cancer statistics, 2002. CA Cancer J Clin 2002; 52:23–47.
2. Smart CR. The results of prostate carcinoma screening in the U.S. as reflected in the surveillance, epidemiology, and end results program. Cancer 1997; 80:1835–1844.
3. Zincke H, Oesterling JE, Blute ML, et al. Long-term (15 years) results after radical prostatectomy for clinically localized (stage T2c or lower) prostate cancer. J Urol 1994; 152:1850–1857.
4. Gerber GS, Thisted RA, Chodak GW, et al. Results of radical prostatectomy in men with locally advanced prostate cancer. Multi-institutional pooled analysis. Eur Urol 1997; 32:385–390.
5. Barry MJ, Albertsen PC, Bagshaw MA, et al. Outcomes for men with clinically nonmetastatic prostate carcinoma managed with radical prostatectomy, external beam radiotherapy, or expectant management: a retrospective analysis. Cancer 2001; 91:2302–2314.
6. Bolla M. Adjuvant hormonal treatment with radiotherapy for locally advanced prostate cancer. Eur Urol 1999; 35(suppl 1):23–26.
7. Pound CR, Partin AW, Eisenberger MA, et al. Natural history of progression after PSA elevation following radical prostatectomy. JAMA 1999; 281:1591–1597.
8. Zincke H, Bergstralh EJ, Larson-Keller JJ, et al. Stage D1 prostate cancer treated by radical prostatectomy and adjuvant hormonal treatment. Cancer 1992; 70:311–323.
9. Early Breast Cancer Trialists' Colloborative Group. Systemic treatment of early breast cancer by hormonal, cytotoxic or immune therapy. Lancet 1992; 339:1–14.
10. See WA, McLeod D, Iversen P, Wirth M. The bicalutamide Early Prostate Cancer Program. Demography. Urol Oncol 2001; 6:43–47.
11. Byar DP, Corle DK. Hormone therapy for prostate cancer. Results of the Veterans Administration Cooperative Urological Research Group studies. NCI Monogr 1988; 7:165–170.
12. Daniell HW. Osteoporosis due to androgen deprivation therapy in men with prostate cancer. Urology 2001; 58:101–107.

13. Huggins C, Hodges CV. Studies on prostatic cancer: I. The effect of castration, of estrogen and of androgen injection on serum phosphatases in metastatic carcinoma of the prostate. Cancer Res 1941; 1:293–297.

14. Kolvenbag GJC, Iversen P, Newling DWW. Antiandrogen monotherapy: a new form of treatment for patients with prostate cancer. Urology 2001; 58(suppl 2A):16–23.

15. Iversen P, Tyrrell CJ, Kaisary AV, et al. Bicalutamide monotherapy compared with castration in patients with nonmetastatic locally advanced prostate cancer: 6.3 years of followup. J Urol 2000; 164:1579–1582.

16. Boccardo F, Rubagotti A, Barichello M, et al. Bicalutamide monotherapy versus flutamide plus goserelin in prostate cancer patients: results of an Italian Prostate Cancer Project study. J Clin Oncol 1999; 17:2027–2038.

17. Tyrrell CJ, Kaisary AV, Iversen P, et al. A randomised comparison of 'Casodex' (bicalutamide) 150 mg monotherapy versus castration in the treatment of metastatic and locally advanced prostate cancer. Eur Urol 1998; 33:447–456.

18. Laufer M, Pound CR, Carducci MA, Eisenberger MA. Management of patients with rising prostate-specific antigen after radical prostatectomy. Urology 2000; 55:309–315.

19. Klotz L. Hormone therapy for patients with prostate carcinoma. Cancer 2000; 88:3009–3014.

20. Grossfeld GD, Small EJ, Lubeck DP, et al. Androgen deprivation therapy for patients with clinically localized (stages T1 to T3) prostate cancer and for patients with biochemical recurrence after radical prostatectomy. Urology 2001; 58(2 suppl 1):56–64.

21. The Medical Research Council Prostate Cancer Working Party Investigators Group. Immediate versus deferred treatment for advanced prostatic cancer: initial results of the Medical Reseach Council trial. Br J Urol 1997; 79:235–246.

22. Kirk D, on behalf of the Medical Research Council Prostate Cancer Working Party Investigators Group. Immediate versus deferred hormone treatment for prostate cancer: how safe is androgen deprivation? BJU Int 2000; 86:220 [abstract].

23. Wei JT, Dunn RL, Sandler HM, et al. Comprehensive comparison of health-related quality of life after contemporary therapies for localized prostate cancer. J Clin Oncol 2002; 20:557–566.

24. Epstein JI, Partin AW, Sauvageot J, Walsh PC. Prediction of progression following radical prostatectomy. A multivariate analysis of 721 men with long-term follow-up. Am J Surg Pathol 1996; 20:286–292.

25. Kupelian P, Katcher J, Levin H, et al. Correlation of clinical and pathologic factors with rising prostate-specific antigen profiles after radical prostatectomy alone for clinically localized prostate cancer. Urology 1996; 48:249–260.

26. Tyrrell CJ. Adjuvant and neoadjuvant hormonal therapy for prostate cancer. Eur Urol 1999; 36:549–558.

27. Bolla M, Gonzalez D, Warde P, et al. Improved survival in patients with locally advanced prostate cancer treated with radiotherapy and goserelin. N Engl J Med 1997; 337:295–300.

28. Pilepich MV, Caplan R, Byhardt RW, et al. Phase III trial of androgen suppression using goserelin in unfavourable prognosis carcinoma of the prostate treated with definitive radiotherapy – report of RTOG protocol 85-31. J Clin Oncol 1997; 15:1013–1021.

29. Lawton CA, Winter K, Murray K, et al. Updated results of the phase III radiation therapy oncology group (RTOG) trial 85-31 evaluating the potential benefit of androgen suppression following standard radiation therapy for unfavorable prognosis carcinoma of the prostate. Int J Radiat Oncol Biol Phys 2001; 49:937–946.

30. Granfors T, Modig H, Damber JE, Tomic R. Combined orchiectomy and external radiotherapy versus radiotherapy alone for nonmetastatic prostate cancer with or without pelvic lymph node involvement: a prospective randomized study. J Urol 1998; 159:2030–2034.

31. Arcangeli G, Saracino B, Micheli A, et al. Radiotherapy with or without androgen deprivation in the treatment of localized adenocarcinoma of the prostate. Am J Clin Oncol 1998; 21:1–5.

32. Hanks GE, Lu J, Machtay M, et al. RTOG Protocol 92-02. A phase III trial of the use of long-term androgen suppression following neoadjuvant hormonal cytoreduction and radiotherapy in locally advanced carcinoma of the prostate. Proc ASCO 2000; 19:327a [abstract].

33. Wirth M, Tyrrell C, Wallace M, et al. Bicalutamide (Casodex) 150 mg as immediate therapy in patients with localized or locally advanced prostate cancer significantly reduces the risk of disease progression. Urology 2001; 58:146–151.

34. Pollack A, Zagars GK. Androgen ablation in addition to radiation therapy for prostate cancer. Is there a true benefit? Semin Radiat Oncol 1998; 8:95–106.

35. Pilepich MV, Winter K, John MJ, et al. Phase III radiation therapy oncology group (RTOG) trial 86-10 of androgen deprivation adjuvant to definitive radiotherapy in locally advanced carcinoma of the prostate. Int J Radiat Oncol Biol Phys 2001; 50:1243–1252.

36. Schröder FH, van den Ouden D. Management of locally advanced prostate cancer. 2. Radiotherapy, neoadjuvant endocrine treatment, update 1997–1999. World J Urol 2000; 18:204–215.

37. Seay TM, Blute ML, Zincke H. Long-term outcome in patients with pTxN+ adenocarcinoma of prostate treated with radical prostatectomy and early androgen ablation. J Urol 1998; 159:357–364.

38. Messing EM, Manola J, Sarosdy M, et al. Immediate hormonal therapy compared with observation after radical prostatectomy and pelvic lymphadenectomy in men with node-positive prostate cancer. N Engl J Med 1999; 341:1781–1788.

39. Wirth M, Frohmüller H, Marx F, for the study group. Adjuvant antiandrogenic treatment after radical prostatectomy in stage C prostate cancer – preliminary results of a randomized controlled multicenter trial. J Urol 1997; 157(suppl):1308 [abstract].

40. Prayer-Galetti T, Zattoni F, Capizzi A, et al. Disease free survival in patients with pathological "C stage" prostate cancer at radical retropubic prostatectomy submitted to adjuvant hormonal treatment. Eur Urol 2000; 38(suppl 4):504 [abstract].

41. Zincke H, Lau W, Bergstralh, Blute ML. Role of early adjuvant hormonal therapy after radical prostatectomy for prostate cancer. J Urol 2001; 166:2208–2215.

42. Eisenberger MA, Walsh PC. Early androgen ablation for prostate cancer? N Engl J Med 1999; 341:1837–1838.

43. Wirth MP, Froehner M. Perspectives in adjuvant treatment of prostate cancer. Urol Int 2002; 85:1–5.

44. Wirth M, Froehner M. A review of studies of hormonal adjuvant therapy in prostate cancer. Eur Urol 1999; 36(suppl 2):14–19.

45. Wirth M. Delaying/reducing the risk of clinical tumor progression after primary curative procedures. Eur Urol. 2001; 40(suppl 2):17–23.

46. Paulson DF, Moul JW, Robertson JE, Walther PJ. Postoperative radiotherapy of the prostate for patients undergoing radical prostatectomy with positive margins, seminal vesicle involvement and/or penetration through the capsule. J Urol 1990; 143:1178–1182.

47. Valicenti RK, Gomella LG. Durable efficacy of adjuvant radiation therapy for prostate cancer: will the benefit last? Semin Urol Oncol 2000; 18:115–120.

48. Grossfeld GD, Tigrani VS, Nudell D, et al. Management of a positive surgical margin after radical prostatectomy. Decision analysis. J Urol 2000; 164:93–99.

49. Leibovich BC, Engen DE, Patterson DE, et al. Benefit of adjuvant radiation therapy for localized prostate cancer with a positive surgical margin. J Urol 2000; 163:1178–1182.

50. Tiguert R, Forman JD, Hussain M, Wood DP. Radiation therapy for a rising PSA level after radical prostatectomy. Semin Urol Oncol 1999; 17:141–147.

51. Ornstein DK, Oh J, Herschman JD, Andriole GL. Evaluation and management of the man who has failed primary curative therapy for prostate cancer. Urol Clin North Am 1998; 23:591–601.

52. American Society for Therapeutic Radiology and Oncology Consensus Panel. Consensus statements on radiation therapy of prostate cancer: guidelines for prostate re-biopsy after radiation and for radiation therapy with rising prostate-specific antigen levels after radical prostatectomy. J Clin Oncol 1999; 17:1155–1162.

12

Antisense therapy in oncology: current status

Martin E Gleave, Hideaki Miyaki and Burkhard Jansen

Introduction

Accelerated identification and characterization of cancer-relevant molecular targets has sparked considerable interest in the development of new generations of anticancer agents that specifically inhibit a progression-relevant target. These agents may be small molecules, antibodies or antisense oligonucleotides, and promise to show enhanced specificity for malignant cells and a more favorable side-effect profile due to well-defined and tailored modes of action. Antisense oligonucleotides – short synthetic stretches of chemically modified DNA capable of specifically hybridizing to the mRNA of a chosen cancer-relevant target gene – are close, after decades of challenges, to fulfilling their promise in the clinical setting. Although not all of the challenges have been met to date, emerging clinical evidence supports the premise that antisense oligonucleotides stand a realistic chance of emerging as major partners of rationally designed anticancer agents. The status of antisense targeting of several genes, including Bcl-2, Bcl-xL, clusterin, androgen receptor and insulin-like growth factor binding proteins (IGFBPs), relevant to prostate and other genitourinary (GU) cancers, are reviewed.

High throughput technological platforms have been developed in the last few years and are now accessible to rapidly and cost effectively produce an entire 'transcriptome', 'genome'- or 'proteome'-wide view of tumor biology. Integrated gene and protein expression data gathered from these high throughput technologies and mined by advanced bioinformatics will dramatically transform our understanding and approach to human malignancies. Medicine is poised to make the next leap, from the foundation of tumor classification derived from pathologic and molecular profiles to individualized prognostication and treatment based on the unique genetic aspects of individual tumors. As therapeutics is developed to address specific genetic abnormalities, custom therapeutic protocols will become the standard of care. Already specific aberrantly expressed genes in cancers have been directly targeted, such as in the case of antisense Bcl-2, Gleevec and Herceptin, and are leading the way into specialized and customized therapeutic approaches according to the tumor's aberrations, with low toxicity.

Elucidation of the pathogenic role of candidate genes implicated in tumor progression is a rapidly progressing field of cancer research and has provided a steadily growing list of candidates. Known nucleotide sequences of cancer-relevant genes offer the possibility to design tailored anticancer agents which lack many of the toxic side effects displayed by conventional therapeutics. The focus of this review is to address the development and recent progress in the use of antisense oligonucleotides (ASOs) as potential therapeutics in oncology, with an emphasis on those of specific relevance to urologic cancers. An ASO is designed to target the complementary sequence within a given RNA species, and once delivered into the target cell, hybridize with its RNA complement to inhibit translation of the disease-relevant protein. In contrast to the use of plasmid-derived endogenous expression of antisense RNA which has failed to overcome inefficient plasmid delivery, the oligonucleotide approach has overcome many of the hurdles on the way to successful clinical application. While the idea behind oligonucleotide-based antisense therapy is appealing and dates back more than 30 years,[1–3] recent advances in nucleic acid chemistry, along with the advent of automated DNA synthesis, has accelerated progress in the use of this technology for target validation and therapy.

Mechanisms of ASO-induced inhibition of protein expression

DNA is a 'double helix', a duplex of entwined strands of nucleotide base pairs. In each duplex, the bases or nucleotides – namely adenine (A), thymidine (T), guanine (G), cytosine (C) – are weakly bound or 'paired' by hydrogen bonds to complementary nucleotides on the other strand (A to T, G to C). This highly specific complementary base pairing is essential for accurate information transfer from DNA to its intermediary, messenger RNA (mRNA). During transcription of information from DNA into mRNA, the two complementary strands of the DNA partly uncoil. The 'sense' ($5'\rightarrow3'$) strand separates from the 'antisense' ($3'\rightarrow5'$) strand. The 'antisense' strand of DNA is used as a template for transcribing enzymes to assemble mRNA – a process called 'transcription'. The unpaired, single-stranded mRNA nucleotides are 'read' by transfer RNA anticodons as the ribosome proceeds to translate the message into protein synthesis (a process referred to as 'translation'). RNA can, however, form duplexes in the same way that DNA does and this is the basis of the mechanism of action of ASOs. ASOs are com-posed of short (hence the term 'oligo') lengths of 15–20 deoxynucleotides such as those in DNA and their sequence is $3'\rightarrow5'$, complementary to the sense sequence of a molecule of its target mRNA; for example the ASO sequence 5'–GGT-GTA-GAC-GCC-GCA-CG–3' hybridizes to 5'–CG-TGC-GGC-GTC-TAC-ACC–3' mRNA.

ASOs bind to a selected target mRNA by Watson–Crick base pairing, with subsequent inhibition of mRNA processing or translation by a variety of mechanisms including prevention of mRNA transport, splicing or translational arrest (Fig. 12.1). For such Watson–Crick base pairing to occur, nucleic acid drugs must be (almost completely) complementary to the exposed regions in their target RNAs and must co-localize with them. The specificity of this approach is based on the estimate that any sequence of at least 13 bases in RNA and 17 bases in DNA is represented only once within the human genome. While small molecules designed for therapeutic use generally recognize a specific protein target based on its molecular domain structure, an ASO recognizes a specific mRNA based on its sequence. Tertiary structures blocking the accessibility of the target mRNA and shared sequence homologies with non-target genes are

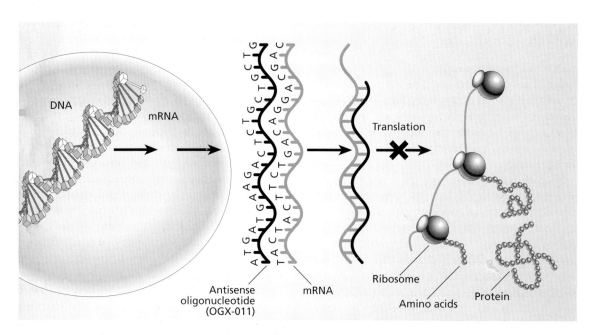

Figure 12.1 Schema illustrating the mechanism of action of antisense oligonucleotide targeting the cell survival gene clusterin.

important issues that need to be considered in the design of ASOs. While ASOs hybridizing to the start codon have been used successfully for a number of target mRNAs, other sites, such as 5′ untranslated regions, may prove to be even more effective under certain conditions.[4-6]

Cleavage of target mRNA by RNase H, a ubiquitous endonuclease usually involved in DNA replication, that cleaves the RNA strand of a DNA–RNA heteroduplex, appears to be the most important mechanism of antisense action. While the exact recognition structure for RNase H is still unknown, oligonucleotides with DNA-like properties as short as tetramers seem to be capable of activating this potent endonucleolytic activity.[7] High affinity oligonucleotides with a 5–7 base homology may provide sufficient overlap for RNase H competency.[8] In early 2001, the first successful use of double-stranded 21-nucleotide small interfering RNAs (siRNAs) that specifically suppress the expression of homologous genes in mammalian cells was described.[9] Although definitely promising as a strategy for the regulation of gene expression in theory, data available to date do not yet allow conclusions on the potential usefulness of this approach in animal models or in the clinic.

Strategies to stabilize ASOs for in vivo application

Initially, the usefulness of ASOs under in vivo conditions was limited by rapid degradation of the original phosphodiester backbone by cellular nucleases. A variety of backbone, sugar and base modifications have been investigated to improve stability characteristics required for clinical applications. Backbone modifications, such as the replacement of the oxygen atom of the phosphodiester (PO) moiety by sulfur (phosphorothioates, PS), a methyl group (methylphosphonates) or amines (phosphoramidates) led to significant improvements. Although these analogs improves backbone stability and resistance to nuclease digestion, only the PS modification has resulted in antisense compounds combining serum stability with reasonable high RNA binding affinity and the ability to elicit RNase H cleavage of the target RNA.[10] Today, after more than a decade of intensive research, PS ASOs still represent the most widely used class of antisense compounds, and several of these analogs are currently being tested in clinical trials and have shown considerable promise. Nevertheless, the overall physicochemical properties of PS oligonucleotides are suboptimal and warrant further study, primarily because of backbone-related issues including complement activation, thrombocytopenia, inhibition of cell–matrix interaction, or immune stimulation related to CpG motifs.[11-13]

To overcome the drawbacks associated with PS oligonucleotides, ongoing research has focused on backbone modifications that provide a more attractive pharmacological profile. The main goal of the modifications investigated so far was to further increase the metabolic stability and enhance the hybridization affinity of PS oligonucleotides for complementary mRNA. The affinity of ASOs to the target mRNA is a measure of stability of the nucleic acid hybrid, and higher affinity translates into higher gene-repressing activity.[8] Among a number of different modifications at the 2′-sugar position, the 2′-O-(2-methoxy)ethyl (2′-MOE) incorporation was identified as enhancing both binding affinity and further resisting degradation by intracellular nucleases.[14] 2′-O,4′-C-ethylene bridge (locked nucleic acid; LNA)[15] render ASOs in an RNA-like C3′-endo conformation also resulting in greatly enhanced affinity. The 2′-MOE modification resulted in decreased binding affinity to RNase H, the principal nuclease that cleaves ASO-bound mRNA. This problem was overcome by the use of 'gapped' ASO such that the 5′ and 3′ ends of the molecule contained 2′-MOE-modified sugar residues and the central portion of the ASO contained 2′-deoxy sugar residues that support RNase H activity.[8,16] This chemical design is usually accompanied with a uniformly modified PS backbone. The incorporation of 2′-MOE modifications into 20-mer PS ASO showed a dramatic effect on the ability of the sequence to hybridize to a target mRNA as a result of the conformation of the sugar and the backbone. Furthermore, 2′-MOE gapmers exhibited substantially increased resistance to intracellular nucleases, compared to conventional PS ASO. Both increased hybridizing affinity toward the targeted mRNA and enhanced resistance toward both serum and intracellular nucleases resulted in a 20-fold increase in activity of 2′-MOE modified ASO.[16,17] The enhanced potency of this new class of ASO did not lead to any decrease in specificity.

Antisense targets

Although only a minority of the 30 000–40 000 gene sequences and about 100 000 mRNAs identified by the Human Genome Project will prove suitable for therapeutic strategies, the potential for the development of tailored treatment approaches is certainly encouraging. The most attractive candidates for antisense therapy regulate cell proliferation,[18] apoptosis,[19] angiogenesis[20] and metastasis.[21] Antisense therapy that targets the apoptotic rheostat in cells or interferes with signaling pathways involved in cell proliferation and growth are particularly promising in combination with conventional anticancer treatments. An overview of key ASOs currently evaluated in clinical trials is provided in Table 12.1. Biologic and clinical studies focusing on candidate genes with potential relevance to prostate cancer progression are discussed in greater detail.

Bcl-2 family

Bcl-2

Bcl-2 is a critical regulator of apoptosis in numerous tissues and part of a growing family of apoptosis regulatory gene products that function as either death antagonists (e.g. Bcl-2, Bcl-xL) or death agonists (Bax, Bcl-Xs, Bad).[22–26] The ratio of death antagonists to death agonists determines how a cell responds to an apoptotic signal. Alterations in this balance that favor cell survival may cause proliferative disorders such as cancer. In the prostate gland, Bcl-2 is expressed in the less differentiated basal cell layer of prostatic acini, but not in benign differentiated luminal cells or androgen-dependent (AD) prostate cancer cells. In prostate cancer cells, Bcl-2 is upregulated within months after androgen withdrawal[27] and remains increased in androgen-independent (AI) tumors.[24,25] Bcl-2 upregulation after androgen withdrawal may be an adaptive mechanism that helps some prostate cancer cells survive castration-induced apoptosis and subsequently progress to androgen independence.[26]

Preclinical efficacy data with Bcl-2 ASO in GU tumor models. Bcl-2 also blocks proapoptotic signals by a variety of chemotherapeutic agents and may contribute to the multidrug-resistant phenotype characteristic of hormone refractory prostate cancer (HRPC) and other cancers. Induction of apoptotic cell death after androgen ablation or chemotherapy may be enhanced through functional inhibition of Bcl-2. Indeed, Bcl-2 ASOs induce apoptosis and enhance chemosensitivity in numerous cancers. Preclinical studies have shown that Bcl-2 ASOs decreased Bcl-2 protein and increased chemosensitivity in models of human melanoma[28] and prostate xenografts.[29–31] In prostate cancer models, Bcl-2 ASO reduced the IC_{50} of paclitaxel, docetaxel, and mitoxanthrone in vitro by a factor of 1 log (Fig. 12.2). Adjuvant in vivo administration of Bcl-2 ASO plus paclitaxel following castration significantly delayed AI progression compared to administration of either

Table 12.1 Key antisense clinical trials in oncology

Phase of clinical trial	Target gene/gene product	Antisense compound/ drug	Company or investigator	ASO size/ chemistry	Target malignancy	Combination treatment
I–III	PKC-alpha	ISIS 3521	ISIS	20-mer/PS	Solid tumors	+
I–II	c-raf	ISIS 5132	ISIS	20-mer/PS	Solid tumors	+
I–II	Ha-ras	ISIS 2503	ISIS	20-mer/PS	Solid tumors	–
III	Bcl-2	Genasense™, G3139	Genta	18-mer/PS	Solid tumors, MM, CLL	+
I–II	Clusterin/TRPM-2	OGX-011	OncoGeneX	21-mer/SGO	Solid tumors ?	+
I–II	PKA-R1-alpha	GEM 231	Hybridon	18-mer/SGO	Solid tumors	–
I–II	c-myb	LR/INX-3001	Gewirtz et al.	24-mer/PS	CML	–
I–II	Ribonucleotide-reductase	GTI-2040	Lorus	21-mer/PS	Solid tumors	–
I–II	DNA methyltransferase	MG98	MethylGene	20-mer/SGO	Solid tumors	+

CLL, chronic lymphatic leukemia, CML, chronic myelogenous leukemia; MM, multiple myeloma; PS, phosphorothioate oligonucleotide; SGO, second generation oligonucleotide.

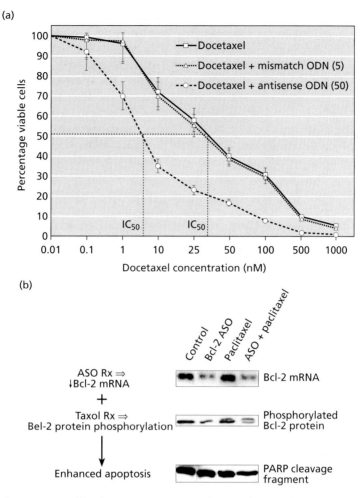

(a)

(b)

Figure 12.2 (a) Bcl-2 ASO treatment enhances docetaxel chemosensitivity in vitro. Shionogi tumor cells were treated with various concentrations of docetaxel and 500 nM antisense or control oligodeoxynucleotide (ODN). Cell viability was measured using the MTT assay. Bcl-2 ASOs increased the cytotoxic effects of docetaxel in vitro, shifting the dose–response curve to the left, reducing the IC_{50} by 80%. (b) After treatment of Shionogi cells with Bcl-2 ASO, paclitaxel, or both, Bcl-2 mRNA and protein levels were analyzed by Northern blotting (top), by Western blotting with an anti-Bcl-2 antibody (middle), or Western blotting with an antipoly PARP (poly-adenosine 5'-diphosphate-ribose polymerase) (bottom). Apoptosis, as measured by PARP cleavage, was detected with combined treatment with Bcl-2 ASO and paclitaxel.

agent alone.[29–31] Furthermore, paclitaxel-induced regression of established AI Shionogi[30] or LNCaP[32] tumors was synergistically enhanced when combined with Bcl-2 ASO. Synergistic activity between Bcl-2 ASO and taxanes results from ASO-induced decreases in Bcl-2 mRNA and protein levels and taxol-induced Bcl-2 phosphorylation.

The uptake and effect of antisense Bcl-2 ASO has also been evaluated in bladder tumor cells and in an ex vivo bladder tumor model.[33,34] ASO-induced downregulation of the Bcl-2 protein and chemosensitization was cell-line dependent and did not always translate into enhanced chemosensitivity. Chemosensitization by Bcl-2 ASO was most apparent in the T24/83[33] and T24[33] cell lines, suggesting that the apoptotic pathway in T24 and T24/83 cells is Bcl-2 dependent. In contrast, there was no synergistic effect in three other bladder cancer cell lines. These data illustrate that alternative pathways that resist or bypass the apoptosis initiation are cell-line specific. Alternatively, chemoresistance could be the result of other anti-apoptotic proteins substituting for Bcl-2 after its downregulation, such as Bcl-xL, clusterin, or members of the inhibitors of apoptosis protein family (i.e. survivin). Fluorescein isothiocyanate-conjugated (FITC) antisense oligonucleotide sequences have also been used to confirm uptake in RT4 bladder cancer cells, normal pig urothelium and fresh human urothelial tumors in an ex vivo model.[33,34]

Clinical trial experience with Bcl-2 ASO

Initial data of a phase I clinical study evaluating single-agent Bcl-2 ASO G3139 (Genasense, Table 12.1), a 18-mer phosphorothioate oligonucleotide targeting the Bcl-2 translation initiation site, was reported in 21 patients with non-Hodgkin's lymphoma (NHL) in 1997[36] (updated in 2000[37]). The dose-limiting toxicity in the initial study was thrombocytopenia; one complete response and two minor responses were seen. In nine patients the disease stabilized and nine patients showed disease progression. However, reduction in Bcl-2 protein by ASO treatment was observed in only ~50% of evaluable patients. A second single agent phase I study in men with HRPC at Memorial Sloan-Kettering Cancer Center used a 14-day continuous intravenous infusion schedule of Genasense.[38] Dose escalations to 5.3 mg/kg/day for 14 days were well tolerated. Pharmacokinetic studies demonstrated that dose levels of 2–4 mg/kg/day achieve linear plasma concentrations between 1–4 µg/ml. Toxicity was mild in most patients, with a single patient experiencing Grade IV leukopenia which resolved in one day. Bcl-2 expression in peripheral blood lymphocytes was significantly decreased by day 7.

In a phase I/II trial in patients with metastatic melanoma conducted in Vienna, Austria, Genasense was safely administered by continuous intravenous infusion in combination with full-dose dacarbazine (DTIC).[39] This trial demonstrated that Genasense downregulated Bcl-2 protein in serial melanoma biopsies, and that this biologic activity was associated with major clinical responses. Overall survival of the entire group of advanced-stage patients has exceeded 1 year. Transient thrombocytopenia at 12 mg/kg/day was dose limiting in patients who also received full-dose DTIC treatment. An international, phase III, randomized trial is currently ongoing in patients with advanced melanoma using a 5-day pretreatment regimen of Genasense administered by continuous intravenous infusion at a dose of 7 mg/kg/day, followed by DTIC at 1000 mg/m^2.

A dose escalation study of combined Genasense plus mitoxantrone was recently completed in Vancouver.[40] Twenty-six patients with HRPC were treated at seven dose levels receiving Genasense at a dose ranging from 0.6 to 5.0 mg/kg/day and mitoxantrone ranging from 4 to 12 mg/m^2. Genasense was administered as a 14-day intravenous continuous infusion every 28 days with mitoxantrone given as an intravenous bolus on day 8. No dose limiting toxicities were observed. Hematologic toxicities were transient and included neutropenia, thrombocytopenia and lymphopenia. Non-hematologic toxicities included cardiac dysfunction, fatigue, arthralgias and myalgias, none of which was severe. Two patients had > 50% reductions in prostate specific antigen (PSA). One patient who received Genasense at 1.2 mg/kg/day and a low dose (4 mg/m^2) of mitoxantrone also had symptomatic improvement in bone pain, receiving a total of six cycles. The other patient also had measurable disease with a documented partial response and received eight cycles. Bcl-2 expression in peripheral blood lymphocytes decreased in all patients treated at the 5 mg/kg/day of Genasense. Results from this trial suggest that biologically active doses of Genasense are well tolerated in combination with mitoxantrone without significant additional toxicity.

A phase II trial is now underway in San Antonio and Vancouver to determine activity of combination docetaxel plus G3139 Bcl-2 ASO in men with HRPC. Additional controlled multicenter trials in multiple myeloma, chronic lymphatic leukemia (CLL), lung cancer and other indications (Table

12.1) with the goal to enhance the efficacy of available and experimental treatment strategies are ongoing.

Bcl-xL

Alternative splicing of the Bcl-x pre-mRNA results in two distinct mRNAs, Bcl-xL which codes for the antiapoptotic protein and Bcl-xS that codes for the proapoptotic variant.[41] Bcl-xL ASOs have been reported to induce apoptosis in various tumor cells and sensitize tumor cells to chemotherapy.[42–44] In the androgen-dependent Shionogi xenograft model, Bcl-xL expression increased threefold postcastration and remained elevated in recurrent AI tumors, and could be decreased by Bcl-xL ASO treatment.[45] Although treatment of Shionogi cells with Bcl-xL ASO marginally enhanced chemo-sensitivity and delayed AI progression, combined adjuvant treatment using Bcl-xL and/or Bcl-2 ASO plus paclitaxel acted synergistically to further enhance chemotherapy and delay time to AI progression beyond that of either agent alone. These findings illustrate that combinatory regimens that inhibit two or more specific gene targets can produce additive effects and provide the basis for identifying additional antiapoptotic genes that may serve as targets in a multiagent approach to enhance the activity of existing chemo- and hormonal therapies.

The issue about which of the antiapoptotic Bcl-2 family members may prove to be the most important survival factor in a given malignancy has sparked considerable interest since many tumor cells coexpress the Bcl-2, Bcl-xL, as well as other Bcl-2 family members. Although Bcl-2 and Bcl-xL are functionally similar, there is evidence in support of distinct biological roles of these proteins in protecting from apoptosis induced by different stimuli.[46] Together with the finding that the Bcl-2 and the Bcl-xL mRNA share homology regions with high sequence identity, it would be potentially advantageous to design an ASO which targets these two key inhibitors of apoptosis. The design and preclinical testing of a Bcl-2/Bcl-xL bispecific antisense oligonucleotide was reported recently.[46,47] This 20-mer MOE gapmer oligonucleotide efficiently downregulated Bcl-2 expression simultaneously with Bcl-xL, and induced apoptosis in tumor cells of diverse histological origins in vitro and in vivo.

Clusterin

Clusterin, also known as testosterone-repressed prostate message-2 (TRPM-2), or sulfated glyco-protein-2, was first isolated from ram rete testes fluid and has been implicated in tissue remodeling, lipid transport, reproduction, complement regulation and apoptotic cell death. Although clusterin was initially reported as an androgen-repressed gene in prostate tissue, the functional role of clusterin in apoptosis was poorly defined. Because clusterin binds to a wide variety of biological ligands,[48] and the recent identification of a 14 bp element in its promoter that is recognized by transcription factor HSF1 (heat shock factor 1),[49] an emerging view suggests that clusterin functions like small heat shock proteins (Hsp) to chaperone and stabilize protein conformations at times of cell stress. Indeed, clusterin is substantially more potent than other small heat shock proteins at inhibiting stress-induced protein precipitation.

Increased clusterin levels have also been documented in renal cell,[50–52] urothelial[53,54] and ovarian[55] cancers relative to benign tissues, and correlates with poor outcome. Clusterin levels increase following androgen ablation in androgen dependent Shionogi[56] tumors, and following chemotherapy and other cell death triggers in other cancer lines.[50,54,57,58] Immunostaining of prostate tissue arrays spotted with hormone naive and post neoadjuvant hormone therapy (NHT)-treated specimens confirmed that clusterin is highly expressed in specimens after NHT, but low or absent in untreated specimens.[59] To investigate the functional significance of clusterin upregulation after androgen withdrawal, the effects of clusterin overexpression on time to AI progression after androgen ablation was evaluated by stably transfecting LNCaP cells with a clusterin/TRPM-2 cDNA expression vector. Tumor volume and serum PSA levels increased fourfold faster after castration in clusterin over-expressing LNCaP tumors compared to control tumors. Furthermore, LNCaP tumors overexpressing clusterin were more resistant to paclitaxel chemotherapy,[57] and to radiotherapy.[60] The upregulation of clusterin in human prostate cancer tissues after castration and the accumulating findings implicating clusterin in protection of apoptosis suggested that targeting the clusterin upregulation precipitated by androgen ablation may enhance castration-induced apoptosis and delay AI progression.

To this end, clusterin ASOs were designed that reduced mRNA levels in a dose-dependent and sequence-specific manner in several cancer cell lines.[17,50,54,57,58] Adjuvant treatment with clusterin ASO after castration decreased clusterin mRNA levels by 70% and resulted in earlier onset and more rapid apoptotic tumor regression, with significant delay in recurrence of AI Shionogi tumors.[56] Clusterin ASOs also increased the cytotoxic effects of mitoxantrone, docetaxel, and paclitaxel in vitro, reducing the IC_{50} by 75–90% in human prostate PC3 cells and tumors[7,58] Although treatment with single-agent clusterin ASOs had no effect on the growth of established tumors, clusterin ASOs synergistically enhanced chemotherapy-induced regression of prostate,[17,57,58] renal[50] and urothelial tumors.[54]

In human bladder cancer KoTCC-1 cells, clusterin mRNA was increased in a dose-dependent manner by cisplatin treatment, and could be inhibited by clusterin ASO.[54] Although clusterin ASO had no significant effect on growth of KoTCC-1 cells, they significantly enhanced cisplatin chemosensitivity of KoTCC-1 cells in a dose-dependent manner, reducing the IC_{50} by more than 50%. Moreover, in vivo systemic administration of clusterin ASO and cisplatin significantly decreased tumor volume compared with mismatch control oligos plus cisplatin. Furthermore, after the orthotopic implantation of KoTCC-1 cells, combined treatment with clusterin ASO plus cisplatin significantly inhibited the growth of primary KoTCC-1 tumors as well as the incidence of lymph node metastasis.

Renal cell cancer (RCC) is a chemoresistant disease with no active chemotherapeutic agent achieving objective response rates higher than 15%. Immunohistochemistry of normal and malignant kidney tissue sections of 67 patients demonstrated positive clusterin staining for almost all RCC (98%) and an overexpression, compared to normal tissue, in a majority of RCC (69%).[50] Overexpression of clusterin in human RCC cells increased their resistance to cytotoxic chemotherapy through inhibition of apoptosis both in vitro and in vivo, while clusterin ASO decreased clusterin mRNA expression in Caki-2 cells in a dose-dependent and sequence-specific manner and significantly enhanced chemosensitivity to paclitaxel in vitro and in vivo.[50]

A second generation 2′-MOE ASO targeting the translation initiation site of the clusterin gene (OGX-011, Table 12.1, Fig. 12.3) more potently suppressed clusterin mRNA compared to phosphorothioate ASO, and had a significantly longer (5 days vs 0.5 days) in vivo tissue half-life.[17] Weekly administration of OGX-011 was equivalent to daily phosphorothioate clusterin ASO in enhancing paclitaxel efficacy in vivo, with no additional side effects. These results support the use of 2′-MOE-modified ASO over conventional phosphorothioate ASO by potentially increasing potency and allowing longer dosing intervals in clinical trials. A Phase I/II clinical trial to determine the serum and tissue pharmacokinetics and biologic activity (i.e. the ability of clusterin ASOs to inhibit the upregulation of clusterin after androgen ablation) of OGX-011 when combined with neoadjuvant hormone therapy prior to radical prostatectomy began in December 2002.

Androgen receptor

Androgens act to regulate the expression of specific genes by binding to the androgen receptor (AR), a ligand responsive transcription factor. Androgen ablation causes prostate cancer cell death through apoptosis, but despite high initial response rates, remissions are temporary because surviving tumor cells eventually recur. Failure of endocrine therapy and tumor progression is characterized by androgen-independent growth despite high levels of AR expression in recurrent disease. Furthermore, the androgen-independent (AI) phenotype is characterized by the upregulation of genes that initially required androgens for expression, such as PSA, but become constitutively re-expressed in the absence of androgens.[60] Indeed, PSA may be a sentinel of other androgen-regulated genes that likewise become re-expressed in the absence of androgens during AI progression. Accumulating data implicate the AR as a key transcription factor activated in a ligand-independent manner during AI progression. How androgen-regulated genes become dysregulated during AI progression remains incompletely understood, but potential mechanisms include aberrant phosphorylation of the AR via growth factor activated pathways, expression of coactivator, or mutations in the ligand-binding domain allowing activation by other steroids.[61] It is clear from

(a)

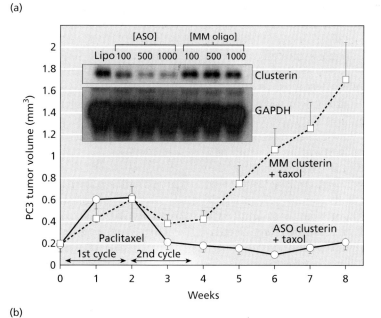

(b)

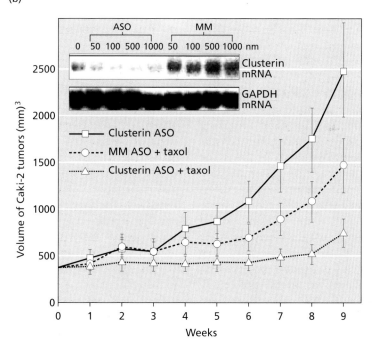

Figure 12.3 (a) Human-specific clusterin ASO enhances taxol-induced apoptosis and delays tumor progression in human androgen-independent PC3 tumors. Insert shows dose-dependent and sequence specific inhibition of clusterin levels in PC3 cells in vitro. (b) Human-specific clusterin ASO enhances taxol-induced apoptosis and delays tumor progression in human renal cell carcinoma (Caki-2) tumors. Insert shows dose-dependent and sequence specific inhibition of clusterin levels in Caki-2 cells in vitro. GAPDH, glyceraldehyde-3-phosphate dehydrogenase.

clinical studies that antiandrogens are not able to prevent AI gene expression in prostate tumors in vivo,[62] although these molecules can effectively block AR action in cultured prostate cell lines. This suggests that AI tumor progression is likely independent of the ligand-driven activity of AR.

Antisense inhibition of AR expression may offer one method to inhibit ligand-independent activation of the AR. Eder et al[63] inhibited AR expression in LNCaP prostate tumor cells by using a 15-mer AR ASO targeting the CAG repeats encoding the polyglutamine region of the AR (as750/15). Treatment of LNCaP cells with as750/15 significantly reduced AR expression and resulted in significant cell growth inhibition, strongly reduced secretion of the androgen-regulated PSA, and an increase in apoptotic cells. Antisense inhibition was also very efficient in LNCaP-abl cells, a subline established after long-term androgen ablation of LNCaP cells, resulting in inhibition of AR expression and cell proliferation that was similar to that seen for parental LNCaP cells. This study suggests AR ASOs may be one method of inhibiting AI progression and warrants further investigation.

IGF-1 and IGF binding proteins

(IGF)-1 plays an important role in the pathophysiology of prostatic disease. The biological response of cells to IGFs, a potent mitogen for prostate cells, is regulated by various factors in the microenvironment, including the IGF-binding proteins (IGFBPs).[64] After castration, the expression levels of certain IGFBPs change rapidly in the rat ventral prostate.[65] Differences in expression of various IGFBPs in benign and malignant prostatic epithelial cells have also been reported, with increases in IGFBP-2 and IGFBP-5, and decreases in IGFBP-3 in malignant versus benign cells.[66] Increased IGFBP-5 levels after castration have been shown to be an adaptive cell survival response that helps potentiate the antiapoptotic and mitogenic effects of IGF-1, thereby accelerating AI progression.[67,68] Forced overexpression of IGFBP-5 stimulated LNCaP cell proliferation, with corresponding increases in PI3K activity. In vivo, IGFBP-5 overexpressing LNCaP tumors progressed significantly faster to androgen independence after castration compared to controls. PI3K inhibitor-induced apoptosis could be prevented by IGF-1 treatment of IGFBP-5 transfectants, suggesting

that high IGFBP-5 levels can potentiate the anti-apoptotic effects of IGF-1. Systemic administration of IGFBP-5 ASOs in mice bearing Shionogi tumors after castration attenuated castration-induced increases in IGFBP-5 and significantly delayed time to AI progression. IGFBP-2 levels also increase in LNCaP and human prostate tumors after castration and during AI progression and, like IGFBP-5, appear to accelerate time to AI progression by enhancing IGF-1 responsiveness.[69] IGFBP-2 ASOs decreased IGFBP-2 levels and reduced LNCaP cell growth rates in vitro and in vivo. Increased IGFBP-5 and -2 levels after androgen ablation may represent adaptive responses to potentiate IGF-1-mediated survival and mitogenesis. Use of ASOs to target IGFBP modulation of IGF signaling is a potentially useful antiproliferative therapy that warrants further study.

Inhibitors of apoptosis proteins

The inhibitors of apoptosis proteins (IAPs) regulate apoptosis signaling by directly binding to caspases, thereby blocking their processing and activity. Survivin is a human IAP family member that regulates apoptosis by directly binding and inhibiting certain caspase-family cell death proteases.[70-72] The IAPs have shown a remarkable ability to block apoptosis induced by a wide spectrum of non-related apoptotic triggers.[73] Survivin associates with the mitotic spindle, is involved in cytokinesis, and inhibits apoptosis induced by various apoptotic stimuli.[74-76] A possible oncogenic role for survivin is suggested by its cancer-specific expression and regulation by NF-kappa B transcription factor, the latter exerting its anti-apoptotic effect through upregulation of various Bcl and IAP family members.[73] Survivin is detected in many human cancers but not in adjacent normal cells.[73-79] Survivin expression is prominent and developmentally regulated in embryonic and fetal tissue, is limited to the thymus in normal adult tissues, but has been detected in most lung, breast, colorectal, prostate and pancreas tumor samples and many transformed cell lines.

Although the case for a role for survivin in drug resistance is correlative so far, survivin has been shown to protect against apoptosis induced by various diverse signals. Survivin lacks expression in terminally differentiated tissues but becomes re-expressed during neoplastic transformation, which identifies this IAP as a truly tumor-specific target for antisense therapy. Indeed, ASOs targeting different sites within the survivin mRNA in different cell systems induce apoptosis directly or sensitize cells to additional apoptotic stimuli.[80,81] IAP-mediated antiapoptosis appears to be a highly trigger- and cell type-specific phenomenon, and what is observed in one system may not hold true for another. Hence it remains important to characterize the functional role of survivin in prostate cancer. The functional significance of survivin in in vivo prostate cancer models is unknown and is the subject of ongoing investigations.

The future of antisense therapy: integrated combinatorial regimens

Accumulating evidence demonstrates that ASOs can work in a sequence-specific manner in patients and supports moving this class of target-specific agents through late-stage clinical trial development. The choice of target is critical, and must be biologically and clinically relevant and inhibited in combination with other cell death triggers in an integrated and biologically relevant manner.

While challenges remain, these are most likely easier to overcome in oncology than in any other field of large unmet medical needs. Recent clinical data strongly support the potential of combining ASOs with conventional anticancer treatment modalities. Antisense strategies designed to alter the apoptotic threshold of cancer cells, to hamper tumor microvasculature and to alter signal transduction pathways critical to the survival of cancer cells are certainly among the most promising and most obvious target choices.

Since numerous genes and cellular pathways control the rate of tumor progression, inhibition of a single target gene will likely be insufficient to adequately suppress tumor progression. Exploration of additive or synergistic effects of combination antisense targeting in preclinical models will help guide further clinical protocols. Once target mechanisms and proof of principle for novel agents are established in preclinical model systems, significant methodological challenges confront clinicians, industry and regulatory agencies for development in the clinical arena. The challenges inherent to successful translation of an integrated and combinatory systemic therapy for prostate and other cancers will require close communication and collaboration amongst bench scientists, clinicians, industry and regulatory agencies.

References

1. Belikova AM ZVGN. Synthesis of ribonucleosides and diribonucleosides phosphates containing 2-chloroethylamine and nitrogen mustard residues. Tetrahedron Lett 1967; 37:3357–3362.
2. Paterson BM, Roberts BE, Kuff EL. Structural gene identification and mapping by DNA-mRNA hybrid-arrested cell-free translation. Proc Natl Acad Sci USA 1977; 74:4370–4374.
3. Zamecnik PC, Stephenson ML. Inhibition of Rous sarcoma virus replication and cell transformation by a specific oligodeoxynucleotide. Proc Natl Acad Sci USA 1978; 75:280–284.
4. Bacon TA, Wickstrom E. Walking along human c-myc mRNA with antisense oligodeoxynucleotides: maximum efficacy at the 5′ cap region. Oncogene Res 1991; 6:13–19.
5. Monia BP, Johnston JF, Geiger T, et al. Antitumor activity of a phosphorothioate antisense oligodeoxynucleotide targeted against C-raf kinase. Nat Med 1996; 2:668–675.
6. Ziegler A, Luedke GH, Fabbro D, et al. Induction of apoptosis in small-cell lung cancer cells by an antisense oligodeoxynucleotide targeting the Bcl-2 coding sequence. J Nat Cancer Inst 1997; 89:1027–1036.
7. Donis-Keller H. Site specific enzymatic cleavage of RNA 2. Nucleic Acids Res 1979; 7:179–192.
8. Monia BP, Lesnik EA, Gonzalez C, et al. Evaluation of 2′-modified oligonucleotides containing 2′-deoxy gaps as antisense inhibitors of gene expression. J Biol Chem 1993; 268:14514–14522.
9. Elbashir SM, Harborth J, Lendeckel W, et al. Duplexes of 21-nucleotide RNAs mediate RNA interference in cultured mammalian cells. Nature 2001; 411:494–498.
10. Crooke ST. Molecular mechanisms of antisense drugs: RNase H. Antisense Nucleic Acid Drug Dev 1998; 8:133–134.
11. Galderisi U, Cascino A, Giordano A. Antisense oligonucleotides as therapeutic agents 4. J Cell Physiol 1999; 181:251–257.
12. Agrawal S. Importance of nucleotide sequence and chemical modifications of antisense oligonucleotides. Biochim Biophys Acta 1999; 1489:53–68.
13. Krieg AM, Yi AK, Hartmann G. Mechanisms and therapeutic applications of immune stimulatory cpG DNA. Pharmacol Ther 1999; 84:113–120.
14. Altmann KH, Dean NM, Fabbro D, et al. Second generation of antisense oligonucleotides: from nuclease resistance to biological efficacy in animals. Chimia 1996; 50:168–176.
15. Wahlestedt C, Salmi P, Good L, et al. Potent and nontoxic antisense oligonucleotides containing locked nucleic acids. Proc Natl Acad Sci USA 2000; 97:5633–5638.
16. Baker BF, Lot SS, Condon TP, et al. 2′-O-(2-methoxy)ethyl-modified anti-intercellular adhesion molecule 1 (ICAM-1) oligonucleotides selectively

increase the ICAM-1 mRNA level and inhibit formation of the ICAM-1 translation initiation complex in human umbilical vein endothelial cells. J Biol Chem 1997;272:11994–12000.

17. Zellweger T, Miyake H, Monia B, et al. Efficacy of antisense clusterin oligonucleotides is improved in vitro and in vivo by incorporation of 2′-o-(2-methoxy) ethyl chemistry. J Pharmacol Exp Ther 2001; 298(3):934–940.

18. Hanahan D, Weinberg RA. The hallmarks of cancer. Cell 2000; 100:57–70.

19. Adams JM, Cory S. The Bcl-2 protein family: arbiters of cell survival. Science 1998; 281:1322–1326.

20. Folkman J. The role of angiogenesis in tumor growth. Semin Cancer Biol 1992; 3:65–71.

21. John A, Tuszynski G. The role of matrix metalloproteinases in tumor angiogenesis and tumor metastasis. Pathol Oncol Res 2001; 7:14–23.

22. Tsujimoto Y, Croce CM. Analysis of the structure, transcripts, and protein products of bcl-2, the gene involved in human follicular lymphoma. Proc Natl Acad Sci USA 1986; 83:5214–5218.

23. Sato T, Hanada M, Bodnig S, et al. Interactions among members of the bcl-2 protein family analysed with a yeast two-hybrid system. Proc Natl Acad Sci USA 1994; 91:9238–9242.

24. McDonnell TJ, Troncoso P, Brisby SM, et al. Expression of the protooncogene Bcl-2 in the prostate and its association with emergence of androgen-independent prostate cancer. Cancer Res 1992; 52:6940–6944.

25. Colombel M, Symmans F, Gil S, et al. Detection of the apoptosis-suppressing oncoprotein Bcl-2 in hormone-refractory human prostate cancers. Am J Pathol 1993; 143:390–400.

26. Raffo AJ, Periman H, Chen MW, et al. Overexpression of bcl-2 protects prostate cancer cells from apoptosis in vitro and confers resistance to androgen depletion in vivo. Cancer Res 1995; 55:4438–4445.

27. Paterson R, Gleave M, Jones E, et al. Immunohistochemical analysis of radical prostatectomy specimens after 8 months of neoadjuvant hormone therapy. Mol Urol 1999; 3:277–286.

28. Jansen B, Schlagbauer-Wadl H, Brown BD, et al. bcl-2 antisense therapy chemosensitizes human melanoma in SCID mice. Nat Med 1998; 4:232–234.

29. Miyake H, Tolcher A, Gleave ME. Antisense Bcl-2 oligodeoxynucleotides delay progression to androgen-independence after castration in the androgen dependent Shionogi tumor model. Cancer Res 1999; 59:4030–4034.

30. Miyake H, Tolcher A, Gleave ME. Antisense Bcl-2 Oligodeoxynucleotides enhance taxol chemosensitivity and synergistically delay progression to androgen-independence after castration in the androgen dependent Shionogi tumor model. JNCI 2000; 92:34–41.

31. Gleave ME, Tolcher A, Miyake H, et al. Progression to androgen-independence is delayed by antisense Bcl-2 oligonucleotides after castration in the LNCaP prostate tumor model. Clin Cancer Res 1999; 5:2891–2898.

32. Leung S, Miyake H, Jackson J, et al. Polymeric micellar paclitaxel phosphorylates Bcl-2 and induces apoptotic regression of androgen-independent LNCaP prostate tumors. Prostate 2000; 44:156–163.

33. Duggan BJ, Maxwell P, Kelly JD, et al. The effect of antisense Bcl-2 oligonucleotides on Bcl-2 protein expression and apoptosis in human bladder transitional cell carcinoma. J Urol 2001; 166:1098.

34. Duggan BJ, Cotter FE, Kelly JD, et al. Antisense Bcl-2 oligonucleotide uptake in human transitional cell carcinoma. Eur Urol 2001; 40:685.

35. Bilim V, Kasahara T, Noboru H, et al. Caspase involved synergistic cytotoxicity of bcl-2 antisense oligonucleotides and adriamycin on transitional cell cancer cells. Cancer Lett 2000; 155:191.

36. Webb A, Cunningham D, Cotter F, et al. Bcl-2 antisense therapy in patients with non-Hodgkin-lymphoma. Lancet 1997; 349:1137–1141.

37. Waters JS, Webb A, Cunningham D, et al. Phase I clinical and pharmacokinetic study of bcl-2 antisense oligonucleotide therapy in patients with non-Hodgkin's lymphoma. J Clin Oncol 2000; 18:1812–1823.

38. Morris MJ, Tong WP, Cordon-Cardo C, et al. Intravenous Bcl-2 antisense alone and in combination with paclitaxel in patients with advanced cancer. Clin Cancer Res. 2002; 8(3):679–683.

39. Jansen B, Wacheck V, Heere-Ress E, et al. Chemosensitisation of malignant melanoma by BCL2 antisense therapy. Lancet 2000; 356:1728–1733.

40. Chi KN, Gleave ME, Klasa R, et al. A phase I dose-finding study of combined treatment with an antisense Bcl-2 oligonucleotide (Genasense) and mitoxantrone in patients with metastatic hormone-refractory prostate cancer. Clin Cancer Res 2001; 7(12):3920–3927.

41. Boise L, Gonzaalez-Garcia M, Postema C, et al. bcl-x, a bcl-2-related gene that functions as a dominant regulator of apoptotic cell death. Cell 1993; 74:597–608.

42. Leech SH, Olie RA, Gautschi O, et al. Induction of apoptosis in lung-cancer cells following bcl-xL anti-sense treatment. Int J Cancer 2000; 86:570–576.

43. Simoes-Wust AP, Olie RA, Gautschi O, et al. Bcl-xl antisense treatment induces apoptosis in breast carcinoma cells. Int J Cancer 2000; 87:582–590.

44. Lebedeva I, Rando R, Ojwang J, et al. Bcl-xL in prostate cancer cells: effects of overexpression and down-regulation on chemosensitivity 1. Cancer Res 2000; 60:6052–6060.

45. Miyaki H, Monia B, Gleave ME. Antisense Bcl-xL and Bcl-2 Oligodeoxynucleotides synergistically enhance taxol chemosensitivity and delay progression to androgen-independence after castration in the androgen dependent Shionogi tumor model. Int J Cancer 2000; 86:855–862.

46. Zangemeister-Wittke U, Leech SH, Olie RA, et al. A novel bispecific antisense oligonucleotide inhibiting both bcl-2 and bcl-xL expression efficiently induces apoptosis in tumor cells. Clin Cancer Res 2000; 6:2547–2555.

47. Gautschi O, Tschopp S, Olie RA, et al. Activity of a novel bcl-2/bcl-xL-bispecific antisense oligonucleotide against tumors of diverse histologic origins. J Natl Cancer Inst 2001; 93:463–471.

48. Koch-Brandt C, Morgans C. Clusterin: a role in cell survival in the face of apoptosis? Prog Mol Subcell Biol 1996; 16:130–149 [Review].

49. Wilson MR, Easterbrook-Smith SB. Clusterin is a secreted mammalian chaperone. Trends Biochem Sci 2000; 25:95–98.

50. Zellweger T, Miyake H, July LV, et al. Chemosensitization of human renal cell cancer using antisense oligonucleotides targeting the antiapoptotic gene clusterin. Neoplasia 2001; 3:360–367.

51. Hara I, Miyake H, Gleave ME, Kamidono S. Introduction of clusterin gene into human renal cell carcinoma cells enhances their resistance to cytotoxic chemotherapy through inhibition of apoptosis both in vitro and in vivo. Jpn J Cancer Res 2001; 92(11):1220–1224.

52. Miyake H, Hara S, Zellweger T, et al. Acquisition of resistance to fas-mediated apoptosis by overexpression of clusterin in human renal-cell carcinoma cells. Mol Urol 2001; 5(3):105–111.

53. Miyake H, Gleave M, Kamidono S, Hara I. Overexpression of clusterin in transitional cell carcinoma of the bladder is related to disease progression and recurrence. Urology 2002; 59(1):150–154.

54. Miyake H, Hara, I Kamidono S, Gleave ME. Synergistic chemsensitization and inhibition of tumor growth and metastasis by the antisense oligodeoxynucleotide targeting clusterin gene in a human bladder cancer model. Clin Cancer Res 2001; 7(12):4245–4252.

55. Gleave ME, Akbari, M, and Gilks B. Unpublished data.

56. Miyake H, Rennie P, Nelson C, et al. Testosterone-repressed prostate message-2 (TRPM-2) is an antiapoptotic gene that confers resistance to androgen ablation in prostate cancer xenograft models. Cancer Res 2000; 60:170–176.

57. Miyake H, Rennie P, Nelson C, Gleave ME. Acquisition of chemoresistant phenotype by overexpression of the antiapoptotic gene, testosterone-repressed prostate message-2 (TRPM-2), in prostate cancer xenograft models. Cancer Res 2000; 60:2547–2554.

58. Miyake H, Chi KN, Gleave ME. Antisense TRPM-2 oligodeoxynucleotides chemosensitize human androgen-independent PC-3 prostate cancer cells both in vitro and in vivo Clin Cancer Res 2000; 6:1655–1663.

59. July LV, Akbari M, Zellweger T, et al. Clusterin expression is significantly enhanced in prostate cancer cells following androgen withdrawal therapy. Prostate. 2002; 50(3):179–188.

60. Gregory CW, Hamil KG, Kim D, et al. Androgen receptor expression in androgen-independent prostate cancer is associated with increased expression of androgen regulated genes. Cancer Res 1998;58:5718–5724.

61. Feldman BJ, Feldman D. The development of androgen-independent prostate cancer. Nature Rev 2001; 1:34–45.

62. Denis L, Murphy GP. Overview of phase III trials on combined androgen treatment in patients with metastatic prostate cancer. Cancer 1993; 72:3888–3895.

63. Eder IE, Culig Z, Ramoner R, et al. Inhibition of LNCaP prostate cancer cells by means of androgen receptor antisense oligonucleotides. Cancer Gene Ther 2000; 7(7):997–1007.

64. Jones JI, Clemmons DR. Insulin-like growth factors and their binding proteins: biological actions. Endocrinol Rev 1995; 16:3–34.

65. Nickerson T, Pollak M, Huynh H. Castration-induced apoptosis in rat ventral prostate is associated with increased expression of genes encoding insulin-like growth factor binding proteins 2, 3, 4 and 5. Endocrinology 1998; 139:807–810.

66. Figueroa JA, De Raad S, Tadlock L, et al. Differential expression of insulin-like growth factor binding proteins in high versus low Gleason score prostate cancer. J Urol 1998; 159:1379–1383.

67. Miyake H, Nelson C, Rennie P, Gleave ME. Overexpression of insulin-like growth factor binding protein-5 helps accelerate progression to androgen-independence in the human prostate LNCaP tumor model through activation of phosphatidylinositol 3'-kinase pathway. Endocrinology 2000; 141:2257–2265.

68. Miyake H, Pollak M, Nelson C, Gleave ME. Antisense insulin-like growth factor binding protein-5 oligodeoxynucleotides inhibit progression to androgen-independence after castration in the Shionogi tumor model via negative modulation of insulin-like growth factor-I action. Cancer Res 2000; 60:3058–3064.

69. Kiyama S, Zellweger T, Akbari M, et al. Antisense oligonucleotides inhibit castration-induced increases in insulin-like growth factor-binding protein-2 and delay progression to androgen-independence in the human prostate LNCaP tumor model. (Submitted)

70. Roy N, Deveraux Q, Takahashi R, et al. The c-IAP and c-IAP-2 proteins are direct inhibitors of specific caspases. EMBO J 1997; 16:6914–6925.

71. Deveraux Q, Takahashi R, Salvesen GS, Reed JC. X-linked IAP is a direct inhibitor of cell-death proteases. Nature 1997; 17:300–304.

72. Deveraux Q, Leo E, Stennicke HR, et al. Cleavage of human inhibitor of apoptosis protein XIAP results in fragments with distinct specificities for caspases. EMBO J 1999; 18:5242–5251.

73. Lacasse EC, Baird S, Korneluk RG, Mackenzie AE. The inhibitors of apoptosis (IAPs) and their emerging role in cancer. Oncogene 1998; 17:3247–3259.

74. Li F, Ambrosini G, Chu EY, et al. Control of apoptosis and mitotic spindle checkpoint by survivin. Nature 1998; 396:580–583.

75. Ambrosini G, Adida C, Altieri DC. A novel anti-apoptosis gene, survivin, expressed in cancer and lymphoma. Nature Med 1997; 3:917–921.

76. Tamm I, Wang Y, Sausville E, et al. IAP-family protein survivin inhibits caspase activity and apoptosis induced by Fas, Bax, and anticancer drugs. Cancer Res 1998; 58:5315–5320.

77. Lu CD, Altieri DC, Tanigawa N. Expression of a novel antiapoptosis gene, survivin, correlated with tumor cell apoptosis and p53 accumulation in gastric carcinomas. Cancer Res 1998; 58:1808–1812.

78. Kawasaki H, Altieri DC, Lu CD, et al. Inhibition of apoptosis by survivin predicts shorter survival rates in colorectal carcinoma. Cancer Res 1998; 58:5071–5074.

79. Adida C, Berrebi D, Peuchmaur M, et al. Anti-apoptosis gene, survivin, and prognosis of neuroblastoma. Lancet 1998; 351:882–883.

80. Olie RA, Simoes-Wust AP, Baumann B, et al. A novel antisense oligonucleotide targeting survivin expression induces apoptosis and sensitizes lung cancer cells to chemotherapy. Cancer Res 2000; 60:2805–2809.

81. Chen J, Wu W, Tahir SK, et al. Down-regulation of survivin by antisense oligonucleotides increases apoptosis, inhibits cytokinesis, and anchorage-independent growth. Neoplasia 2000; 2(3):235–241.

13

Bisphosphonates: a potential new treatment strategy in prostate cancer

Jonathan P Coxon and Grenville M Oades

Introduction

In 1998 prostate cancer was the most commonly registered new malignant diagnosis and the second most commonly registered cause of cancer related death amongst men, after lung cancer, in southeast England.[1] Together with cancers of the breast, lung, thyroid and kidney, it accounts for more than 80% of metastatic bone disease. At the time of diagnosis approximately one-quarter of men with prostate cancer in the UK will have distant metastases and around 90% of these individuals will have bone involvement.[2]

In addition to their frequency of occurrence, bone metastases in prostate cancer are frequently symptomatic and often responsible for considerable deterioration of quality of life in those with advanced disease, being the most frequent cause of morbidity. In prostate cancer, the metastases are primarily osteoblastic in nature, in contrast to most other cancers which tend to produce osteolytic lesions. Despite this, bone loss is a major contributory factor behind these various presentations of metastatic prostate cancer, as is discussed further later.

Current treatment of the prostate cancer patient with bony metastases is primarily palliative, with a reduction in bone pain being a particularly important goal in aiming towards improved quality of life and performance status. Once primary hormonal therapy has failed, management can be extremely difficult as the response to any further hormonal or cytotoxic therapy is poor. Given a median survival of around only 6 months in hormone-refractory patients with painful metastases, the side effects of any chosen therapy should be minimal, with optimal efficacy.[3]

This chapter focuses on current thinking on the interaction of prostate cancer with bone, providing the background to introduce the potential role of bisphosphonates in the treatment and prevention of prostate cancer metastasizing to bone.

Clinical aspects of bone metastases

Before considering the pathophysiology of the interaction of prostate cancer with bone, and the consequential potential role for bisphosphonates, a brief further background on the clinical impact of this problem is outlined.

The predilection of prostate cancer for the bones is well known. Unsurprisingly, clinical stage and Gleason grading correlate well with the long-term development of bone metastases. Considering patients treated with active surveillance, patients with T1/T2 disease develop metastases in 3–41% of cases at 10 years, in contrast to 12–55% of T3/T4 cases. Patients with well, moderately or poorly differentiated tumors develop metastases at 10 years in 2.7–10%, 13–57% and 42–80%, respectively (reviewed in Carlin & Andriole[4]).

The formation of bony metastases after radical prostatectomy is rare. One large study followed around 2000 men for a median of 5 years postoperation, without adjuvant treatment; 15% developed biochemical recurrence, and 5% developed bony metastases. The median actuarial time from prostate specific antigen (PSA) recurrence to metastasis was 8 years.[5] There is a similar picture after radiotherapy treatment, with one study finding 29% of patients developing PSA recurrence at a mean follow up of 4 years, and a total of 6% developing bony metastases.[6]

Bony spread from the prostate tends to be focused on axial areas of the skeleton with a good blood supply, especially the vertebral column, ribs, skull and proximal ends of long bones. Preferential seeding to the spinal column has been explained by the Batson venous plexus, which provides a low-pressure system for accessing the vertebral veins.

Radiographic evaluation

As the risk of bony metastases is well appreciated, radiographic evaluation forms an integral part of the initial work-up of many newly diagnosed cases of prostate cancer. Radionuclide imaging remains the most commonly used modality to aid diagnosis of bony metastases. Focal increases in the uptake of radiotracers, which are based on the bisphosphonate structure and so strongly localize to bone, are noted as suspicious. While the bone scan is a very sensitive investigation, specificity is less impressive and further evaluation is then needed – usually as a plain radiograph of the region in question to further evaluate any pathology. This helps to distinguish metastases from other lesions such as arthritic changes, osteoporosis and old fractures. Some centers propose the use of magnetic resonance imaging (MRI) for assessing bony involvement, but this is not widely practiced.

Skeletal complications

Potential skeletal complications from prostate cancer spread are numerous, and include intermittent or constant bone pain, pathological fractures, vertebral collapse, spinal cord compression and occasionally bone marrow suppression, leukopenia or derangements in calcium metabolism. Palliative treatment essentially comprises initiating hormone manipulation therapy (through testicular or total androgen ablation), with or without focal radiotherapy. Approximately 80% of men with bony metastases will have symptomatic improvement with androgen deprivation alone. The median survival for patients with bony metastases treated with hormonal therapy is 30–35 months, though this is longer for those with a solitary metastasis.[7] When the cancer develops into a hormone-refractory state, available treatment options for the patient, and in particular for his bony metastases, are few. Hence there is a great deal of interest in seeking out alternative therapies for this widespread problem.

Pathophysiology of bone metastases in prostate cancer

In adults normal bone is being continually remodeled, under the influence of systemic hormones and local bone-derived growth factors. The rich milieu of cytokines and growth factors in bone matrix provide a favorable soil for seeding of metastases from certain circulating tumor cells.[8] Metastatic bone lesions can interfere with normal bone homeostasis by causing the abnormal release of cytokines and growth factors that can alter the bone microenvironment. Activation of normal bone cells plays a central role in the initiation and growth of metastatic bone lesions. The normal process of bone remodeling and the inherent coupling of resorption with formation is altered by the presence of tumor resulting in increased bone resorption and/or increased bone formation.

Cancer metastasizing to bone often causes bone destruction or osteolysis. It is believed that prostate cancer, despite producing typically osteosclerotic lesions, initially also causes focal resorption, as well as generalized osteolysis, as is discussed below. There is substantial evidence to show that the increased bone resorption in many bone metastases is mainly osteoclast mediated and, whilst locally activated by tumor, is not mediated by cancer cells themselves. Histomorphometric measurements of bone biopsies from patients with metastatic breast cancer have shown that the number of osteoclasts is significantly increased in bone immediately adjacent to tumor as well as within metastases. Parathyroid hormone related protein (PTHrP) is a major factor responsible for osteoclast-mediated bone resorption at the site of bone metastases. Its expression is far more common in bone metastases than in metastases at other sites and levels are positively correlated to the presence of bony metastases and hypercalcemia in patients with breast cancer (reviewed in Guise & Mundy[8]). PTHrP is widely expressed in prostate cancer.[9]

Parathyroid hormone related protein (PTHrP)

The molecular mechanisms by which PTHrP stimulates bone resorption have now been elucidated (Fig. 13.1). The osteoclast is a specialized macrophage whose differentiation is principally regulated by macrophage colony-stimulating factor (M-CSF), receptor activator of nuclear factor kappa B ligand (RANKL) and osteoprotegerin.[10] RANKL is secreted by osteoblasts and induces terminal differentiation of osteoclast precursors by binding to its receptor, RANK, located on osteoclast precursor cells. RANK and RANKL, together

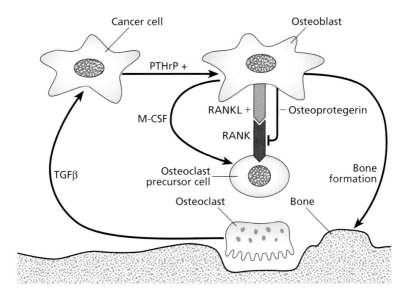

Figure 13.1 Mechanisms of bone metastasis development in prostate cancer. Parathyroid hormone related peptide (PTHrP) produced by metastatic prostate cancer cells induces osteoblasts to stimulate osteoclastogenesis by increasing the expression of receptor activator of NF-kappa B ligand (RANKL) which acts via the receptor activator of NF-kappa B (RANK) on the osteoclast. This activity can be limited by the binding of RANKL by osteoprotegerin. Paracrine factors from prostate cancer cells and the release of agents such as transforming growth factor beta (TGFβ) from bone by osteoclastic activity alter the bone microenvironment and cause osteoblastic activation. MCS-F, macrophage-colony stimulating factor.

with M-CSF (which initiates differentiation of uncommitted precursors), are sufficient for osteo-clastogenesis. Osteoclast differentiation from precursor cells is inhibited in a dose-dependent manner by recombinant osteoprotegerin. It has been shown that osteoprotegerin can bind to RANKL, limiting its biological actions. Cancer cells are unable to act as surrogate osteoblasts as they do not express RANKL and are therefore unable to directly stimulate osteoclastogenesis.[11] Rather, they act through induction of osteoblast signaling. When MCF-7 breast cancer cells overexpressing PTHrP are added to co-cultures of murine osteo-blasts and undifferentiated hemopoietic cells, osteoclast formation results without addition of any other osteotropic agents.[11] This suggests that cancer cells facilitate the lytic potential of osteoclasts via the action of cancer cell-derived PTHrP on osteoblasts, which causes the release of osteoclastogenic factors.

Transforming growth factor beta
The enhancement of osteoclast numbers and activity in bone metastases results in pronounced osteolysis with the subsequent release of bone-derived growth factors such as transforming growth factor beta (TGF-beta). TGF-beta has been demonstrated to decrease RANKL mRNA and enhance osteoprotegerin mRNA levels in osteo-blasts, a sequence of events that normally would usefully limit osteoclastogenesis and aid remodel-ing in normal bone. In bone containing metastatic cells, however, the microenvironment is changed and TGF-beta also acts on cancer cells, stimulating production of cytokines and growth factors that induce osteoclast activity. TGF-beta has been shown to significantly stimulate PTHrP expression in human breast cancer cells.[8] TGF-beta may therefore be an important factor in the establish-ment and progression of cancer metastases to bone.

Sclerotic metastases

As prostate cancer is more frequently associated with sclerotic metastases, prostate cancer cells must possess properties different from those of other tumors commonly associated with lytic metastases. The cellular and molecular mechanisms underlying this phenomenon are largely unknown. This is due at least in part to a lack of appropriate models to address these questions experimentally, which is in stark contrast to breast cancer, behind which research in the prostate cancer field is lagging. Sclerotic metastases are likely to be due to the production of soluble factors that can stimulate bone formation. A number of osteoblastic factors have been identified in prostate carcinoma tissue, including insulin-like growth factors, prostate specific antigen, fibroblast growth factor, bone morphogenic protein, urokinase-type plasminogen activator and endothelin-1.[12] Despite the osteoblastic tendencies in sclerotic metastases there is much evidence to suggest that osteolysis is a regular feature of prostate cancer bone disease. Indeed, osteolysis may be a necessary part of tumor invasiveness in bone.

Histological studies

Histological studies have shown that indices of bone resorption as well as bone-forming surfaces and active osteoblast numbers are increased in skeletal sites adjacent to metastatic prostate tumor tissue. In a series of 78 iliac crest biopsies of patients with prostate cancer bone metastases, the fraction of eroded trabecular surfaces was consistently high and proportional to the severity of tumor invasion.[13] Eroded surfaces have been shown to be greatest within metastases but are associated with increased bone volume due to replacement of the existing trabecular tissue with osteoid and abnormal weakened woven bone, giving an overall appearance of sclerosis. In vivo evidence exists showing the induction of osteolysis by prostate cancer. When the androgen insensitive prostate carcinoma cell line PC3 is injected intracardially into athymic male mice, an early response is the induction of extensive osteolysis, detected radiologically. These cells express known bone resorbing factors such as M-CSF and PTHrP.[14] Similar observations have been made following the systemic administration in nude mice of a breast carcinoma cell line that forms sclerotic metastases. The first event in this model was an increase in osteoclast-mediated bone resorption followed later by an increase in bone formation at the same sites.[15]

Clinical studies

Evidence of osteoclastic activity in metastatic prostate cancer also comes from clinical studies. Increased biochemical indices of bone resorption are consistently found in patients with bone metastases. Ikeda et al[16] showed that prostate carcinoma patients with active bone metastases had a higher urinary excretion of pyridinoline and deoxypyridinoline, specific markers of bone resorption, than did patients with benign prostatic hyperplasia (BPH), with localized disease or with bone metastases well controlled on hormonal therapy. Urinary levels of these collagen breakdown products correlated with the extent of bone metastases.[29] That increased osteoblastic activity may be associated with increased osteoclastic activity in patients with metastatic prostate cancer was also suggested by work showing serum alkaline phosphatase activity to be positively correlated to urinary hydroxyproline excretion, suggesting a link between bone formation and resorption.[13] However, the slope of this correlation deviated from the line of identity, representing the predominance of the osteoblastic component.

Taken together these observations indicate that osteolysis plays a crucial role in the appearance and growth of prostate cancer bone lesions. The classic sclerotic bone lesions seen in prostate cancer represent an uncoupling of normal bone resorption and deposition shifting the balance towards new matrix formation and mineralization. The presence of osteoclastic bone resorption associated with prostate cancer bone metastasis provides one rationale for the use of bisphosphonates in the treatment of patients with advanced prostate cancer.

Bisphosphonates

Bisphosphonates are potent inhibitors of osteoclastic bone resorption. For this reason, these drugs are established therapeutic options in the treatment of diseases involving osteoclast overactivity, such as Paget's disease, postmenopausal osteoporosis and general tumor-associated bone disease. They can be considered to be ideal drugs for use in a palliative setting because of their low incidence of side effects and complications. Oral preparations have to be taken in relatively high doses, due

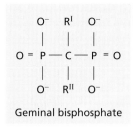

Figure 13.2 Geminal bisphosphonate structure.

to their very poor absorption and complexing with any calcium in food, and are sometimes associated with gastrointestinal side effects such as dyspepsia.

Bisphosphonates are analogs of natural inorganic pyrophosphates, in which the oxygen bridge between phosphate groups has been replaced by a carbon atom. This alteration creates a molecule highly resistant to hydrolysis, and so clinically more viable. The addition of different carbon side chains has generated a diverse group of compounds based on a geminal bisphosphonate structure (Fig. 13.2). The R^I side chain is usually a hydroxyl group but the R^{II} side chain varies considerably and accounts for the widely differing potencies of these compounds. Early, first generation, bisphosphonates – lacking nitrogen atoms in the R^{II} chain – include clodronate and etidronate. A longer R^{II} chain generally provides greater potency, as does the addition of a primary (e.g. pamidronate), secondary (e.g. ibandronate) or tertiary amine group (e.g. zoledronate), in increasing order of potency. These latter compounds are termed the aminobisphosphonates.

Bisphosphonates form a 3-dimensional structure that binds with high avidity to divalent ions. It is the strong binding with calcium that underlies the bone targeting properties of this compound. The ability to adsorb to bone mineral in vivo, to exposed hydroxyapatite crystals, selectively delivers bisphosphonates to sites of active bone remodeling, and explains their rapid disappearance from the circulation. In particular, they appear to localize to sites of osteoclast activity. The binding to bone forms the basis for the use of these compounds as skeletal markers in nuclear medicine when linked to 99m-technetium. Once bisphosphonates are bound to the skeleton they will be released only when bone is destroyed in the course of turnover or metastatic erosion. The ability to chelate Ca^{2+} ions is reduced at low pH. Therefore,

in the acidic environment of the resorption lacuna, bisphosphonates are released and their local concentrations may reach several hundred micromolar.[12] This may be extremely relevant when considering various in vitro effects of bisphosphonates, achieved at varying concentrations, as discussed below.

As recently described, the action of bisphosphonates on bone can be considered at tissue, cellular and molecular levels.[17] At the tissue level the principal action of all bisphosphonates is to decrease bone turnover. There is good evidence that the first step in this process is a reduction in bone resorption as shown by a reduction in urinary excretion of bone resorption markers such as cross-linked collagen peptides containing pyridinoline. Decreased bone formation is secondary to inhibition of resorption and reflects reduced bone remodeling. Bisphosphonates do not directly suppress bone formation. At the cellular level the principal site of action of bisphosphonates in normal bone is the osteoclast. In vitro and in vivo evidence supports at least four ways in which bisphosphonates can inhibit osteoclast activity: inhibition of early osteoclast differentiation; inhibition of osteoclast maturation; inhibition of activity of mature osteoclasts and induction of apoptosis (reviewed in Rodan[18]). This is particularly interesting when one learns that initial information from the pharmaceutical industry ruled out any cytotoxic effects.

Direct effects of bisphosphonates on osteoclasts and cancer cells

Bisphosphonates were well known to inhibit osteoclast activity, and for a long time it was thought that any improvements in cancer patient outcomes were due uniquely to this action on osteoclasts. This may explain why so few studies have previously looked at survival as an outcome with bisphosphonate treatment. An exciting oncological development came with observations that direct effects could also be observed in tumor cells – namely myeloma, breast and prostate cancer cells.

Induction of apoptosis

There is now substantial evidence to show that bisphosphonates induce osteoclast apoptosis both in vitro and in vivo.[19] The resultant decrease in osteoclast number on the bone surface thus reduces osteoclastic resorption. Since osteoclasts are highly endocytic, it seemed likely that bisphosphonates in the resorption lacunae would be internalized by the osteoclast and hence have intracellular mechanisms of action. At the molecular level the definitive targets responsible for bisphosphonate inhibition of osteoclastic bone resorption, including induction of apoptosis, are beginning to be identified. There is increasing evidence to suggest that not all bisphosphonates act through similar mechanisms. The aminobisphosphonates may exert different intracellular effects from the earlier, less potent forms. Importantly, it appears that the molecular effects on osteoclasts are replicated in some tumor cells.

Mammalian cells metabolize clodronate to a non-hydrolyzable adenosine triphosphate (ATP) analog.[20] It is likely that any growth-inhibitory and cytotoxic effects of bisphosphonates such as clodronate are the result of cytoplasmic accumulation of these toxic metabolites. These compete with ATP in enzymatic reactions, ultimately resulting in cell death. Non-hydrolyzable ATP analogs cannot, however, be detected in mammalian cells after 24-hour treatment with aminobisphosphonates. A different mechanism of action has recently been proposed for these drugs. Aminobisphosphonates can inhibit enzymes of the mevalonate pathway.[21] This biosynthetic pathway is responsible for the production, from mevalonate, of various steroids, including cholesterol and isoprenoid lipids such as farnesyl pyrophosphate and geranylgeranyl pyrophosphate. These latter compounds are required for the post-translational modification (isoprenylation) of a number of important cellular proteins, such as laminins and small guanosine triphosphate binding proteins (G proteins), including Ras, Rho and Rac. These modifications are essential for cytoskeletal integrity and intracellular signaling by allowing these proteins to localize to the plasma membrane (Fig. 13.3). Hence inhibition of the pathway can lead to loss of cell viability, or apoptosis.

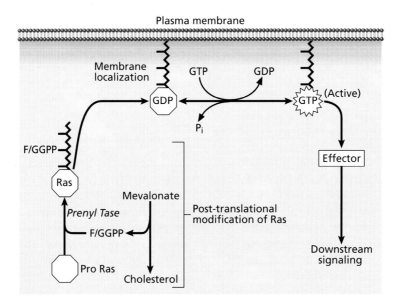

Figure 13.3 Post-translational modification, membrane localization and activation of Ras. Farnesyl pyrophosphate and geranylgeranyl pyrophosphate (F/GGPP) are transferred to cysteine residues on proteins such as Ras by prenylprotein transferases (*Prenyl Tase*). This allows association of the Ras protein with the inner surface of the plasma membrane, an essential step for its activation. GDP, guanosine 5'-diphosphate; GTP, guanosine 5'-triphosphate; Pi, inorganic phosphate

Inhibition of the mevalonate pathway has been identified as a possible target for anticancer therapy. Phenylacetate, an inhibitor of farnesyl transferase, inhibits protein isoprenylation including Ras farnesylation in LNCaP prostate cancer cells, resulting in apoptosis in this cell line.[22] While the initial actions of aminobisphosphonates on the mevalonate pathway were described using macrophages, it appears they are capable of inducing apoptosis in other cell lines in a similar way. Studies in other cancer cell lines have shown aminobisphosphonates can induce apoptosis.[23] It has been observed that inhibition of the mevalonate pathway and prevention of protein prenylation does occur.[24] Growth inhibitory effects of the aminobisphosphonates pamidronate and zoledronic acid on the prostate carcinoma cell lines LNCaP, PC3 and DU145 have previously been demonstrated[25] and zoledronic acid has been shown to induce apoptosis by inhibition of the mevalonate pathway in prostate cancer.[26] A good deal of support for this comes from demonstrating reversal of the effects on apoptosis by adding geranylgeraniol, a cell-permeable form of geranylgeranyl pyrophosphate, which bypasses the inhibition of the pathway by the bisphosphonate.[26]

Interruption of the metastatic cascade

Bisphosphonates have the ability to prevent tumor-induced osteolysis and delay progression of metastasis in rodent models of prostate cancer.[27] Treatment with bisphosphonates suppressed and delayed the development of hind leg paralysis in male Copenhagen rats using the intravenous injection of MLL tumor cells and concomitant caval vein clamping as a model for causing lumbar metastasis. Metastasis of tumor cells to bone is a complex cascade involving angiogenesis, loss of tumor cell adhesion, invasion of the vasculature, embolism, evasion of host defense, arrest at a distant site, extravasation and establishment of new growth.[8] There is preclinical evidence that bisphosphonates may interrupt this pathway in prostatic bone metastasis at a number of points.

Angiogenesis

In order for a tumor to grow beyond a size of $1-2$ mm^3 and metastasize, it must develop a new vascular network and angiogenesis is therefore an integral part of the metastatic cascade. Preliminary evidence suggests that bisphosphonates may have antiangiogenic potential. Zoledronate has been shown to inhibit proliferation and induce apoptosis in human umbilical vein endothelial cells in vitro. In a subcutaneous murine growth factor implant model, zoledronate dose-dependently inhibited the angiogenic response induced by fibroblast growth factor.[28]

Invasion

Tumor cell invasion may also be a target for bisphosphonate action. Boissier et al[29] showed that preincubation with bisphosphonates inhibited breast and prostate cancer cell line invasion in a Matrigel invasion assay. Inhibition of invasion was through a specific action on tumor cells. Tumor cell invasion requires digestion of the basement membrane matrix, by matrix metalloproteinases (MMPs). These enzymes may also have a role in tumor-mediated osteolysis. A possible mechanism by which bisphosphonates may affect invasion is via inhibition of the proteolytic activity of MMPs.[29] Unpublished work from France, using breast cancer cells, has provided good evidence that inhibition of invasion is modulated via inhibition of prenylation and subsequent membrane localization of the G protein Rho, at concentrations of zoledronate considerably lower than those required for apoptosis. Rho is known to play a central role in cytoskeletal trafficking.

Adhesion to bone

The localization and subsequent growth of a tumor metastasis in the skeleton depends on the ability of tumor cells to adhere to specific ligands on endothelial cells, bone marrow stroma and the extracellular matrix. Bossier et al[30] evaluated direct effects of various aminobisphosphonates on the ability of prostate and breast cancer cells to adhere to unmineralized and mineralized bone matrices. Pretreatment of these cells subsequently inhibited adhesion, providing evidence for a direct cellular effect of bisphosphonates in preventing tumor cell adhesion to bone.[30] The bisphosphonates used in this study – ibandronate, NE-10244 (an analog of risedronate), pamidronate and clodronate – did not exert any cytotoxic effects following 24 hours' treatment at concentrations used to inhibit tumor cell adhesion.

Bisphosphonates as a treatment of choice in prostate cancer

Preclinical studies indicate a potential role for bisphosphonates not only for the treatment, but also for the prevention of bone metastases due to prostate cancer. A number of trials have been conducted to investigate the clinical potential of bisphosphonate therapy. However, there are disappointingly relatively few randomized controlled trials – in comparison to breast cancer, for example.

Before outlining some of the clinical work that has been done, it is useful to consider a number of issues regarding the evidence for use of bisphosphonates in managing patients with prostate cancer:[14]

1. It should be appreciated that there has been a great deal of skepticism at times regarding the use of bisphosphonates for treating predominantly osteoblastic lesions.
2. In contrast to cancers producing osteolytic lesions, prostate cancer tends to be associated with fewer of the hard endpoints for progression of metastasis, such as hypercalcemia, pathological fractures and vertebral collapse. Studies therefore need to rely more on outcomes such as pain and quality of life, which are notoriously more difficult to accurately assess objectively.
3. Assessing the progression of the extent of metastatic bone disease in response to treatment can be very difficult, especially as patients with prostate carcinoma who may be deemed suitable for bisphosphonate treatment often have a baseline of extensive skeletal involvement. It is not surprising then that, in comparison to breast carcinoma, fewer studies have looked at the efficacy of bisphosphonates in prostate cancer. Consequently, the overall picture is less clear cut, but some encouraging results have been reported.

Bone pain

It is thought that tumor-induced bone resorption is a major contributory factor causing bone pain in advanced cancer with skeletal metastasis.[8] Bisphosphonates have been shown to reduce pain in women with advanced breast cancer and clinically evident bone metastasis.[31] Patients with prostate cancer metastatic to the skeleton show acute metabolic changes following bisphosphonate administration that are very similar to those observed in other malignancies associated with osteolytic lesions. Thus it follows that bisphosphonates may also lessen bone pain in metastases from prostate cancer.

In an uncontrolled study in 1985 it was reported for the first time that treatment with intravenous clodronate induced sustained pain relief, and allowed mobilization of some bedridden patients with advanced prostate cancer.[32] This was followed by a number of open studies showing reductions in pain in metastatic prostate cancer patients receiving i.v. clodronate.[33,34] Unfortunately these results have not been supported by randomized trials of oral[35] or intravenous followed by oral[36] clodronate. No significant decrease in pain could be demonstrated in the treated groups, although all favored clodronate treatment. Experience from open trials with other bisphosphonates, such as etidronate, olpadronate and pamidronate[37,38] is similar, with encouraging results, especially for the later generation compounds. No meta-analysis has so far been performed.

The lack of confirmed efficacy of bisphosphonates in randomized studies for pain control, compared to studies in other malignancies, is disappointing though they are few in number. There are a number of possible explanations, in addition to the problem of measuring a subjective outcome. The studies were often small and may have been of insufficient power to determine a significant difference in symptomatic improvement. The potency of the compounds, mode of administration and dose and duration of treatment may also all play a role. It is hoped that more continuous administration of the newer generation bisphosphonates will provide more reproducible encouraging results.

Bone pain secondary to metastases has a complex etiology and tumor-induced osteolysis is not the only cause. Many other factors may also play a role. The pain in bone metastatic lesions may be partly due to immune responses. There is evidence indicating that inflammatory mediators, such as prostaglandins, can cause hyperalgesia in bone. Microfractures due to mechanical stress are also associated with bone pain, as are changes in intraosseous pressure.[39] Osteoporosis caused by androgen deprivation in patients with advanced prostate cancer may significantly contribute to bone pain and skeletal fracture.[40] Bisphosphonates, due to their primary effect on the osteoclast, would not be expected to have an effect on all these causes of bone pain.

Reduction of skeletal related events

Skeletal related events are complications of metastatic disease and include pathological fractures, the need for radiation or surgery to bone, spinal cord compression and hypercalcemia. A number of studies in other cancers have addressed the issue of attempting to limit skeletal morbidity with the prophylactic use of bisphosphonates once bony metastasis has been diagnosed. The results of two large, prospective randomized controlled trials in a total of 754 women with osteolytic metastasis secondary to breast cancer have recently been collated. Intravenous pamidronate (90 mg) every 3–4 weeks in addition to normal treatments significantly reduced skeletal morbidity.[41] Such are the deemed benefits of bisphosphonates in reducing skeletal-related morbidity in women with osteolytic metastases from breast cancer, that guidelines from the American Society of Clinical Oncology (ASCO) state that bisphosphonates should be routinely considered in these patients.[42]

This issue has been addressed less extensively in patients with prostate cancer, partly due to the conception that such events are much less common. However, encouraging evidence is emerging. An important double-blind, multicenter randomized study examined effects of zoledronic acid (4 or 8 mg via infusion every 3 weeks) in men with hormone-refractory prostate cancer and a history of metastatic bone disease. Treatment with 4 mg led to a significant reduction in skeletal related events (mainly pathological fracture and radiation therapy to bone) at 15 months, and a significant increase in the time to first skeletal related event. Pain scores were also decreased. Urinary markers of bone resorption were confirmed to be lower in the treated patients.[44] Zoledronic acid has now become the first and only bisphosphonate licensed for prevention of cancer-related bone complications in the UK. The MRC are currently conducting a phase III double-blind, placebo-controlled trial of oral clodronate in men with metastatic prostate cancer commencing or responding to standard hormonal treatment (Trial Pr05). By July 1998,

311 patients had been randomized and preliminary results showed that clodronate delayed progression to symptoms.[43]

To date, no survival advantage of bisphosphonates in the treatment of patients with metastatic disease has been demonstrated although the newer more potent aminobisphosphonates have yet to be extensively tested.

Bisphosphonates as adjuvant therapy

At present, treatment for metastatic bone disease and its associated complications is highly unsatisfactory and purely palliative. The idea of being able to achieve early prevention of bone disease, especially in patients at high risk of subsequent skeletal metastasis such as those with locally advanced prostate cancer, is therefore very appealing. Most early clinical studies for the use of bisphosphonates in prostate cancer were limited to patients in whom bone metastases were well established, as in many hormone-refractory cases. Such patients already have extensive tumor disease in bone, and tumor-free skeletal tissue may be very osteoporotic. This obviously provides less potential for impressive clinical effects than if treatment was started before the onset of the bone disease, using bisphosphonates in a preventative role before the skeleton has suffered irreparable damage. Preclinical laboratory work such as that outlined above, discussing effects on adhesion, invasion and apoptosis, contributes towards the rationale for such trials. Animal models have also shown delayed formation of bony metastases following administration of bisphosphonates (reviewed in Diel et al[45]).

Again, work with breast cancer patients precedes that with prostate cancer. Three separate randomized, placebo-controlled trials started around the same time, using oral clodronate (1600 mg daily) in addition to standard adjuvant therapy in patients with early breast cancer, have been inconsistent in their results. Diel et al[46] have reported a 2-year study in 302 patients with stage 1–3 breast cancer and confirmed micrometastatic bone marrow invasion. There was a significant decrease in the incidence of bony metastases in the treatment group.[46] Similar results have been reported in abstract form in a larger study with around 1000 patients[47] but the third – a conflicting study in 299 patients – showed no difference in the incidence of bone metastasis at 5 years.[48]

The results of similar studies in prostate cancer are eagerly awaited. The MRC is running a further double-blind, placebo-controlled trial to assess the possibility of using oral clodronate over a 5-year period to delay time to symptomatic bone metastases in patients who have locally advanced, non-metastatic adenocarcinoma of the prostate (Trial Pr04). Recruitment closed at the end of 1997 with 508 patients randomized. A similar placebo-controlled multicenter randomized trial investigating zoledronate in the prevention of bone metastases is also underway, in patients with biochemically recurrent prostate cancer who have rising PSA levels despite androgen deprivation (Novartis, Protocol 704).

The results of these studies and others in the future will be very useful in determining the best place for bisphosphonates in our armamentarium of treatment options in advanced prostate cancer. To gain results more quickly, studies should aim to enroll patients at high risk for early metastasis, namely those with regional lymph node involvement, local progression, or those with raised concentrations of specific prognostic factors for bone metastasis.

Calcium homeostasis and prostate bone metastasis

Malignancy related hypercalcemia is a serious metabolic disturbance associated with a number of cancers. The usual mechanism of this hypercalcemia is an increased release of calcium from diseased bone, although there may also be a humoral component via the actions of PTHrP on osteoclast activation. Intravenous fluid rehydration and bisphosphonate therapy is the standard treatment for severe, symptomatic hypercalcemia. Symptomatic hypercalcemia in men with metastatic prostate cancer is, however, uncommon. The low risk of hypercalcemia in these men could be explained by the increase in osteoblastic activity in most metastases, preventing the release of calcium from bone. It has, however, been established in this chapter that there is a generalized increase in osteoclastic activity in these patients. Histological findings suggest that prostatic cancer induces *generalized* loss of trabecular bone with *focal* increased deposition in the metastases.[16] This situation may minimize disturbances in plasma calcium homeostasis but could also contribute to

skeletal morbidity. It is also of interest to note that PSA cleavage of PTHrP can regulate the biological activity of this peptide, which may have a stabilizing effect on potential malignant hypercalcemia caused by this hormone.[9,19]

In contrast to most malignancies, hypocalcemia can be associated with metastatic prostate cancer. It is thought to be caused by calcium entrapment in bone as a consequence of excessive osteoblast activity in sclerotic metastasis ('bone hunger syndrome'). There have been a number of reports of low serum calcium levels in patients with advanced prostate cancer. Secondary hyperparathyroidism may occur frequently, and may contribute to the generalized osteoclastic activity in patients with focal osteoblastic metastases.[49] This may worsen any skeletal disease secondary to androgen deprivation. The progression of prostate cancer often accelerates once it has spread to the bone, supporting the theory that the bone microenvironment may provide stimulating factors for prostate cancer progression. A dangerous positive feedback could be set up in which elevated PTH levels could stimulate osteoclasts, increasing bone resorption and releasing bone-derived growth factors that may stimulate progression of prostate cancer. This would, in turn, cause further deposition of calcium in sclerotic metastases and consequently a further elevation in PTH.[49] There is a risk that bisphosphonate treatment in such patients, inhibiting resorption, could result in further falls in serum calcium and further worsening of secondary hyperparathyroidism, which could in turn lessen the effectiveness of treatment. Vitamin D or calcium supplementation may be a wise precaution in some individuals with sclerotic metastases in whom bisphosphonate therapy is being considered.

Preservation of bone mineral density during hormone therapy

It is well recognized that androgens have an important role in maintaining skeletal mass in men. Androgen deprivation therapy is the mainstay of treatment for metastatic prostate cancer. Evidence from the MRC trial looking at immediate versus deferred treatment has shown that early androgen deprivation may improve outcome in patients with locally advanced, non-metastatic disease.[50] Adjuvant hormone therapy starting at the beginning[51] or end[52] of radiotherapy for locally advanced prostate cancer and continuing for 3 years or more has also been reported to give a significant advantage in local and biochemical disease control, with a reduction in the risk of development of metastases at 5 years. There was also a significant survival advantage in these trials. Immediate antiandrogen therapy after radical prostatectomy and pelvic lymphadenectomy has also been shown to improve survival and reduce risk of recurrence in patients with node-positive prostate cancer.[53]

Taken together, these observations suggest that androgen deprivation therapy for prostate cancer is going to be used earlier in the natural history of the disease, often some time before the onset of metastases, and given for longer periods. This increased use of hormonal therapy may have important consequences, including possible increases in osteoporotic complications, as well as considerations of cost and other side effects including decreased energy levels, libido and muscle mass.

It is now realized that osteoporosis is an important potential complication of androgen deprivation therapy. It has been shown to rapidly accelerate bone loss and decrease bone mineral density in men with prostate cancer. A study in 235 men showed an osteoporotic fracture rate of 13.6% in patients treated with hormonal therapy, compared to 1.1% in a control group of age-matched men without prostate cancer (a 12.2-fold relative risk). In this study osteoporotic fractures were much more common than pathologic fractures (due to metastasis) or those due to major trauma. Bone mineral density studies confirmed a significant deterioration in those treated with hormone ablation, and this worsened with length of treatment.[40] There is consequently an important need for treatment strategies to be developed that do not diminish the antitumorigenic effectiveness of androgen ablation but which minimize skeletal complications.

Thus, there is a further indication for the potential use of bisphosphonates in prostate cancer. One study randomized 47 men with locally advanced prostate cancer receiving a gonadotropin releasing hormone (GnRH) agonist to receive pamidronate 60 mg i.v. every 12 weeks or placebo. There were significant differences between the two groups in mean changes in bone mineral density in the hip and spine, favoring pamidronate.[54] In females, similar effects on bone mineral density are known to be associated with large decreases in risk of fracture.

Conclusion

There is experimental evidence to suggest that bisphosphonates may have a role in the treatment and prevention of bone metastases secondary to prostate cancer. They have been shown to induce apoptosis in prostate cancer cells and interrupt the metastatic cascade by inhibiting angiogenesis, tumor cell invasion and adhesion to bone. Clinical evidence has emerged supporting a role for zoledonic acid in minimizing the development of skeletal complications in patients with established metastases. At present there is insufficient evidence from randomized trials to support the use of bisphosphonates for the preventation of bony metastases. Osteoporosis and its complications caused by androgen deprivation can be prevented by the use of bisphosphonates which justifies the early use of these agents in patients receiving this type of treatment. The newer, more potent bisphosphonates such as zoledronic acid warrant further study in large, randomized trials to assess treatment and prevention of bone metastases in prostate cancer.

References

1. Cancer in South East England 1998. London: Thames Cancer Registry; 2001.
2. Bubendorf L, Schopfer A, Wagner U, et al. Metastatic patterns of prostate cancer: an autopsy study of 1,589 patients. Hum Pathol 2000; 31:578–583.
3. Smith JA Jr, Soloway MS, Young MJ. Complications of advanced prostate cancer. Urology 1999; 54:8–15.
4. Carlin BI, Andriole GL. The natural history, skeletal complications, and management of bone metastases in patients with prostate cancer. Cancer 2000; 88:2989–2994.
5. Pound CR, Partin AW, Eisenberger MA, et al. Natural history of progression after PSA elevation following radical prostatectomy. JAMA 1999; 281:1591–1597.
6. Zagars GK, Pollack A, von Eschenbach AC. Serum testosterone: a significant determinant of metastatic relapse for irradiated localized prostate cancer. Urology 1997; 49:327–334.
7. Prostate Cancer Trialists' Collaborative Group. Maximum androgen blockade in advanced prostate cancer: an overview of 22 randomised trials with 3283 deaths in 5710 patients. Lancet 1995; 346:265–269.
8. Guise TA, Mundy GR. Cancer and bone. Endocrinol Rev 1998; 19:18–54.
9. Deftos LJ. Prostate carcinoma: production of bioactive factors. Cancer 2000; 88:3002–3008.

10. Teitelbaum SL. Bone resorption by osteoclasts. Science 2000; 289:1504–1508.

11. Thomas RJ, Guise TA, Yin JJ, et al. Breast cancer cells interact with osteoblasts to support osteoclast formation. Endocrinology 1999; 140:4451–4458.

12. Sato M, Grasser W, Endo N, et al. Bisphosphonates action. Alendronate localization in rat bone and effects on osteoclast ultrastructure. J Clin Invest 1991; 88:2095–2105.

13. Clarke NW, McClure J, George NJ. Morphometric evidence for bone resorption and replacement in prostate cancer. Br J Urol 1991; 68:74–80.

14. Papapoulos SE, Hamdy NA, van der Pluijm G. Bisphosphonates in the management of prostate carcinoma metastatic to the skeleton. Cancer 2000; 88:3047–3053.

15. Yi B, Williams PJ, Niewolna M, et al. Tumor-derived platelet-derived growth factor-BB plays a critical role in osteosclerotic bone metastasis in an animal model of human breast cancer. Cancer Res 2002; 62:917–923.

16. Ikeda I, Miura T, Kondo I. Pyridinium cross-links as urinary markers of bone metastases in patients with prostate cancer. Br J Urol 1996; 77:102–106.

17. Fleisch H. Bisphosphonates: mechanisms of action. Endocrinol Rev 1998; 19:80–100.

18. Rodan GA. Mechanisms of action of bisphosphonates. Annu Rev Pharmacol Toxicol 1998; 38:375–388.

19. Hughes DE, Wright KR, Uy HL, et al. Bisphosphonates promote apoptosis in murine osteoclasts in vitro and in vivo. J Bone Miner Res 1995; 10:1478–1487.

20. Frith JC, Monkkonen J, Blackburn GM, et al. Clodronate and liposome-encapsulated clodronate are metabolized to a toxic ATP analog, adenosine 5'-(beta, gamma-dichloromethylene) triphosphate, by mammalian cells in vitro. J Bone Miner Res 1997; 12:1358–1367.

21. Amin D, Cornell SA, Gustafson SK, et al. Bisphosphonates used for the treatment of bone disorders inhibit squalene synthase and cholesterol biosynthesis. J Lipid Res 1992; 33:1657–1663.

22. Danesi R, Nardini D, Basolo F, et al. Phenylacetate inhibits protein isoprenylation and growth of the androgen-independent LNCaP prostate cancer cells transfected with the T24 Ha-ras oncogene. Mol Pharmacol 1996; 49:972–979.

23. Senaratne SG, Pirianov G, Mansi JL, et al. Bisphosphonates induce apoptosis in human breast cancer cell lines. Br J Cancer 2000; 82:1459–1468.

24. Senaratne SG, Colston KW. Mechanisms involved in aminobisphosphonate-induced apoptosis in breast cancer cells. Proc Am Assoc Cancer Res 2001; [Abstract 2377].

25. Lee MV, Fong EM, Singer FR, Guenette RS. Bisphosphonate treatment inhibits the growth of prostate cancer cells. Cancer Res 2001; 61:2602–2608.

26. Oades GM, Senaratne SG, Clakre I, et al. Mechanisms of bisphosphonate induced apoptosis in prostate cancer. Eur Urol 2002; 1(suppl):158 [Abstract].

27. Sun YC, Geldof AA, Newling DW, Rao BR. Progression delay of prostate tumor skeletal metastasis effects by bisphosphonates. J Urol 1992; 148:1270–1273.

28. Wood J, Schnell JR, Green JR. Zoledronic acid (Zometa), a potent inhibitor of bone resorption, inhibits proliferation and induces apoptosis in human endothelial cells in vitro and is anti-angiogenic in a murine growth factor implant model. ASCO 2000; [Abstract 2620].

29. Boissier S. Ferreras M, Peyrichaud O, et al. Bisphosphonates inhibit breast and prostate carcinoma cell invasion, an early event in the formation of bone metastases. Cancer 2000; 60:2949–2954.

30. Boissier S, Magnetto S, Frappart L, et al. Bisphosphonates inhibit prostate and breast carcinoma cell adhesion to unmineralized and mineralized bone extracellular matrices. Cancer Res 1997; 57:3890–3894.

31. Pavlakis N, Stockler M. Bisphosphonates in breast cancer (Cochrane Review). Cochrane Database Syst 1992; CD003474.

32. Adami S, Salvagno G, Guarrera G, et al. Dichloromethylene-diphosphonate in patients with prostatic carcinoma metastatic to the skeleton. J Urol 1985; 134:1152–1154.

33. Voreuther R, Heidenrich A, Engelmann UH. Bisphosphonates in the treatment of bone metastases in prostate cancer. J Urol 1998; 159:335A.

34. Cresswell SM, English PJ, Hall RR, et al. Pain relief and quality-of-life assessment following intravenous and oral clodronate in hormone-escaped metastatic prostate cancer. Br J Urol 1995; 76:360–365.

35. Elomaa I, Kylmala T, Tammela T, et al. Effect of oral clodronate on bone pain. A controlled study in patients with metastatic prostatic cancer. Int Urol Nephrol 1992; 24:159–166.

36. Kylmala T, Taube T, Tammela TL, et al. Concomitant i.v. and oral clodronate in the relief of bone pain – a double-blind placebo-controlled study in patients with prostate cancer. Br J Cancer 1997; 76:939–942.

37. Clarke NW, Holbrook IB, McClure J, George NJ. Osteoclast inhibition by pamidronate in metastatic prostate cancer: a preliminary study. Br J Cancer 1991; 63:420–423.

38. Pelger RC, Lycklama a Nijeholt AA, Papapoulos SE. Short-term metabolic effects of pamidronate in patients with prostatic carcinoma and bone metastases. Lancet 1989; 2:865.

39. Haegerstam GA. Pathophysiology of bone pain: a review. Acta Orthop Scand 2001; 72:308–317.

40. Daniell HW. Osteoporosis after orchiectomy for prostate cancer. J Urol 1997; 157:439–444.

41. Lipton A, Theriault RL, Hortobagyi GN, et al. Pamidronate prevents skeletal complications and is effective palliative treatment in women with breast carcinoma and osteolytic bone metastases: long term follow-up of two randomized, placebo-controlled trials. Cancer 2000; 88:1082–1090.

42. Hillner BE, Ingle JN, Berenson JR, et al. American Society of Clinical Oncology guidelines on the role of bisphosphonates in breast cancer. J Clin Oncol 2000; 18:1378–1391.

43. Dearnaley DP, Sydes MR. Preliminary evidence that oral clodronate delays symptomatic progression of bone metastasis from prostate cancer: First results of the MRC Pr05 trial. ASCO 2001; [Abstract 693].

44. Saad F, Gleason DM, Murray R, et al. A randomized, placebo-controlled trial of zoledronic acid in patients with hormone-refractory metastatic prostate carcinoma. J Natl Cancer Inst 2002; 94:1458–1468.

45. Diel IJ, Solomayer E-F, Bastert G. Bisphosphonates and the prevention of metastasis. Cancer 2000; 88:3080–3088.

46. Diel IJ, Solomayer EF, Costa SD, et al. Reduction in new metastases in breast cancer with adjuvant clodronate treatment. N Engl J Med 1998; 339:357–363.

47. Powles TJ, Paterson AHG, Nevantaus A, Legault S. Adjuvant clodronate reduces the incidence of bone metastases in patients with primary operable breast cancer. Proc Am Soc Clin Oncol 1998; 17:123 [Abstract 468].

48. Saarto T, Blomqvist C, Virkkunen P, Elomaa I. Adjuvant clodronate treatment does not reduce the frequency of skeletal metastases in node-positive breast cancer patients: 5-year results of a randomized controlled trial. J Clin Oncol 2001; 19:10–17.

49. Murray RM, Grill V, Crinis N, et al. Hypocalcemic and normocalcemic hyperparathyroidism in patients with advanced prostatic cancer. J Clin Endocrinol Metab 2001; 86:4133–4138.

50. The Medical Research Council Prostate Cancer Working Party Investigators Group. Immediate versus deferred treatment for advanced prostatic cancer: initial results of the Medical Research Council trial. Br J Urol 1997; 79:235–246.

51. Bolla M, Gonzales D, Warde P, et al. Improved survival in patients with locally advanced prostate cancer treated with radiotherapy and goserelin. N Engl J Med 1997; 337:295–300.

52. Pilepich MV, Caplan R, Byhardt RW, et al. Phase III trial of androgen suppression using goserelin in unfavorable-prognosis carcinoma of the prostate treated with definitive radiotherapy: report of Radiation Therapy Oncology Group Protocol 85-31. J Clin Oncol 1997; 15:1013–1021.

53. Messing EM, Manola J, Sarosdy M, et al. Immediate hormonal therapy compared with observation after radical prostatectomy and pelvic lymphadenectomy in men with node-positive prostate cancer. N Engl J Med 1999; 341:1781–1788.

54. Smith MR, McGovern FJ, Zietman AL, et al. Pamidronate to prevent bone loss during androgen-deprivation therapy for prostate cancer. N Engl J Med 2001; 345:948–955.

14

Immunotherapy for prostate cancer
Rebecca Greenhalgh, Matthew Perry and Erik Havranek

Introduction

Along with surgery, radiotherapy and chemotherapy, immunotherapy has evolved into an accepted therapeutic strategy for many cancers. Initial approaches were rather non-specific using agents to trigger antitumor responses in the tumor-bearing host. The most successful of these approaches have been the use of bacillus Calmette–Guérin (BCG) in the treatment of superficial bladder cancer and the use of interleukin-2 (IL-2) in renal cell carcinoma.[1–3] Over the last decade, a number of discoveries have led to a more targeted immune-based approach to immunotherapy. This has come about from improving our knowledge of how T cells recognize tumors, the discovery of tumor-associated antigens and identifying potential mechanisms for breaking immune tolerance.[4] A number of novel immune-based strategies are currently being pursued and this number is continuing to increase. In this chapter, we aim to give an overview of tumor immunology and current immunotherapeutic techniques and trials being investigated in the treatment of prostate cancer.

Immune surveillance

In 1970, Burnet described the theory of immune surveillance; he proposed that tumor growth in vivo might be controlled by the immune system.[5] If a clone of tumor cells evolves which express antigens that are immunogenic, an intact immune system would recognize and clear these clones.[6] Thereby the immune system can be seen as the frontline active protection against the development of cancer.[5–7] This surveillance could be overcome if the immune system was depressed as in the use of immunosuppressives or by increased aggressiveness with which tumor cells grow.

Human tumors take many years to develop from the time of the first mutation to clinical problem. This may be due to a number of factors:

- Malignant transformation is a multistep process involving mutational events in tumor suppressor genes, transcriptional regulatory genes, and proto-oncogenes leading to it becoming free of the normal growth control.[8]
- It may take time for a population of growth-transformed cells that have lost the expression of tumor-associated antigens (TAAs) to emerge.[7] The tumor cells that become apparent are therefore fully growth transformed and non-immunogenic, as the immune system would have cleared the immunogenic tumor cells during development of the tumor, positively selecting for the non-immunogenic cells.

This is a simplified view of the immune system and tumor growth, the final tumor population that grows in vivo and is clinically relevant:

1. contains immunogenic cells that cannot be cleared fast enough by the immune system (the immune response cannot keep up with tumor growth)
2. contains cells that are neither antigenic nor immunogenic (they are not recognized by the immune system)
3. contains cells that are antigenic but are only poorly immunogenic (an immune response is raised but is not strong enough to reject the tumor)
4. contains a heterogeneous mixture of cells from 1, 2 and 3.

Mechanisms of tumor recognition and clearance

Effector T cells

The critical first step in the effector arm of immune surveillance is the activation of antigen specific T cells (Fig. 14.1). For an antigen to be recognized by T-cells, it must be presented within the context of either class I or class II major histocompatibility complex (MHC) molecules, either on the tumor cell itself or on a professional antigen presenting cell (APC). Class I molecules are expressed on nearly all mammalian cells whereas class II is expressed on B cells, phagocytes, dendritic cells, subsets of T cells and certain epithelial cells.

Class I MHC molecules generally present antigens from intracellular sources and class II MHC present exogenous antigens.

In tumor cells, endogenously synthesized antigen is cleaved in the proteasome complex into short peptide chains 8–10 amino acids in length;

these chains then bind to the molecular groove conformation of the class I MHC. This MHC–peptide complex is presented at the cell surface where it undergoes high affinity binding to a T-cell receptor (TCR) on CD8+ cytotoxic T lymphocytes (CTLs), which causes target cell lysis.[9]

Professional APCs, of which dendritic cells are the most potent, are concentrated in lymph nodes and peripheral lymphoid tissues, where they process and present peptide fragments to CD4+ T helper cells. Extracellular or soluble tumor antigens of proteins endocytosed via phagocytosis are processed by class II MHC molecules. These antigens associate with class II MHC molecules within the endosomes, which transport them to the cytoplasmic membrane where they are presented on the surface of the APC.[10,11] T helper cells recognize these MHC class II/antigen complexes, become activated and begin to secrete cytokines. This in turn can activate other cells of the adaptive immune system.

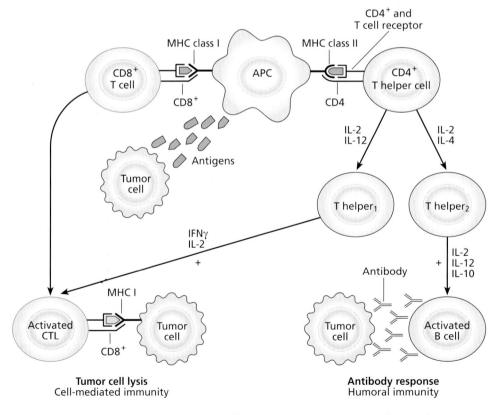

Figure 14.1 Immune response to tumor cells. APC, antigen presenting cell; CTL, cytotoxic T lymphocyte; MHC, major histocompatibility complex.

The immune response requires coordination, and this is achieved by chemical modulators or cytokines. Conventionally, these are divided into two groups based on the subset of T helper cells that produce them. T helper 1 (T_H1) cells broadly promote cytotoxic responses (inflammatory responses, viral immunity and allograft rejection), for example CTL induction, and include interleukin-2 (IL-2), interferon gamma (IFN-gamma) and IL-12. T helper 2 (T_H2) cells produce cytokines including IL-4, IL-5, IL-6 and IL-10, which mainly promote B lymphocyte activation and antibody production or humoral responses.[12] It is generally considered that shifting the balance from T_H2 to T_H1 is beneficial in many chronic infections and solid tumors.[13]

Natural killer (NK) cells

NK cells are large granular lymphocytes that arise in the bone marrow and do not depend on the thymus for maturation. Unlike T cells they do not have target cell specificity and lyse T cells in a non-MHC restricted way. NK cells recognize self-MHC class I on target cells through the KIR receptor, which act as inhibitory signal for cytotoxicity. The NK cell therefore has two opposing sets of receptors, one inhibiting and one stimulating cytotoxicity against cells bearing self-MHC class I ligand. In the presence of high-dose IL-2 in vivo, NK cells, which are able to recognize and kill only a limited number of tumor cells, are activated to become lymphokine-activated killer cells that can recognize and kill most tumor cells.[14]

Tumor-associated macrophages (TAMs)

TAMs express high levels of MHC class II molecules thereby stimulating CD4+ helper T cells at the tumor site. Activation of macrophages to generate TAMs occurs in the context of IFN-alpha and tumor cell contact.[15] Their mechanisms of killing include the secretion of cytotoxic cytokines, reactive oxygen intermediates, proteases and nitric oxide. TAM cytokines recruit secondary immune cells to the tumor site to augment cytotoxicity.[16]

Tumor-associated antigens

The concept of active immunotherapy of cancer is based on the theory that tumors possess specific antigens – tumor-associated antigens (TAAs) – which

can be recognized by the immune system,[17,18] i.e. they are antigenic. However, these antigens may not be sufficient to stimulate an effective immune response, i.e. they are not immunogenic.[19] TAAs can arise from:

- normal differentiation antigens (gp100 in melanoma)
- cancer-testes antigens (MAGE-1 in melanoma)
- overexpressed 'self-antigen' (HER2/neu in breast and ovarian cancer)
- point mutations (beta-catenin in melanoma)
- non-self-antigens such as viral proteins derived from oncogenic viruses (E6 and E7 epitopes on cervical cancers form human papillomavirus). These proteins, aberrantly expressed by tumors, can activate cytotoxic T lymphocytes, thus breaking tolerance.[20]

TAAs such as the MAGE family proteins were first used in the development of antitumor vaccinations in malignant melanoma.[21] A range of new antigens have been shown to be present in metastatic prostate cell lines such as GAGE 7, PAGE,[22] TAG-72,[23] prostate carcinoma-associated glycoprotein complex (PAC),[24] oncogenic antigen 519,[25] and mucin.[26]

Prostate specific antigen (PSA) and prostate specific membrane antigen (PSMA) are TAAs and certain peptide regions can invoke CTL responses to increase proliferation of these cells and increase tumor cell killing.[27] PSA peptide sequences 49–63 and 64–78 have been shown to promote CTL proliferation via T helper cell pathways while sequence 68–77 showed strong induction of CTL cell-mediated killing.[28] PSMA may be a particularly attractive target, as it is overexpressed by prostate cancer, compared to benign prostate[20] and peptide sequences 347–356 and 557–566 induce strong CTL specific killing which is stronger than that induced by PSA.[28] PSMA is also one of the few antigens which has been shown to occur exclusively in prostate epithelium.[29]

The immune system and prostate cancer

Cases of spontaneous regression in both renal cell carcinoma and melanoma supports the theory that the immune system can be capable of delaying tumor progression and may even be able to eliminate tumors completely. However, spontaneous regression of prostate cancer is unknown, and the prostate gland was thought to be an immunologically privileged site[30] due to the lack of lymphatics within the gland. There is now evidence that the prostate has lymphatics and can mount an inflammatory response.[31,32] Recent evidence suggests that the immune response in prostate cancer is associated with prognosis. In a Finnish series of 325 patients with prostate cancer the density of tumor infiltrating lymphocytes (TIL) was a prognostic marker, patients with absent or a low density of TIL were associated with a high risk of tumor progression.[33]

Patients with advanced prostate cancer are known to have defective cell-mediated immunity.[34] They also have lower levels of interferon gamma (IFN-gamma) in mitogen-stimulated blood cell cultures than controls or patients with localized disease.[35] Patients with advanced prostate cancer have also been shown to have a largely T_H2 cell cytokine profile within peripheral blood mononuclear cells with relatively fewer cells producing IFN-gamma and IL-2 and more secreting IL-4.[36] This promotes antibody-based rather than cellular-based immunity.

Defective antigen presentation is one method by which prostate cancer may evade the immune system. Reduction of MHC-I expression has been shown in 34% of primary prostate cancers and 80% tumors associated with lymph node metastases.[37] Defective MHC-I surface expression has been demonstrated in two of five cell lines from human metastatic prostate cancer: one was due to defective expression of TAP-2, a key mediator of antigen transport and MHC class I assembly; the other, to defective post-transcription processing.[38]

Other causes of impaired tumor detection by the immune system in prostate cancer include secretion of inhibitory substances, for example IL-10, transforming growth factor beta (TGF-beta),[39,40] abnormal T lymphocyte signal transduction[41] and expression of *Fas* ligand, which may enable tumor cells to induce apoptosis in *Fas*-expressing tumor infiltrating lymphocytes (TILs).[42]

Passive immunotherapy

Passive immunotherapy is defined as an administration of activated immune system effector components into cancer patients.[43] They confer specific antitumor immunity, but do not stimulate the patient's own immune system to raise an immune response and therefore do not provide long term immunity. Two strategies for passive immunization are antibody therapy and adoptive immunotherapy.

Antibody therapy

Monoclonal antibodies can mediate tumor cell death by both direct and indirect methods. Direct killing includes binding to calcium channels resulting in increased induction of apoptosis and binding to growth factors resulting in inhibition of ligand binding and suppression of transcription factors within the tumor cell.[44,45] Tumor cells are killed indirectly by antibody-dependent cell-mediated cytotoxicity and complement-dependent cytotoxicity.[46]

Original enthusiasm for monoclonal antibody waned as initial clinical trials proved disappointing. During the last decade, molecular advancements have been made to overcome these early failures. Chimeric human/mouse and fully humanized mouse monoclonals should overcome human antimouse activity (HAMA) against the therapeutic monoclonal antibody.[46] In breast cancer, a humanized antibody targeting the oncoprotein HER-2/neu has shown a clinical response rate of 15% in clinical trials.[47]

Conjugation to more potent toxins and radioisotopes should improve tumor penetrance and lethality.[48] A phase I study of radioactive $^{111}In/$$^{90}Y$-2IR-BAD-m170 has shown this monoclonal antibody to be well tolerated, targeting metastases in prostate cancer and temporarily relieving pain.[49] CC49, a murine IgG1 antibody specific for TAG-72 (a tumor-associated mucin expressed on a number of adenocarcinomas including prostate) has been investigated in a number of clinical trials. A phase II study with ^{131}I-CC49 was carried out in 15 men with prostate cancer. Adverse events included thrombocytopenia and bone marrow suppression, and although six out of ten men experienced a decrease in bone pain, none reached PSA or radiographic criteria for an objective response.[50]

Bispecific constructs are artificial antibodies containing two variable regions and can recognize more than one antigen.[51] Bispecific monoclonal antibodies, such as a combination of anti-CD3 and antitumor-associated antigen antibody, redirect cytotoxic T lymphocytes to malignant cells; in vitro experiments are ongoing.[52] A phase I pilot trial of a bispecific antibody in patients with prostate cancer expressing HER-2/neu has shown it to be well tolerated, with only mild malaise or fever. Monocyte-derived cytokine tumor necrosis factor alpha (TNF-alpha) and IL-6 levels decreased and PSA levels were stable for 40 days in five out of six patients.[53]

Future trials of monoclonal antibodies will concentrate on their application in conjunction with chemotherapy, in low-volume disease and as adjuvants.[51] Targeting vascular endothelial factor[54] and necrotic tumors[55] are also new avenues of research. New types of delivery, ensuring optimum concentrations – such as intratumor injection and intraperitoneal delivery in ovarian cancer – are showing promising results.[56,57]

Adoptive immunotherapy

Adoptive immunotherapy delivers biological agents with antitumor activity, most commonly by intravenous infusion of activated immune cells.[4] This involves removal of lymphocytes and other immune cells from the patient and increasing their antitumor activity ex vivo. This activation can be brought about by growing the cells in culture with cytokines and by transfection of genes encoding for cytokines or immunostimulatory molecules designed to increase immune recognition of cancer cells or to kill tumors directly.[58] These cells are then grown in large numbers and readministered to the patient.

Lymphokine-activated killer cells
Lymphokine-activated killer cells (LAK) closely resemble non-MHC restricted NK cells; they are generated from autologous lymphocytes isolated from patients' blood and grown with IL-2. In the Dunning rat model of prostate cancer, LAK cells generated from splenocytes of rats bearing tumors and given with IL-2 prolonged survival over controls.[59] Human trials in renal cell carcinoma have been disappointing where LAK cells given with IL-2 when compared to IL-2 alone showed no significant difference in response rates or survival.[1]

Tumor infiltrating lymphocytes
Other adoptive immunotherapy approaches include tumor infiltrating lymphocytes (TILs) isolated from tumors or lymph nodes draining the tumor, cultured with IL-2 and readministered to the patient. These infusions contain both CD4+ and CD8+ cells. Clinical trials in renal cell carcinoma have been disappointing with no improvement over IL-2 alone.[60] Autolymphocyte therapy uses an infusion of T lymphocytes cultured in vitro with IL-2 and OKT3 (a monoclonal antibody thought to activate cells exposed to TAAs). In activated T cell therapy, lymphocytes are harvested from peripheral blood, stimulated with IL-2 and incubated with anti-CD3 and anti-CD28 antibodies. The CD3 activates the signal transduction of the T-cell receptor and the CD28 stimulates the co-stimulatory pathway activating T cells previously exposed to tumor.[61] The results of clinical trials in prostate cancer are awaited.

Active immunotherapy

Active cancer immunotherapy involves vaccination of patients to elicit activation of tumor specific T cells.[43] This can be achieved by delivery of antigens or immune system components that stimulate the body's own mechanisms to generate antitumor immunity.

Cytokine therapy

Cytokines have shown promise in vitro and in animal models. Cytokines (including IFN-alpha, -beta, -gamma; TNF-alpha, -beta; IL-1, IL-2, IL-4 and IL-12) have been shown to have antitumor activity.[62] Augmenting such cytokine levels can increase the acquisition of cellular immunity.[63] Granulocyte–macrophage colony stimulating factor (GM-CSF) is a monomeric glycoprotein that enhances the expansion of macrophages, neutrophils and eosinophils.[64] It promotes dendritic cell (DC) migration, development and longevity[65] and directly mediates antitumor activity by stimulating macrophages and stimulating the release of TNF. In the Dunning rat model of prostate cancer, tumor onset was delayed and survival increased by treating the rats with GM-CSF before tumor challenge with Mat-Ly-Lu cells.

GM-CSF has been used as a stand-alone agent in a phase I/II clinical trial in hormone escape prostate cancer. One group received GM-CSF for

14 days of a 28-day cycle; a second group received GM-CSF for 14 days followed by ongoing three times weekly injections. There was minimal toxicity, consisting of transient malaise and fever with erythema and swelling at the site of injection. A majority of patients in both groups demonstrated descending PSA when on the therapy and increasing PSA when discontinued. Only one patient had a continued response (> 14 months) decline in PSA > 50% and an improvement in bone scans.[66]

In rats with induced subcutaneous Dunning carcinoma cells, subcutaneous peritumoral administration of IFN-gamma and TNF-alpha has been reported to demonstrate antitumor effect.[67] Several human trials have been carried out using interferon treatment in advanced metastatic prostate cancer: low response rates (0–5%) were observed and toxicity led to dose reduction.[68–70] Maffezzini et al[71] carried out a pilot study looking at IFN-gamma and IL-2 administered subcutaneously in 13 patients with D3 prostate cancer having failed secondary treatment. Four patients showed a partial clinical response; side effects, including fever and nausea, were experienced by all patients.[71]

Direct injection of IL-2, IL-1beta, GM-CSF, IFN-gamma and TNF-alpha, derived from normal donor buffy-coat mononuclear cells (leukocyte interleukin), into primary prostate tumor under ultrasound guidance to ensure highest concentrations in the target organ, has been examined. Five patients underwent injection, tolerating the treatment well, with dysuria as a side effect in two. No identifiable decrease in serum PSA levels was detected. Only two patients showed inflammation in their post-treatment biopsy.[63] The relative failure of this regimen was thought to be indicative of a general problem with this type of therapy since injections were too infrequent to initiate and maintain inflammation. A newly designed study is planned, possibly using some form of slow release vehicle. A similar clinical study on six patients, omitting the administration of IL-1 and IL-2, led to an inflammatory cellular infiltrate with mononuclear cells with some tumor necrosis.[72]

Vaccines

Protein and peptide vaccines

A vaccine directed against TAAs attempts to trigger the autoimmune destruction of the prostate gland. The limited physiological role of the prostate in men of an advanced age group[63] means this does little harm but is still effective in destroying the tumor both within the prostate and at distant sites.

The first vaccines directed against TAAs were trialed in melanoma, an immunologically responsive tumor in which the existence of CTL targeting of tumor antigens can be demonstrated.[18]

MUC-1 is a glycoprotein which is highly expressed in glandular organs; in malignant cells, an over-glycosylated form of mucin is overexpressed on the surface of the cell.[73] Twenty patients with increasing PSA values observed after primary therapies were treated with MUC-1 peptide conjugated to a carrier molecule, KLH together with QS-21. All patients generated IgM and IgG responses after three immunizations.[74]

OncoVax-P[63,75] is a PSA vaccine manufactured by purifying recombinant PSA using a murine monoclonal anti-PSA antibody. Systemic immunization trials with OncoVax-P show that natural tolerance to PSA can be overcome by manufacturing liposomes containing recombinant PSA and the strong T_H1 adjuvant lipid A.[63] Immunoenhancement with combinations of BCG, GM-CSF, IL-2 and cyclophosphamide were also tested in this study. Forty-five patients were entered into a total of six trials. No serious side effects were shown in all forms of administration, with the exception of intravenous use, after which two patients were transiently confused, one of whom also had blurred vision. PSA antibody titers were taken as measures of immune response.[63] Cellular immunity was tested by delayed type skin hypersensitivity reactions. Antibody and cellular responses were detected in regimens incorporating adjuvants. Further trials are planned with a larger sample size[63] to determine whether there may be treatment benefit.

The identification of immunodominant T-cell epitopes from tumor antigens has led to the design of peptide-based vaccines. This peptide therapy offers a new and exciting avenue of research since it may be possible to combine multiple epitopes within a single vaccine. It has been shown that subpopulations of T cells can be activated by certain peptide sequences within PSA and PSMA.[27,28,76] In vitro and in vivo studies have also demonstrated that peptides derived from PSA can trigger cytotoxic T-cell response and specific cytokine secretion.[76-78] While much development remains to be carried out, this approach offers an interesting and potentially useful method of directly stimulating the immune system.[43,79,80]

Glycoprotein vaccines

Globo-H is a carbohydrate with high expression on primary and metastatic prostate cancer. Globo-H has been conjugated to KLH and given with the adjuvant QS-21 in a phase I trial of 18 prostate cancer patients with biochemical relapse after local therapy or metastatic disease.[81] Anti-Globo-H antibody responses, predominantly IgM, were demonstrated in almost all the patients. Clinical benefit was limited to a decreasing slope of PSA rise in two of the five patients with biochemical only disease who did not receive subsequent hormone therapy. No significant toxicity was recorded. Further trials are underway.

DNA vaccines

DNA vaccines consist of a stretch of nucleic acids containing the gene encoding for a specific antigen inserted downstream of a viral promoter into a plasmid. This DNA can be delivered into human tissues and translated into antigen, generating an immune response. Dendritic cells are important in this response; they can take up the DNA either directly by endocytosis or indirectly by phagocytosis of apoptotic or necrotic cells that express the delivered antigen. This leads to dendritic cell activation and to generation of both CD8+ and CD4+ T-cell responses.[82]

The route of administration of DNA has been shown to be of great importance, one of the most successful routes being intramuscular. This may be because professional APCs are attracted to sites of muscle 'injury' from inoculation.[83] There are a number of methods of delivery of DNA vaccines including injection of naked DNA, transfection into attenuated strains of Salmonella which can be given orally and in recombinant viruses modified to contain certain antigens in their genome.

PSA has been considered an attractive target for DNA vaccination. In Rhesus macaques immunized with a DNA-based PSA vaccine, PSA-specific humoral responses, IFN-gamma secretion and PSA-specific lymphoproliferative responses were observed.[86]

PROSTVAC™, a commercially developed vaccine, is a recombinant vaccinia virus expressing human PSA (rV-PSA). In a phase I study, 33 men with biochemical progression after local therapy or with locally advanced disease or metastatic disease, received escalating doses of PROSTVAC™ at 4-week intervals. One group also received GM-CSF. Stable disease was achieved in 14 men for at least 6 months. Higher vaccine dose and addition of GM-CSF tended to produce more patients with stable disease.[84] Phase II trials are underway.

Prokaryotic DNA has been shown to be a very good adjuvant; it contains the unmethylated form of a DNA motif, CpG-DNA, which is not found in human DNA.[85] This CpG-DNA motif binds to DCs via a Toll-like receptor leading to DC maturation and generation of immune responses.

Whole cell vaccination

This technique involves injection of replication incompetent tumor cells into the patient with an adjuvant to stimulate an immune response to both the injected cells and the patient's own tumor. This method of vaccination presents all the TAAs from a tumor and not just one or two as in peptide- and DNA-based vaccines. There are two types of whole cell vaccines: autologous and allogeneic (Fig. 14.2).

Autologous whole cell vaccines

This involves the use of the patient's own tumor cells as a vaccine. Cells can be collected from biopsy or tumor resection and grown in tissue culture. The vaccine may be developed from these cells by a variety of methods, including spontaneous outgrowth, viral transformation and possibly transfection.[86] These cells are then irradiated to make them replication deficient and injected back into the patient. These cells have the advantage of being MHC matched to the patient and can present antigen directly to CTLs. Transfection of the tumor vaccine cells with genes encoding cytokines avoids the toxic effects of systemic cytokine infusion and delivers the cytokines directly to the site of antigen presentation. A number of cytokines have been transfected in a variety of models, mainly in melanoma.[87-89] Vaccination of mice with these autologous modified tumor cells resulted in rejection of the injected tumor. In some cases, mice were shown to generate measurable systema-

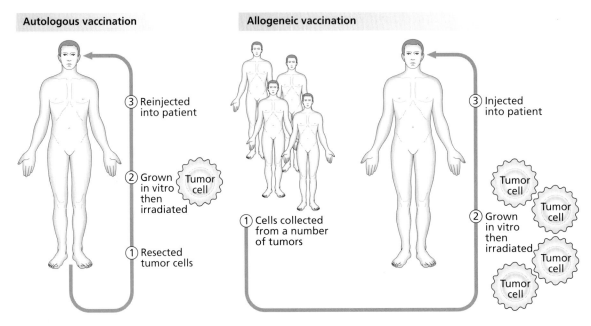

Figure 14.2   Principles of autologous and allogeneic vaccination.

tic antitumor responses, and in a limited number of cases, immunization with such cells resulted in the elimination of reduced growth of pre-existing tumor. IL-2, GM-CSF and IFN-gamma have been evaluated in prostate cancer models. Autologous MAT-Ly-Lu vaccines secreting IL-2, IFN-gamma and GM-CSF were compared in the Dunning rat model of prostate cancer.[90,91] Transfection with IL-2 led to prolonged survival in rats with pre-existing tumors with cure rates of up to 100% in some experiments. This compared with a cure rate of 40% when a GM-CSF vaccine was used and a modest effect with IFN-gamma cells. Rats cured of their tumors were resistant to a second challenge of live tumor cells.

In a phase I trial at the Johns Hopkins Oncology Center, eight immunocompetent prostate cancer patients were treated with autologous, GM-CSF-secreting, irradiated tumor vaccines prepared from ex vivo retroviral transduction of surgically harvested cells. Vaccine site biopsies manifested infiltrates of dendritic cells and macrophages among prostate tumor vaccine cells. Vaccination activated new T-cell and B-cell immune responses against prostate cancer antigens. These findings suggest that both T-cell and B-cell immune

responses to human prostate cancer can be generated by treatment with irradiated, GM-CSF gene-transduced autologous vaccines.[92]

Unfortunately it is very difficult to grow prostate cancer cell lines in vitro;[93] the technique is labor intensive and is not always successful, as this can significantly delay treatment, allogeneic whole cell vaccine is an alternative approach.

Allogeneic whole cell vaccine
It was previously assumed that whole tumor cell vaccines needed to be autologous, because antigen was presented directly to the CD8+ T cell by autologous MHC class I. However, there is evidence in mice that there is no detectable presentation of class I-restricted tumor antigens by the tumor itself. Tumor antigens appear to be presented by bone marrow derived cells[94] and therefore human leukocyte antigen (HLA) matching may be unnecessary as TAAs which are present on allogeneic tumor cells are taken up by autologous DCs and thereby presented by autologous MHC. In addition, the T-cell receptors of allospecific T cells recognize allogeneic MHC-presenting peptide and are known to cross-react with autologous MHC-presenting foreign peptide antigen.[95] It is

also thought that allogeneic molecules themselves provide immune stimuli, which act as an adjuvant and enhance the immunogenicity of TAAs.

Several experiments have shown that using allogeneic cell vaccination may actually be superior to autologous vaccination. This is true in murine malignant melanoma models[96] and in the rat model of prostate cancer,[97] although this remains to be proven in the human system. Currently, the best available clinical evidence in favor of allogeneic cell-based vaccine comes from a large non-randomized phase II study of a polyvalent allogeneic melanoma cell vaccine that reported reduction of measurable disease and a threefold increase in 5-year survival compared with historical controls.[98]

In a phase I/II study in men with hormone refractory prostate cancer (HRPC) using an allogeneic whole-cell vaccine,[99] 60 men were randomly allocated to four groups and treated with three cell lines intradermally (from a bank of four) every 2 weeks initially and then monthly. The vaccine was administered with the immunostimulant *Mycobacterium vaccae*. The vaccine was safe and well tolerated with no major side effects. No patient had a significant drop in PSA that could be attributed solely to the vaccine. However, the immunological data were more encouraging, with several patients having an increase in cytokine production, increases in specific antibodies and evidence of T-cell proliferation in response to the vaccine. The failure of the vaccine to produce a PSA response was felt to be in keeping with high disease burden in this group of patients.

In most ongoing trials, antitumor vaccines are being tested on patients with advanced disease. Their tumor load is already very high and immunological response weakened. Immunization for cancer may well be more beneficial in the treatment of minimal residual disease, for example in prevention of metastases after initial surgery.[100] However obtaining ethics committee approval for trials in less advanced disease is difficult.

Suicide gene therapy

Suicide gene therapy[20,75] involves inserting genes encoding enzymes that convert a prodrug to a toxic metabolite that kills the target cell into which the gene has been placed. This insertion of genetic material is most commonly carried out using an adenoviral vector.

The most studied of these systems is the *Herpes simplex* virus thymidine kinase (HSVtk)/ganciclovir (GCV) system. The HSVtk converts the antiviral drug GCV to a monophosphorylated form that is then metabolized to the toxic triphosphate form by cellular kinases. GCV-triphosphate interacts with the cellular DNA polymerase, causing interference with DNA synthesis and thereby leading to the death of dividing cells.

Another example is bacterial and fungal cytosine deaminase, which has been widely studied in colorectal and hepatocellular carcinoma, but is now being tested for use in prostate cancer. 5-Fluorocytosine (5-FC) is a fungicidal drug, which is metabolized to 5-fluorouracil (5-FU), a cytotoxic agent. 5-FU is further phosphorylated to 5-FU mono- and triphosphate. These inhibit thymidilate synthesis and mRNA transcription, resulting in cell death.[101]

One of the most exciting aspects of suicide gene therapy is the bystander effect (BE). The activated drug not only kills the cell in which the drug was produced but also neighboring cells. Up to 100 times the predicted cell kill can be seen.[102] This means that only a small number of tumor cells need to be transfected with the suicide gene for tumor elimination. Transfection is usually accomplished using a viral vector, which is administered via intratumor or intravenous injection. The BE works though a number of mechanisms. In the HSV-tk/GCV system the toxic drug metabolites cross gap junctions to affect neighboring cells. In the CD/5-FC system toxic metabolites can cross the cell membrane and diffuse into the surrounding cells.[103] In vitro CD/5-FC has a higher BE than the HSV-tk/GCV system, as the cells do not need to be in contact in the former system.[104] Neighboring cells can also endocytose apoptotic bodies from the killed cells and thus enhance BE. In vivo, distant BE can be seen. In a rat model of prostate cancer, wild type tumors – seeded at a distance from a primary tumor and transfected with HSV-tk – were seen to regress on systemic treatment with GCV, whereas wild type tumors on their own were not affected by GCV.[105] Although the BE has been observed in immunocompromised animals, recent findings suggest that the BE in vivo is largely mediated by the release of cytokines.[106] GCV treatment of carcinomas that contained a mixture of wild type and HSV-tk transfected cells resulted in almost total tumor regression in immuno-competent mice but not in athymic animals of the same strain.

Herman et al[107] at Baylor College of Medicine carried out a phase I study involving 18 patients with recurrence of prostate cancer following radical radiotherapy. They were treated with an intraprostatic injection of a replication deficient adenovirus containing HSV-tk followed by intra-venous administration of ganciclovir. Three patients had a more than 50% decrease in PSA from 45 up to 330 days. Side effects were minimal with one patient developing spontaneously reversible grade 4 thrombocytopenia and grade 3 hepatotoxicity.[107]

In a study carried out by Shalev et al, 52 patients with localized prostate cancer received multiple and/or repeat intraprostatic injections of replication deficient adenovirus containing HSV-tk, followed by intravenous administration of ganci-clovir or oral valaciclovir for 14 days.[108] After receiving ganciclovir, 16 patients had a transient fever and four patients had abnormal liver function tests (LFT), one of whom also experienced grade 4 thrombocytopenia. In a mean follow-up time of 12.8 months, 43% of patients showed a decrease in PSA ranging from 25 to 69% from entry levels.[108]

Ayala et al[109] gave an intraprostatic injection of replication deficient adenovirus containing HSV-tk followed by intravenous ganciclovir to four patients prior to radical prostatectomy. Histological evaluation of the resected prostates revealed tumor reduction by cell lysis and stromal fibrosis with distinctive nuclear changes. The benign tissue showed no cytopathic changes. A dense inflamma-tory infiltrate with B cells was seen in the benign tissue while cytotoxic T cells were most prominent in the areas of adenocarcinoma.[109]

Dendritic cell (DC) vaccines

DCs are the most potent stimulators of T-cell responses and play a crucial role in the initiation of primary immune responses.[110] They represent a heterogeneous population of leukocytes, which are morphologically, functionally and phenotypically different from monocytes and macrophages. They are found not only in peripheral blood, but also in bone marrow, respiratory and gastrointestinal systems and in the epidermal layer of the skin. There are no specific cell surface markers for DCs and they lack the typical markers of other leukocyte populations. They express high levels of class I and class II MHC, co-stimulatory molecules CD80 and CD86, cell adhesion molecules and CD40, and produce cytokines which are involved in T cell activation. DCs are unique in their ability to stim-ulate naive T cells. They have the ability to prime T cells capable of recognizing and killing tumor cells in an antigen specific fashion.[111] The presence of DCs in a number of cancers has been shown to be associated with a favorable prognosis,[112] suggesting they play a role in tumor defense but there is no evidence that DCs capture and process antigens from malignant cells in vivo. This may be because tumor-secreted factors (e.g. IL-10 and vascular endothelial growth factor) decrease DC development and function.[113,114]

New technologies have made possible the generation of large numbers of DCs from either CD14+ progenitors or monocyte precursors in vitro from peripheral blood. This has led to the development of DC vaccines. Autologous DCs grown in culture with tumor antigens in the form of tumor lysate, peptide or total RNA, or geneti-cally modified DCs using viral vectors expressing tumor-associated antigens, can be given as a vaccine (Fig. 14.3). The issues of optimal numbers of DCs, the route of administration (intradermal, intranodal, subcutaneous or intravenous), optimal frequency of immunization and the role of immunological adjuvants remain to be clarified.

A phase I study of 13 HRPC patients treated with autologous DCs exposed ex vivo to a recom-binant protein of human prostatic acid phosphatase (PAP) and GM-CSF showed a PSA decline of > 50% in three patients and no significant side effects.[115] Thereafter, a further phase I/II trial was completed in which 31 patients were treated. T-cell responses were elicited in 38% of patients and T cells collected on completion of the trial se-creted IFN-gamma showing a T_H1-type response. Three patients had a PSA decline of > 50%. No objective regression of the disease was seen.[116] These studies demonstrated the ability to generate an antigen specific T-cell response to a normal tissue antigen.

Following a phase I trial, Tjoa et al[117] carried out a phase II clinical trial in 95 patients with HRPC using autologous DCs pulsed with HLA-A2 PSMA peptides. Patients received six infusions at 6-week intervals; half of the patients also

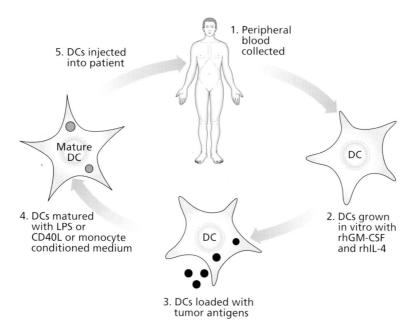

Figure 14.3 Principles of dendritic cell (DC) vaccination. LPS, lipopolysaccharide; rhGM-CSF, recombinant human granulocyte–macrophage colony stimulating factor; rhIL-4, recombinant human interleukin-4. (With kind permission of Mr RJ John, St George's Hospital Medical School, London.)

received GM-CSF as an adjuvant. No significant difference in clinical response was observed between the two groups. A total of three complete responses and 16 partial responses were reported. The median response was approximately 160 days, with 11 responses ongoing for more than 2 years. Investigation into the immune responses in a subset of patients showed that pretreatment immunocompetence was correlated to clinical response.[117] This suggests that immunocompetent patients would benefit from this approach.

Heat shock proteins

A new approach in vaccine development is the use of heat shock protein/peptide complexes. Heat shock proteins (hsps) act as chaperones for peptides and other proteins. Hsps were first recognized in 1962 as a set of molecules reproducibly induced in Drosophila by elevated temperatures.[118] It is now recognized that they are upregulated by a wide range of harmful conditions including heat shock, alcohols, heavy metals and oxidative stress.[119] Hsp overexpression leads to an increased chaperoning of antigenic peptides into a particular

subset of macrophages and other APCs, leading to their efficient presentation via class I or class II pathways.[120,121] The complexes are taken up by DCs via specific receptors (CD91) and processed for antigen presentation. Hsps activate APCs to take up and process the tumor antigens and upregulate expression of co-stimulatory molecules and inflammatory cytokines necessary for T cell activation.[122] Hsps, therefore, chaperone an entire array of antigenic peptides generated by a tumor, instead of one of a few selected antigenic peptides.[123]

Yedavelli et al[124] noted that hsp gp96-peptide complexes derived from Dunning G tumor cells used as a prophylactic vaccination in Copenhagen rats delayed both incidence and growth of tumors. Inhibition of tumor growth was observed when gp96 was administered after tumor induction.[124]

Janetzki et al[125] have carried out a pilot study into the use of autologous tumor derived gp96 preparations. Sixteen patients with advanced malignancies refractory to established therapies were recruited. No unacceptable side effects were observed. MHC-I restricted, tumor specific CD8+

Table 14.1 Examples of ongoing antitumor vaccine trials

Basis [Name (ref)]	Center	Phase
PSA (OncoVax-P)	Jenner Biotherapies, CA	I + II
PSMA/CD86 plasmid	Rockville	I + II
Autologous DC + PSMA peptides		I + II
Autologous ex vivo (MFG-granulocyte colony stimulating factor gene via retrovirus)	Johns Hopkins	I + II
Allogeneic ex vivo (IL-2 + IFN-gamma via retrovirus)	Memorial Sloan Kettering	I + II
Allogeneic whole cell vaccine (Onyvax)	St George's, London, UK	I + II

Allogeneic, based on other individual's tissue; autologous, based on patient's own tissue; DC, dendritic cell; ex vivo, transfection occurred on established cell cultures; PMSA, prostate specific membrane antigen.

T lymphocytes were elicited in 6 of 12 patients and an expansion of the NK cell population was observed in 8 of 13 patients.

Conclusion

It is now known that the prostate is not an immunologically privileged site and that prostate cancer could in fact be a good target for immunotherapy. There are many immunotherapeutic strategies currently being investigated for use in patients with prostate cancer (Table 14.1). Although passive immunotherapy has been used in clinical trials, current evidence that active immunotherapy could be more successful has led to an increase in trials using these methods. Most trials have been in patients with advanced prostate cancer and these patients are often immunocompromised from their disease, indicating that immunotherapy is less likely to be successful. The ideal patients to treat may be those with early disease and high risk of metastasis, where the primary tumor could be removed and any remaining tumor cells (either locally or from distant spread) could be eliminated with immunotherapy.

References

1. Rosenberg SA, Lotze MT, Yang JC, et al. Prospective randomized trial of high-dose interleukin-2 alone or in conjunction with lymphokine-activated killer cells for the treatment of patients with advanced cancer. J Natl Cancer Inst 1993; 85(8):622–632.
2. Herr HW, Wartinger DD, Fair WR, Oettgen HF. Bacillus Calmette–Guerin therapy for superficial bladder cancer: a 10-year followup. J Urol 1992; 147(4):1020–1023.
3. Lamm DL. Long-term results of intravesical therapy for superficial bladder cancer. Urol Clin North Am 1992; 19(3):573–580.
4. Chang AE, Geiger JD, Sondak VK, Shu S. Adoptive cellular therapy of malignancy. Arch Surg 1993; 128(11):1281–1290.
5. Burnet FM. The concept of immunological surveillance. Prog Exp Tumor Res 1970; 13:1–27.
6. Doherty PC, Knowles BB, Wettstein PJ. Immunological surveillance of tumors in the context of major histocompatibility complex restriction of T cell function. Adv Cancer Res 1984; 42:1–65.
7. Kripke ML. Immunoregulation of carcinogenesis: past, present, and future. J Natl Cancer Inst 1988; 80(10):722–727.
8. Vogelstein B, Kinzler KW. The multistep nature of cancer. Trends Genet 1993; 9(4):138–141.
9. Engberg J, Krogsgaard M, Fugger L. Recombinant antibodies with the antigen-specific, MHC restricted specificity of T cells: novel reagents for basic and clinical investigations and immunotherapy. Immunotechnology 1999; 4(3–4):273–278.
10. Neefjes JJ, Hammerling GJ, Momburg F. Folding and assembly of major histocompatibility complex class I heterodimers in the endoplasmic reticulum of intact cells precedes the binding of peptide. J Exp Med 1993; 178(6):1971–1980.
11. Janeway CA Jr, Mamula MJ, Rudensky A. Rules for peptide presentation by MHC class II molecules. Int Rev Immunol 1993; 10(4):301–311.
12. Romagnani S. The Th1/Th2 paradigm. Immunol Today 1997; 18(6):263–266.
13. Yates A, Bergmann C, Van Hemmen JL, et al. Cytokine-modulated regulation of helper T cell populations. J Theor Biol 2000; 206(4):539–560.
14. Matzinger P. An innate sense of danger. Semin Immunol 1998; 10(5):399–415.
15. Mantovani A, Bottazzi B, Colotta F, et al. The origin and function of tumor-associated macrophages. Immunol Today 1992; 13(7):265–270.
16. Bartholeyns J. Monocytes and macrophages in cancer immunotherapy. Res Immunol 1993; 144(4):288–291; discussion 294–298.
17. Boon T, Cerottini JC, Van den Eynde B, et al. Tumor antigens recognized by T lymphocytes. Annu Rev Immunol 1994; 12:337–365.

18. Houghton AN. Cancer antigens: immune recognition of self and altered self. J Exp Med 1994; 180(1):1–4.

19. Pardoll D. New strategies for active immunotherapy with genetically engineered tumor cells. Curr Opin Immunol 1992; 4(5):619–623.

20. Hrouda D, Perry M, Dalgleish AG. Gene therapy for prostate cancer. Semin Oncol 1999; 26(4):455–471.

21. van der Bruggen P, Traversari C, Chomez P, et al. A gene encoding an antigen recognized by cytolytic T lymphocytes on a human melanoma. Science 1991; 254(5038):1643–1647.

22. Chen ME, Lin SH, Chung LW, Sikes RA. Isolation and characterization of PAGE-1 and GAGE-7. New genes expressed in the LNCaP prostate cancer progression model that share homology with melanoma-associated antigens. J Biol Chem 1998; 273(28):17618–17625.

23. Brenner PC, Rettig WJ, Sanz-Moncasi MP, et al. TAG-72 expression in primary, metastatic and hormonally treated prostate cancer as defined by monoclonal antibody CC49. J Urol 1995; 153(5):1575–1579.

24. Wright GL Jr, Beckett ML, Lipford GB, et al. A novel prostate carcinoma-associated glycoprotein complex (PAC) recognized by monoclonal antibody TURP-27. Int J Cancer 1991; 47(5):717–725.

25. Shurbaji MS, Kuhajda FP, Pasternack GR, Thurmond TS. Expression of oncogenic antigen 519 (OA-519) in prostate cancer is a potential prognostic indicator. Am J Clin Pathol 1992; 97(5):686–691.

26. Burchell J, Graham R, Taylor-Papadimitriou J. Active specific immunotherapy: PEM as a potential target molecule. Cancer Surv 1993; 18:135–148.

27. Tjoa B, Boynton A, Kenny G, et al. Presentation of prostate tumor antigens by dendritic cells stimulates T-cell proliferation and cytotoxicity. Prostate 1996; 28(1):65–69.

28. Corman JM, Sercarz EE, Nanda NK. Recognition of prostate-specific antigenic peptide determinants by human CD4 and CD8 T cells. Clin Exp Immunol 1998; 114(2):166–172.

29. Zhang S, Zhang HS, Reuter VE, et al. Expression of potential target antigens for immunotherapy on primary and metastatic prostate cancers. Clin Cancer Res 1998; 4(2):295–302.

30. Gittes RF, McCullough DL. Occult carcinoma of the prostate: an oversight of immune surveillance – a working hypothesis. J Urol 1974; 112(2):241–244.

31. Kelalis PP, Greene LF, Harrison EG Jr. Granulomatous prostatitis. A mimic of carcinoma of the prostate. JAMA 1965; 191(4):287–289.

32. Neaves WB, Billingham RE. The lymphatic drainage of the rat prostate and its status as an immunologically privileged site. Transplantation 1979; 27(2):127–132.

33. Vesalainen S, Lipponen P, Talja M, Syrjanen K. Histological grade, perineural infiltration, tumour-infiltrating lymphocytes and apoptosis as determinants of long-term prognosis in prostatic adenocarcinoma. Eur J Cancer 1994; 12(803):1797–1803.

34. Schellhammer PF, Bracken RB, Bean MA, et al. Immune evaluation with skin testing. A study of testicular, prostatic, and bladder neoplasms. Cancer 1976; 38(1):149–156.

35. Elsasser-Beile U, von Kleist S, Fischer R, et al. Impaired cytokine production in whole blood cell cultures of patients with urological carcinomas. J Cancer Res Clin Oncol 1993; 119(7):430–433.

36. Hrouda D, Baban B, Dunsmuir WD, et al. Immunotherapy of advanced prostate cancer: a phase I/II trial using *Mycobacterium vaccae* (SRL172). Br J Urol 1998; 82(4):568–573.

37. Blades RA, Keating PJ, McWilliam LJ, et al. Loss of HLA class I expression in prostate cancer: implications for immunotherapy. Urology 1995; 46(5):681–686; discussion 686–687.

38. Sanda MG, Restifo NP, Walsh JC, et al. Molecular characterization of defective antigen processing in human prostate cancer. J Natl Cancer Inst 1995; 87(4):280–285.

39. Mukherji B, Chakraborty NG. Immunobiology and immunotherapy of melanoma. Curr Opin Oncol 1995; 7(2):175–184.

40. Huber D, Philipp J, Fontana A. Protease inhibitors interfere with the transforming growth factor-beta-dependent but not the transforming growth factor-beta-independent pathway of tumor cell-mediated immunosuppression. J Immunol 1992; 148(1):277–284.

41. Zier K, Gansbacher B, Salvadori S. Preventing abnormalities in signal transduction of T cells in cancer: the promise of cytokine gene therapy. Immunol Today 1996; 17(1):39–45.

42. Hahne M, Rimoldi D, Schroter M, et al. Melanoma cell expression of Fas(Apo-1/CD95) ligand: implications for tumor immune escape. Science 1996; 274(5291):1363–1366.

43. Tjoa BA, Murphy GP. Progress in active specific immunotherapy of prostate cancer. Semin Surg Oncol 2000; 18(1):80–87.

44. Demidem A, Lam T, Alas S, et al. Chimeric anti-CD20 (IDEC-C2B8) monoclonal antibody sensitizes a B cell lymphoma cell line to cell killing by cytotoxic drugs. Cancer Biother Radiopharm 1997; 12(3):177–186.

45. Pardee AB, Dubrow R, Hamlin JL, Kletzien RF. Animal cell cycle. Annu Rev Biochem 1978; 47:715–750.

46. LoBuglio AF, Saleh MN. Monoclonal antibody therapy of cancer. Crit Rev Oncol Hematol 1992; 13(3):271–282.

47. Cobleigh MA, Vogel CL, Tripathy D, et al. Multinational study of the efficacy and safety of humanized anti-HER2 monoclonal antibody in women who have HER2-overexpressing metastatic breast cancer that has progressed after chemotherapy for metastatic disease. J Clin Oncol 1999; 17(9):2639–2648.

48. Lopes AD, Davis WL, Rosenstraus MJ, et al. Immunohistochemical and pharmacokinetic characterization of the site-specific immunoconjugate CYT-356 derived from antiprostate monoclonal antibody 7E11-C5. Cancer Res 1990; 50(19):6423–6429.

49. O'Donnell RT, DeNardo SJ, Yuan A, et al. Radioimmunotherapy with (111)In/(90)Y-2IT-BAD-m170 for metastatic prostate cancer. Clin Cancer Res 2001; 7(6):1561–1568.

50. Slovin SF, Scher HI, Divgi CR, et al. Interferon-gamma and monoclonal antibody 131I-labeled CC49: outcomes in patients with androgen-independent prostate cancer. Clin Cancer Res 1998; 4(3):643–651.

51. Murray JL. Monoclonal antibody treatment of solid tumors: a coming of age. Semin Oncol 2000; 27(6 suppl 11):64–70; discussion 92–100.

52. Riesenberg R, Buchner A, Pohla H, Lindhofer H. Lysis of prostate carcinoma cells by trifunctional bispecific antibodies (alpha EpCAM _ alpha CD3). J Histochem Cytochem 2001; 49(7):911–917.

53. Schwaab T, Lewis LD, Cole BF, et al. Phase I pilot trial of the bispecific antibody MDXH210 (anti-Fc gamma RI X anti-HER-2/neu) in patients whose prostate cancer overexpresses HER-2/neu. J Immunother 2001; 24(1):79–87.

54. Ryan AM, Eppler DB, Hagler KE, et al. Preclinical safety evaluation of rhuMAbVEGF, an antiangiogenic humanized monoclonal antibody. Toxicol Pathol 1999; 27(1):78–86.

55. Epstein AL, Chen FM, Taylor CR. A novel method for the detection of necrotic lesions in human cancers. Cancer Res 1988; 48(20):5842–5848.

56. Rosenblum MG, Verschraegen CF, Murray JL, et al. Phase I study of 90Y-labeled B72.3 intraperitoneal administration in patients with ovarian cancer: effect of dose and EDTA coadministration on pharmacokinetics and toxicity. Clin Cancer Res 1999; 5(5):953–961.

57. Meredith RF, Partridge EE, Alvarez RD, et al. Intraperitoneal radioimmunotherapy of ovarian cancer with lutetium-177-CC49. J Nucl Med 1996; 37(9):1491–1496.

58. Rosenberg SA. Progress in human tumour immunology and immunotherapy. Nature 2001; 411(6835):380–384.

59. Tjota A, Zhang YQ, Piedmonte MR, Lee CL. Adoptive immunotherapy using lymphokine-activated killer cells and recombinant interleukin-2 in preventing and treating spontaneous pulmonary metastases of syngeneic Dunning rat prostate tumor. J Urol 1991; 146(1):177–183.

60. Figlin RA, Thompson JA, Bukowski RM, et al. Multicenter, randomized, phase III trial of CD8(+) tumor-infiltrating lymphocytes in combination with recombinant interleukin-2 in metastatic renal cell carcinoma. J Clin Oncol 1999; 17(8):2521–2529.

61. Garlie NK, LeFever AV, Siebenlist RE, et al. T cells coactivated with immobilized anti-CD3 and anti-CD28 as potential immunotherapy for cancer. J Immunother 1999; 22(4):336–345.

62. North RJ. Cyclophosphamide-facilitated adoptive immunotherapy of an established tumor depends on elimination of tumor-induced suppressor T cells. J Exp Med 1982; 155(4):1063–1074.

63. Harris DT, Matyas GR, Gomella LG, et al. Immunologic approaches to the treatment of prostate cancer. Semin Oncol 1999; 26(4):439–447.

64. Clark SC, Kamen R. The human hematopoietic colony-stimulating factors. Science 1987; 236(4806):1229–1237.

65. Dranoff G, Jaffee E, Lazenby A, et al. Vaccination with irradiated tumor cells engineered to secrete murine granulocyte–macrophage colony-stimulating factor stimulates potent, specific, and long-lasting anti-tumor immunity. Proc Natl Acad Sci USA 1993; 90(8):3539–3543.

66. Small EJ, Reese DM, Um B, et al. Therapy of advanced prostate cancer with granulocyte macrophage colony-stimulating factor. Clin Cancer Res 1999; 5(7):1738–1744.

67. van Moorselaar RJ, Hendriks BT, van Stratum P, et al. Synergistic antitumor effects of rat gamma-interferon and human tumor necrosis factor alpha against androgen-dependent and -independent rat prostatic tumors. Cancer Res 1991; 51(9):2329–2334.

68. Chang AY, Fisher HA, Spiers AS, Boros L. Toxicities of human recombinant interferon-alpha 2 in patients with advanced prostate carcinoma. J Interferon Res 1986; 6(6):713–715.

69. Bulbul MA, Huben RP, Murphy GP. Interferon-beta treatment of metastatic prostate cancer. J Surg Oncol 1986; 33(4):231–233.

70. van Haelst-Pisani CM, Richardson RL, Su J, et al. A phase II study of recombinant human alpha-interferon in advanced hormone-refractory prostate cancer. Cancer 1992; 70(9):2310–2312.

71. Maffezzini M, Simonato A, Fortis C. Salvage immunotherapy with subcutaneous recombinant interleukin 2 (rIL-2) and alpha-interferon (A-IFN) for stage D3 prostate carcinoma failing second-line hormonal treatment. Prostate 1996; 28(5):282–286.

72. Pulley MS, Nagendran V, Edwards JM, Dumonde DC. Intravenous, intralesional and endolymphatic administration of lymphokines in human cancer. Lymphokine Res 1986; 5(suppl 1):S157–S163.

73. Ho SB, Niehans GA, Lyftogt C, et al. Heterogeneity of mucin gene expression in normal and neoplastic tissues. Cancer Res 1993; 53(3):641–651.

74. Slovin SF, Kelly WK, Scher HI. Immunological approaches for the treatment of prostate cancer. Semin Urol Oncol 1998; 16(1):53–59.

75. Salgaller ML. Prostate cancer immunotherapy at the dawn of the new millennium. Expert Opin Investig Drugs 2000; 9(6):1217–1229.

76. Correale P, Walmsley K, Nieroda C, et al. In vitro generation of human cytotoxic T lymphocytes specific for peptides derived from prostate-specific antigen. J Natl Cancer Inst 1997; 89(4):293–300.

77. Correale P, Walmsley K, Zaremba S, et al. Generation of human cytolytic T lymphocyte lines directed against prostate-specific antigen (PSA) employing a PSA oligoepitope peptide. J Immunol 1998; 161(6):3186–3194.

78. Gotoh A, Ko SC, Shirakawa T, et al. Development of prostate-specific antigen promoter-based gene therapy for androgen-independent human prostate cancer. J Urol 1998; 160(1):220–229.

79. Fernandez N, Duffour MT, Perricaudet M, et al. Active specific T-cell-based immunotherapy for cancer: nucleic acids, peptides, whole native proteins, recombinant viruses, with dendritic cell adjuvants or whole tumor cell-based vaccines. Principles and future prospects. Cytokines Cell Mol Ther 1998; 4(1):53–65.

80. Disis ML, Cheever MA. HER-2/neu oncogenic protein: issues in vaccine development. Crit Rev Immunol 1998; 18(1–2):37–45.

81. Slovin SF, Ragupathi G, Adluri S, et al. Carbohydrate vaccines in cancer: immunogenicity of a fully synthetic globo H hexasaccharide conjugate in man. Proc Natl Acad Sci USA 1999; 96(10):5710–5715.

82. Tuting T. The immunology of cutaneous DNA immunization. Curr Opin Mol Ther 1999; 1(2):216–225.

83. Berlyn KA, Ponniah S, Stass SA, et al. Developing dendritic cell polynucleotide vaccination for prostate cancer immunotherapy. J Biotechnol 1999; 73(2–3):155–179.

84. Eder JP, Kantoff PW, Roper K, et al. A phase I trial of a recombinant vaccinia virus expressing prostate-specific antigen in advanced prostate cancer. Clin Cancer Res 2000; 6(5):1632–1638.

85. Krieg AM, Matson S, Cheng K, et al. Identification of an oligodeoxynucleotide sequence motif that specifically inhibits phosphorylation by protein tyrosine kinases. Antisense Nucleic Acid Drug Dev 1997; 7(2):115–123.

86. Havranek EG, Whelan MA, Greenhalgh R, et al. Advances in prostate cancer immunotherapy. Surg Oncol 2002; 11(1–2):35–45.

87. Asher AL, Mule JJ, Kasid A, et al. Murine tumor cells transduced with the gene for tumor necrosis factor-alpha. Evidence for paracrine immune effects of tumor necrosis factor against tumors. J Immunol 1991; 146(9):3227–3234.

88. Fearon ER, Pardoll DM, Itaya T, et al. Interleukin-2 production by tumor cells bypasses T helper function in the generation of an antitumor response. Cell 1990; 60(3):397–403.

89. Golumbek PT, Lazenby AJ, Levitsky HI, et al. Treatment of established renal cancer by tumor cells engineered to secrete interleukin-4. Science 1991; 254(5032):713–716.

90. Vieweg J, Rosenthal FM, Bannerji R, et al. Immunotherapy of prostate cancer in the Dunning rat model: use of cytokine gene modified tumor vaccines. Cancer Res 1994; 54(7):1760–1765.

91. Moody DB, Robinson JC, Ewing CM, et al. Interleukin-2 transfected prostate cancer cells generate a local antitumor effect in vivo. Prostate 1994; 24(5):244–251.

92. Simons JW, Mikhak B, Chang JF, et al. Induction of immunity to prostate cancer antigens: results of a clinical trial of vaccination with irradiated autologous prostate tumor cells engineered to secrete granulocyte–macrophage colony-stimulating factor using ex vivo gene transfer. Cancer Res 1999; 59(20):5160–5168.

93. Huang AY, Golumbek P, Ahmadzadeh M, et al. Role of bone marrow-derived cells in presenting MHC class I-restricted tumor antigens. Science 1994; 264(5161):961–965.

94. Huang AY, Golumbek P, Ahmadzadeh M, et al. Bone marrow-derived cells present MHC class I-restricted tumour antigens in priming of antitumour immune responses. Ciba Found Symp 1994; 187:229–240.

95. Matis LA, Sorger SB, McElligott DL, et al. The molecular basis of alloreactivity in antigen-specific, major histocompatibility complex-restricted T cell clones. Cell 1987; 51(1):59–69.

96. Knight BC, Souberbielle BE, Rizzardi GP, et al. Allogeneic murine melanoma cell vaccine: a model for the development of human allogeneic cancer vaccine. Melanoma Res 1996; 6(4):299–306.

97. Hrouda D, Todryk SM, Perry MJ, et al. Allogeneic whole-tumour cell vaccination in the rat model of prostate cancer. BJU Int 2000; 86(6):742–748.

98. Morton DL, Foshag LJ, Hoon DS, et al. Prolongation of survival in metastatic melanoma after active specific immunotherapy with a new polyvalent melanoma vaccine. Ann Surg 1992; 216(4):463–482.

99. Eaton JD, Perry MJ, Nicholson S, et al. Allogeneic whole-cell vaccine: a phase I/II study in men with hormone-refractory prostate cancer. BJU Int 2002; 89(1):19–26.

100. Bocchia M, Bronte V, Colombo MP, et al. Antitumor vaccination: where we stand. Haematologica 2000; 85(11):1172–1206.

101. Hilgenfeld RU, Streit M, Thiel E, Kreuser ED. Current treatment modalities in advanced colorectal carcinoma. Recent Results Cancer Res 1996; 142:353–380.

102. Freeman SM, Abboud CN, Whartenby KA, et al. The 'bystander effect': tumor regression when a fraction of the tumor mass is genetically modified. Cancer Res 1993; 53(21):5274–5283.

103. Lawrence TS, Rehemtulla A, Ng EY, et al. Preferential cytotoxicity of cells transduced with cytosine deaminase compared to bystander cells after treatment with 5-flucytosine. Cancer Res 1998; 58(12):2588–2593.

104. Kuriyama S, Mitoro A, Yamazaki M, et al. Comparison of gene therapy with the herpes simplex virus thymidine kinase gene and the bacterial cytosine deaminase gene for the treatment of hepatocellular carcinoma. Scand J Gastroenterol 1999; 34(10):1033–1041.

105. Eaton JD, Perry MJ, Todryk SM, et al. Genetic prodrug activation therapy (GPAT) in two rat prostate models generates an immune bystander effect and can be monitored by magnetic resonance techniques. Gene Ther 2001; 8(7):557–567.

106. Ramesh R, Marrogi AJ, Munshi A, et al. In vivo analysis of the 'bystander effect': a cytokine cascade. Exp Hematol 1996; 24(7):829–838.

107. Herman JR, Adler HL, Aguilar-Cordova E, et al. In situ gene therapy for adenocarcinoma of the prostate: a phase I clinical trial. Hum Gene Ther 1999; 10(7):1239–1249.

108. Shalev M, Kadmon D, Teh BS, et al. Suicide gene therapy toxicity after multiple and repeat injections in patients with localized prostate cancer. J Urol 2000; 163(6):1747–1750.

109. Ayala G, Wheeler TM, Shalev M, et al. Cytopathic effect of in situ gene therapy in prostate cancer. Hum Pathol 2000; 31(7):866–870.

110. Banchereau J, Steinman RM. Dendritic cells and the control of immunity. Nature 1998; 392(6673):245–252.

111. Steinman RM. The dendritic cell system and its role in immunogenicity. Annu Rev Immunol 1991; 9:271–296.

112. Tsujitani S, Kakeji Y, Watanabe A, et al. Infiltration of dendritic cells in relation to tumor invasion and lymph node metastasis in human gastric cancer. Cancer 1990; 66(9):2012–2016.

113. Dummer W, Becker JC, Schwaaf A, et al. Elevated serum levels of interleukin-10 in patients with metastatic malignant melanoma. Melanoma Res 1995; 5(1):67–68.

114. Gabrilovich DI, Chen HL, Girgis KR, et al. Production of vascular endothelial growth factor by human tumors inhibits the functional maturation of dendritic cells. Nat Med 1996; 2(10):1096–1103.

115. Burch PA, Breen JK, Buckner JC, et al. Priming tissue-specific cellular immunity in a phase I trial of autologous dendritic cells for prostate cancer. Clin Cancer Res 2000; 6(6):2175–2182.

116. Small EJ, Fratesi P, Reese DM, et al. Immunotherapy of hormone-refractory prostate cancer with antigen-loaded dendritic cells. J Clin Oncol 2000; 18(23):3894–3903.

117. Tjoa BA, Lodge PA, Salgaller ML, et al. Dendritic cell-based immunotherapy for prostate cancer. CA Cancer J Clin 1999; 49(2):117–128.

118. Ritossa F. Discovery of the heat shock response. Cell Stress Chaperones 1996; 1(2):97–98.

119. Parsell DA, Lindquist S. The function of heat-shock proteins in stress tolerance: degradation and reactivation of damaged proteins. Annu Rev Genet 1993; 27:437–496.

120. Udono H, Levey DL, Srivastava PK. Cellular requirements for tumor-specific immunity elicited by heat shock proteins: tumor rejection antigen gp96 primes CD8+ T cells in vivo. Proc Natl Acad Sci USA 1994; 91(8):3077–3081.

121. Li Z. Priming of T cells by heat shock protein–peptide complexes as the basis of tumor vaccines. Semin Immunol 1997; 9(5):315–322.

122. Suto R, Srivastava PK. A mechanism for the specific immunogenicity of heat shock protein-chaperoned peptides. Science 1995; 269(5230):1585–1588.

123. Wang XY, Kaneko Y, Repasky E, Subjeck JR. Heat shock proteins and cancer immunotherapy. Immunol Invest 2000; 29(2):131–137.

124. Yedavelli SP, Guo L, Daou ME, et al. Preventive and therapeutic effect of tumor derived heat shock protein, gp96, in an experimental prostate cancer model. Int J Mol Med 1999; 4(3):243–248.

125. Janetzki S, Palla D, Rosenhauer V, et al. Immunization of cancer patients with autologous cancer-derived heat shock protein gp96 preparations: a pilot study. Int J Cancer 2000; 88(2):232–238.

15

What's hot and what's not – the medical management of BPH

Simon RJ Bott, Charlotte L Foley and Roger S Kirby

Introduction

Benign prostatic hyperplasia (BPH) has been treated medically for over 20 years. Where once surgery was the treatment of choice, now medical therapy is used as the first line treatment except in complicated bladder outflow obstruction. The number of patients undergoing transurethral resection of the prostate (TURP) in the United States has halved and Europe is gradually mirroring this decline.[1] This is in the context of an ever-aging population, where the incidence of BPH is rising and will continue to do so for the foreseeable future. While currently about 15% of the population in the US is over 65 years old, this figure is expected to rise to 22% by 2025.[2] To compound matters, total populations in developed countries are gradually falling, resulting in fewer younger people to pay for the health care of increasing numbers of elderly patients.

The terminology used to describe symptomatic BPH is variable and therefore the quoted incidence figures also vary depending on the definition used. Overall however, it appears that the incidence of BPH is fairly uniform across the developed world. The American Agency for Health Care Policy and Research (AHCPR) estimates that of 22.5 million white men aged between 50 and 79 years in the US, 5.6 million (25%) would have symptoms of sufficient severity to warrant a discussion of treatment options, according to the AHCPR guidelines. These criteria are an international prostate symptom score (I-PSS) of > 7 and a maximum flow rate of < 15 ml/sec. Community based studies in Europe confirm these figures. For example, in Austria the proportion of men with an I-PSS > 7 is 27.1% in those aged 50–59 years and 36% in those aged 70–79.[3] In the UK, 29–51% of men aged 50 or over have an I-PSS ≥ 8, depending on the age group.[4]

Although the incidence of BPH is similar, the management strategies vary greatly from country to country. In both France and the UK the number of elderly men is about equal (approximately 4 million); however France spends in the order of 180 million euros in ex-factory sales on medical therapies for BPH compared with less than half this value in the UK.[5] This may be due to a variety of reasons. Men in the UK may stoically accept their lower tract urinary symptoms (LUTS) as a feature of aging and be unaware of the risk of prostate cancer and so not seek medical help. Alternatively, within the tight financial confines of the UK's National Health Service doctors may be more willing to advise a 'watch and wait' policy in men with mild or moderate LUTS. Finally, patients in France are more likely to receive phytotherapeutic drugs, which make up nearly 40% of the medicinal market share. As these are perceived as 'natural' and 'harmless' there may be a lower threshold for initiating one of these agents than a standard pharmaceutical product. It is perhaps surprising that despite a large body of evidence defining the role of medical therapies there is not a greater consensus on their respective use. More data are required on the efficacy and safety of phytotherapies, though a management strategy along the lines of the AHCPR guidelines[6] or the International Consultation on BPH[7] would offer a more rational approach to BPH management.

The natural history of BPH

The likely outcome of a watch and wait policy – whether 'prescribed' or incidental – is being addressed by the ongoing longitudinal community trial in Olmsted County, USA. Encompassing over 2000 untreated men and with follow up of up to 11 years, this represents one of the largest and longest studies of its kind. From a randomly selected subset of 25% of patients aged 40–79 years, the I-PSS, peak flow and prostate volume were measured every 18–24 months.[8] The prostate growth rate was 2.4% per year, but was greater in men with higher baseline prostate volumes (> 30 ml) and higher prostate specific antigen (PSA) scores. Prostate growth rate was only mildly related to the symptom score and not related to the baseline peak urinary flow rate. Prostatic enlargement, PSA and age are all associated with an increased risk of developing acute urinary retention (AUR) and requiring BPH related treatment.[9] The Olmsted County trial implies that men with prostates > 30 ml or an elevated PSA in particular should be targeted for treatment as they are more likely to have faster growing BPH and as a result are more likely to require intervention in the future.[8]

The impact of LUTS on sexual function was addressed in a large study by Rosen et al[8a]. They reported on 14 000 European and American men aged 50–79 years who completed the I-PSS, Danish Prostate Symptom Score (DAN-PSSsex) and the international index of erectile function (IIEF-15) questionnaires. They found that across Europe and the US the mean frequency of sexual intercourse/activity in this age group was 5.8 times per month. In men with no LUTS this varied from a mean 8.6 times for a man in his 50s to 4.0 times for a man in his 70s. Notably, men who had moderate or severe LUTS had sexual intercourse/activity, erectile function and sexual desire equivalent to a man a decade their senior. What is more, 78% of men with erectile problems were bothered by their symptoms. This large study exposes the extent and affect that LUTS have on men's sexual function. It would be interesting to see whether by improving these men's LUTS with medical therapy there is a corresponding improvement in their sexual function.

Alpha-adrenergic antagonists

Alpha-blockers remain the gold standard medical therapy for symptomatic BPH taking the largest market share of medical therapies across Europe and the US. The human lower urinary tract contains both alpha-1 and alpha-2 adrenoceptors; prostatic smooth muscle however contains predominantly alpha-1 adrenoceptors.[10] Three alpha-1 adrenoceptors subtypes have been identified: alpha-1A, alpha-1B and alpha-1D; lower urinary tract smooth muscle contraction is mainly mediated through the alpha-1A subtype. Alpha-blockers act by blocking these receptors, interrupting the motor sympathetic adrenergic nerve supply and leading to relaxation of the smooth muscle of the prostatic stroma, capsule and the bladder neck. The first alpha-blocker used in the treatment of symptomatic BPH was phenoxybenzamine, a non-selective alpha-1 and 2 inhibitor.[11] This is now obsolete as alpha-2 receptor blockade resulted in excessive cardiovascular side effects. Subsequently, prazosin (a selective alpha-1 blocker originally used as an antihypertensive agent) was developed for the treatment of BPH. A second generation of alpha-blockers followed including doxazosin, alfuzosin, terazosin and indoramin, marketed as having fewer side effects. With the discovery of the alpha-1 receptor subtypes more recently, a third generation (or alpha 1A-selective) alpha-blocker, tamsulosin, has been developed.

Interestingly, alpha-blockers are particularly effective at treating the irritative symptoms associated with BPH and provide fairly modest improvements in urinary flow rates. Surgery on the other hand, is very effective at relieving obstructive symptoms and improving flow rates but is not as efficient at relieving irritative symptoms. These findings may point to another role of alpha-blockers besides simply smooth muscle relaxation in and around the prostate.[12] Alpha-1 receptors are found in the human bladder and the spinal cord; in contrast to the prostate these are predominantly alpha-1D adrenoceptors. Furthermore, in rats alpha-1D adrenoceptors antagonists, inhibit detrusor instability possibly through inhibition at the levels of the bladder and the spinal cord.[13] The fact that even the relatively selective alpha-1A blocker tamsulosin also has a high affinity for alpha-1D adrenoceptors explains why these agents are as effective as the less selective alpha-1 blockers at relieving irritative symptoms.[12] Moreover, their effect on alpha-1D adrenoceptors may explain why these drugs are useful in some women with irritative voiding symptoms.

Our understanding of how exactly alpha-blockers exert their effect is incomplete; however this should not detract from the large body of evidence supporting their efficacy and safety. Data from large multicenter placebo-controlled trials on all the main alpha-blockers has been available for a number of years and has recently been pooled in several meta-analyses. In one such meta-analysis of 92 phase II and III trials involving 44 000 patients, alpha-blockers were shown to provide superior efficacy when compared with placebo controls.[14] In addition, efficacy was very similar for the different alpha-blockers available. Symptom scores improved by an average 35% on treatment and maximum flow rate increased by between 1.8 and 2.5 ml/sec. The authors concluded that selective alpha-1 blockers significantly reduced the incidence of side effects and that super-selective agents may reduce these unwanted effects still further.

In a separate review, Chapple specifically examined the more specific alpha-blockers with respect to efficacy and safety.[15] Pooling together four studies involving nearly 3000 patients he reported that alfuzosin, terazosin, doxazosin and tamsulosin all significantly improve symptom scores by 17–38% and flow rates by 1.4–2.4 ml/sec.

As all alpha-blockers are largely equally efficacious, their side effect profile dictates which agent is used in a particular patient. In a further meta-analysis Djavan et al[16] reported that the discontinuation rates due to unwanted side effects such as orthostatic hypertension and dizziness were higher in trials involving prazosin, terazosin and doxazosin. These side effects may be beneficial in some patients. Doxazosin has been shown to reduce the blood pressure of hypertensive but not normotensive individuals.[17] This single agent can therefore be used to treat both BPH and hypertension. However, in the majority of men side effects are unwanted and these can be minimized by choosing a more selective agent. The effect of alpha-blockers on sexual function is summarized in Table 15.1.

5 Alpha-reductase inhibitors (5ARIs)

Finasteride, a 5 alpha-reductase type II inhibitor, has been available for over 10 years and although prescribing patterns vary, it commands up to 36% market share in some European countries[5] (Fig. 15.1). Finasteride was one of the first 'designer drugs' with a structure mimicking that of testosterone, so it competitively inhibits 5-alpha reductase, without inhibiting the testosterone receptor. By blocking the enzyme that produces the more potent testosterone analog, dihydrotestosterone (DHT), finasteride reduces gland size and reverses the disease process albeit over several months. Large studies have confirmed its efficacy at reducing LUTS, improving flow rates and reducing the incidence of acute urinary retention and the need for surgical intervention.[18–20] In a meta-analysis of 2600 patients, Boyle et al[21] noted that differences in prostate size accounted for about 85% of the variation in outcome seen between the six randomized trials in this study. Significant benefits over placebo were only seen in men with prostate glands of over 40 ml and these benefits increased with prostate size.[21]

Finasteride inhibits type II 5-alpha reductase only. In an attempt to reduce the levels of DHT still further GlaxoSmithKline pioneered a novel type I and II 5-alpha reductase inhibitor – dutasteride. Recently launched, the first reports of its efficacy and safety were presented at the European Association of Urology and American Urological Association (AUA) annual meetings in 2002.[22] To be included in these phase III multicenter trials, men had to be at least 50 years old, with prostate volumes of 30 ml or over, an I-PSS of 12 points

Table 15.1 The effects of alpha-blockers on sexual function

Alpha-blocker	Impotence (%)		Ejaculation failure (%)		Reduced libido (%)	
	Drug	Placebo	Drug	Placebo	Drug	Placebo
Alfuzosin (n = 358)	2.2	–	0	–	0.6	–
Terazosin (n = 305)	6	5	0.3	1	3	1
Tamsulosin (n = 381)	0.8	1.6	4.5*	1	1	0

p < 0.05. Adapted from Debruyne FMJ. Urology 2000; 56(suppl 5A):20.

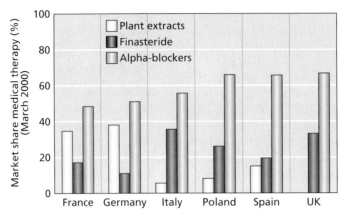

Figure 15.1 Percentage market share (value March 2000) of phytotherapy, finasteride and alpha-1 adrenoceptor agonists in France, Germany, Italy, Poland, Spain and the UK.

or more and a maximum flow rate of 15 ml/sec or less. Men who had large residual volumes (> 250 ml), a history of prostate cancer, previous prostate surgery, an episode of acute urinary retention within 3 months, the use of an alpha-blocker within 4 weeks or any 5ARI, were excluded. Men with a PSA value less than 1.5 ng/ml or greater than 10 ng/ml were also excluded. A minimum prostate volume and PSA level was set as data from finasteride trials demonstrates 5ARIs are most effective in men with glands of 30 ml or more and a serum PSA in excess of 1.5 ng/ml. A total of 4325 patients were randomized in three parallel placebo-controlled trials lasting 24 months. Dutasteride was shown to rapidly lower serum DHT measurements in the majority of men by 90% or more and prostate volume measurements showed a significant corresponding decline from as early as the first month of the trial. However, although the AUA symptom index scores improved in one of the three studies within 3 months, when pooled a significant improvement was not seen until 6 months. At 24 months the treated group experienced a mean improvement of 4.5 points compared with an improvement of 2.3 for the placebo controls (p < 0.001) (Table 15.2).

Flow rate improvements were significantly better from 1 month and thereafter in the treatment arm, up to 2.2 ml/sec compared with 0.6 ml/sec in the placebo group. Interestingly serum PSA levels fell by just over half in the dutasteride group, a similar reduction to that seen with finasteride. There was

a relative risk reduction of 57% for developing AUR and 48% for BPH-related surgical intervention. Dutasteride was well tolerated, although impotence, decreased libido, ejaculation disorder and gynecomastia were significantly greater in the test arm during the first year of the study. The sexual side effects declined in the test arm and were no longer significantly different at 2 years. In addition, the incidence of newly diagnosed prostate cancer was 1.9% in the placebo arm and 1.1% in the dutasteride group. While this represents only a small absolute risk reduction, the relative risk reduction of over 40% has prompted a larger trial to look at its possible role in prostate cancer prevention.

Dutasteride is clearly very effective at rapidly lowering serum DHT and shrinking the prostate, particularly the transition zone. Despite its dual action its efficacy and side effect profile is similar to finasteride.[18] While we will not know whether the additional effect of antagonizing both isoenzymes is better than type II alone until a comparative study is performed, this agent appears at least as good as finasteride and offers an alternative medication for the treatment of men with larger glands.

Combination therapy

The concept of combining an alpha-blocker, which relaxes the smooth muscle in the bladder neck and prostate, with a 5 alpha-reductase

Table 15.2 Results of placebo controlled clinical trials on dutasteride22

	Dutasteride	Placebo	p value
Median change in serum DHT	−90.2%	+9.6%	p < 0.001
Total prostate volume (ml)	−14.6 ± 13.5	0.8 ± 14.3	p < 0.001
Change in symptom score	−4.5 ± 6.6	−2.3 ± 6.8	p < 0.001
Change in Qmax ml/sec	+2.2 ± 5.2	+0.6 ± 4.7	p < 0.001
Patients with AUR	39 (1.8%)	90 (4.2%)	p < 0.001, relative risk reduction 57%
Patients requiring BPH related surgery	47 (2.2%)	89 (4.1%)	p < 0.001, relative risk reduction 48%

AUR, acute urinary retention; BPH, benign prostatic hyperplasia; DHT, dihydrotestosterone.

Table 15.3 Summary of the results of the MTOPS trial

	Placebo	Doxazosin	Finasteride	Combination
Reduction in median AUA SS	4.0	6.0	5.0	7.0
Increase in median maximum flow rate	1.4	2.5	2.2	3.7
Disease progression (crude event rate per 100 patient years)	4.5	2.7	2.9	1.5
Risk reduction compared to placebo	–	39%	34%	67%
AUR rate (per 100 patient years)	0.6	0.4	0.2	0.1
Rate of invasive therapy for BPH (per 100 patient years)	1.3	1.2	0.5	0.4

AUA SS, American Urological Association symptom score; AUR, acute urinary retention; BPH, benign prostatic hyperplasia.

inhibitor, which by acting on the epithelial component reverses the natural progression of BPH, seems sound. Yet, until recently, large randomized placebo-controlled studies failed to show a significant difference when finasteride was added to either the alpha-blocker terazosin[23] or doxazosin.[24] Perhaps this was not surprising, as the mean prostate size in these two studies was below the 40 ml cut-off at which finasteride has been shown to provide a significant improvement. Furthermore the follow-up period in each of these two trials was for only 1 year. It is conceivable that the small number of men with prostates over 40 ml did not have sufficient treatment time to benefit fully from finasteride.

Recently however, the Medical Therapy of Prostate Symptoms (MTOPS) trial has been reported[24a]. The aim of this study was to determine whether medical therapy prevents or delays the clinical progression of BPH. This multicenter, randomized, placebo-controlled, double-blind study assigned 3047 men to receive doxazosin (4–8 mg), finasteride (5 mg), doxazosin plus finasteride, or placebo. The primary outcome was the time to clinical progression after a minimum follow up of 4 years and a mean follow up of 5 years. Mean baseline patient characteristics were I-PSS 17.0 (range 12.0–21.0), Qmax 10.6 ml/sec (range 8.5–12.3) and prostate size 36 ml (± 20 ml).

In all study arms, a total of 350 men progressed to one of the predefined clinical endpoints; 78% of these were an I-PSS rise > 4 points, 12% developed acute urinary retention, 9% incontinence, 1% urinary infection and none developed renal insufficiency secondary to BPH.

Monotherapy with either doxazosin or finasteride produced an equivalent but significant reduction in the incidence of BPH progression compared with placebo, while combination therapy was substantially more effective when compared with monotherapy (Table 15.3).

Interestingly, finasteride alone was equally effective at preventing AUR as combination therapy, with an overall risk reduction of 70–80%. The alpha-blockers postponed the time to occurrence of AUR, although over the whole course of the trial there was no reduction in risk of AUR in the doxazosin monotherapy arm. Likewise, finasteride and combination therapy significantly reduced the incidence of an invasive procedure; doxazosin alone delayed the occurrence but not the overall rate of invasive procedures.

The authors emphasized that combination therapy was particularly beneficial with respect to symptom score and flow rate improvements over the longer term. The prostate volume increased in both the placebo and the doxazosin arms by an average 4.5% per annum, while in the finasteride and combination arms a mean reduction of 13 and 16% respectively, was reported.

The incidence of adverse events was similar to other series. McConnell concluded that combination therapy in selected patients might be the most effective way of improving symptom score and flow rate as well as reducing the risk of clinical progression with its associated sequelae[24a].

Other approaches to combination therapy have also been reported. Alpha-blockers provide rapid relief of symptomatic BPH, although this may not be maintained over the longer term. 5ARIs on the other hand take longer to achieve symptomatic relief, but sustain this relief over a period of many years by modifying the disease process. Diamond et al[25] therefore took the logical step and randomized 120 patients to receive an alpha-blocker in combination with a 5ARI and after 24 weeks withdrew the alpha-blocker in the test arm. This double-blind trial used the super-selective alpha-blocker tamsulosin and the 5ARI finasteride in group one and tamsulosin and placebo in second parallel control group. In both groups tamsulosin was stopped at 6, 9 and 12 months and patients were re-evaluated 1 month after discontinuation of treatment. It should be emphasized all 120 patients in this trial had prostates of > 40 g, I-PSS > 17 and Q_{max} < 15 ml/sec and so reflect the moderate–severe end of the BPH spectrum.

At 6 months, 55% of patients from the first group reported no change in symptom scores after discontinuing tamsulosin and their Q_{max} maintained an increase of 2.5 ml/sec compared with 20% of men in the control arm. By 9 months 80% of group 1 men successfully discontinued tamsulosin compared with 25% in the control group and at 12 months 85% of group 1 were successfully discontinued compared with 20% in group 2. This study concluded that finasteride maintains the subjective and objective effects of combination therapy after 9–12 months in patients with enlarged prostate and LUTS.

A similar study by Baldwin et al used the alpha-blocker doxazosin rather than tamsulosin in combination with finasteride.[26] They reported no worsening of symptom score in 13–15% of men who discontinued doxazosin at 3 months, 40–48% at 6 months, 73–84% at 9 months and 84–87% at 12 months.

Similarly the Symptom Management After Reducing Therapy (SMART) trial randomized 327 men with I-PSS ≥ 12 and prostate volumes ≥ 30 ml in a prospective, multicenter, double-blind study involving combination therapy followed by withdrawal.[27] Initially, all patients received the new 5ARI dutasteride in combination with tamsulosin for a period of 24 weeks. In the study arm, the tamsulosin was then withdrawn and replaced by placebo and the trial continued for a further 12 weeks. In the men in whom the alpha-blocker was discontinued, 77% felt their symptoms were the same or better 6 weeks after stopping tamsulosin and this was maintained in 93% of patients at the end of the study period.

In a subsidiary part of the SMART trial there was a close correlation between the I-PSS and the how the patient felt. Patients who 'felt better' had a decrease (improvement) in I-PSS of –2.0 (median: interquatile range –4.00 to 0.00). Conversely, men who 'felt worse' had an increase in their I-PSS of 4.0 (2.0–9.5) and in patients who 'felt the same' there was little or no change in their I-PSS (0.0, –1.0 to 2.0). This is contrary to the findings from the Olmsted County trial.[28] In this untreated population of men, aged between 40 and 79 years old, I-PSS gradually deteriorated with advancing age, increasing from a median 0.02 units per annum for men in their 40s to 0.43 units per annum for men in their 60s. Importantly, there was no change in the bother score across all ages (median change = 0, –0.30, 0.29). This reflects the selection criteria for patients receiving active treatment. Men with BPH tend to consult a doctor either because they are troubled by their LUTS or because they are concerned with the possibility that they might have prostate cancer. As the treated patients are bothered or at least aware of their symptoms, they are more likely to notice a change in their LUTS.

The role of combination therapy in the management of symptomatic BPH has yet to be defined.

Adding two therapies together not only increases the costs of treatment but also the incidence of side effects. Moreover, both finasteride and dutasteride are only effective in men with prostates of more than 40 ml, so the value of combination therapy in men with glands smaller than this is questionable. Nevertheless, in men with larger glands, combination therapy may be the best option, particularly in patients where surgery would be best avoided. It offers rapid and lasting symptom relief, enhanced quality of life and a reduced risk of complications secondary to BPH. While MTOPS suggested an additive effect with regard to efficacy in combination therapy, most other studies have not. It may be possible to maintain symptom and quality of life improvements by using combination therapy at least for 6–12 months and then discontinue the alpha-blocker without a resultant worsening in symptoms.

Phytotherapy

Men have used phytotherapies for centuries for the treatment of a variety of ailments, including symptomatic BPH. Though not a new medical therapy, the rapid expansion of this market in recent years has focused our attention to these products. Now over 90% of men in the US referred with lower urinary tract symptoms have tried or are using an alternative/complementary therapy.[29] The market for these treatments has increased dramatically, rising in the US from $500 000 in 1996 to over $1 billion today.[29] In Europe, the use of phytotherapies is variable. They are the first line therapy of choice in Germany, Austria, France and Spain and make up over 90% of all drugs prescribed for BPH in Austria and Germany. In the UK, Italy and Poland their share of the BPH medicines market is less than 10%.[5]

Phytotherapies are derived from roots, seeds, bark, fruits, flowers and leaves. They are sold either as monopreparations or in combination. Several manufacturers supply a combination of different plant extracts to create their own 'prostate health pill'; this can then be registered whereas single-plant monopreparations have no patent protection. Furthermore, combinations may have enhanced marketability by having a 'unique formula' or 'enhanced efficacy'.

The trouble with performing studies to investigate these compounds is not only the variability of the combinations but also the varying dose of active ingredients obtained from the plant. The same plant species may produce different amounts of active product depending on the conditions in which it grows as well as the technique used in the extraction process. As the 'active' compound is frequently unknown, quantifying the optimal dosing may be little more than guesswork. Indeed, when the National Consumer Laboratory in the US analyzed the free fatty acid content, the presumed active ingredient, in 27 different saw palmetto products,[30] they found this to vary by 0–95%, with only 17 of the products containing the 'standard' 85% dose.

Studies aimed at investigating the mechanism of action of phytotherapies are almost all performed in vitro on tissue cultures and with supraphysiologic doses, which do not reflect the in vivo effects.[31] The mechanisms of action most commonly suggested include anti-inflammatory, 5 alpha-reductase inhibition and growth factor alteration. Until recently, very little reliable safety or efficacy data were available on these compounds. Even now, properly performed studies are scarce and limited by the complexity and uncontrolled nature of these substances.

Despite these reservations, these products have stood the test of time and the fact that so many men go out and buy them is perhaps testimony to their efficacy even if they have not passed through the rigorous scrutiny of conventional pharmacological agents. Although they are perceived as natural and therefore presumed safe, this remains to be demonstrated objectively in large scale trials.

Serenoa repens

Serenoa repens is the most popular and best studied of the phytotherapies used in BPH. It is also known as saw palmetto, American dwarf palm, *Sabal serrulatum* (its botanical name) and Permixon (its trade name). The mechanism of action of *Serenoa repens* is probably by inhibition of the enzyme 5 alpha-reductase,[32] although there may be other mechanisms including an anti-inflammatory effect via inhibition of cyclooxygenase synthesis,[32] inhibition of the growth factors b-FGF and EGF[33] or antiestrogenic effects.[34] Interestingly, *Serenoa repens* does not reduce serum PSA levels, unlike finasteride, and therefore its mechanism of action, though antiandrogenic, may differ from the highly selective 5 alpha-reductase inhibitors.[35,36]

There have been a large number of trials considering the efficacy of *Serenoa repens*; however, the vast majority are uncontrolled, open label studies. Of those that are placebo controlled, none meets the accepted criteria for assessing treatment in men with LUTS developed by the International Consultation on BPH[37] since they involved small patient numbers, limited follow up or lack of standardized symptom scoring.

Two large meta-analyses have been performed in an attempt to combine the results of these limited trials and to derive the best information available. The first by Wilt et al[38] combined 21 randomized trials involving 3139 men receiving *Serenoa repens* either as monotherapy or in combination. They concluded that *Serenoa repens* provided a mild to moderate improvement in urinary symptoms (weighted mean difference −1.41 points, 95% CI = −2.52, −0.30) and urinary flow (weighted mean difference 1.86 ml/sec, 95% CI = 0.60, 3.12). In two studies that compared *Serenoa repens* with finasteride there were similar improvements with both agents. Side-effects were mild and infrequent, occurring in 9% of men compared with 11% in the two studies involving finasteride (not significantly different).

In the second meta-analysis on *Serenoa repens* performed by Boyle et al,[39] 13 trials were combined incorporating 2859 men receiving Permixon only. Only two of the 13 trials used the standard I-PSS questionnaire, so the only common endpoints were nocturia and peak flow rates with the latter not given in two studies. Although some heterogeneity existed between trials, Permixon significantly reduced the mean number of episodes of nocturia by an additional 0.50 ± 0.012 episodes per night and the flow rate by an additional 2.20 ± 0.51 ml/sec over and above the placebo effect.

No valuable data were accrued by either meta-analysis with regard to the effects of *Serenoa repens* on the incidence of acute urinary retention or the need for surgical intervention.

Meta-analyses are by design inherently flawed due to the heterogeneity of studies incorporated, each with their different patients, different design populations and different outcome measures.

These findings may not reflect the results of future long-term, randomized, placebo-controlled trials, though in the meantime they may reassure us that *Serenoa repens* is safe and probably effective at least to some extent. The results of two ongoing large placebo-controlled trials sponsored and coordinated by the National Institute of Health and the United States National Institute of Diabetes and Diseases of the Kidney should provide a more objective, unbiased assessment of *Serenoa repens*.

Published more recently and therefore not included in these meta-analyses was a study over a period of 12 months comparing Permixon with the alpha-blocker tamsulosin.[35] This double-blind, multicenter European trial involved 811 men with I-PSS ≥ 10. Both drugs produced very similar improvements in the I-PSS (decreased by 4.4 in both groups) and maximum flow rates (increased by 1.8 ml/sec Permixon, 1.9 ml/sec tamsulosin). Both compounds were well tolerated. This is the first valid comparison of *Serenoa repens* with an alpha-blocker, although further studies and longer follow up are required before these two products can be considered equally efficacious.

The use of *Serenoa repens* in combination with tamsulosin was addressed in a study by Glémain et al.[40] Over 300 patients with I-PSS ≥ 13 were randomized to receive either 0.4 mg tamsulosin monotherapy or tamsulosin in combination with 160 mg *Serenoa repens*. While tamsulosin monotherapy improved I-PSS by a mean −5.2 units (SD 6.4), combination with *Serenoa repens* had no additional benefit (I-PSS improvement −6.0 SD 6.0, p = 0.286).

Pygeum africanum

Pygeum africanum (African plum) is believed to act by modulating growth factor induced cell growth and proliferation.[33] Its effects on the bladder were elegantly demonstrated by Levin et al[41] using a rabbit model with surgically induced partial bladder outflow obstruction. They showed that increases in the bladder wall mass and decreases in compliance caused by partial outflow obstruction could be reduced by treatment with *Pygeum africanum*.

Although numerous, clinical trials on this compound are largely inadequate and to date none has met the criteria of the International Consultation on BPH for assessing treatment in men with

LUTS.[37] Studies currently underway include the Tadenam–I-PSS study and the United States National Institute of Diabetes and Diseases of the Kidney sponsored trials. The results of these are awaited before meaningful efficacy and safety conclusions can be drawn about this product.

Hypoxis rooperi

Also known as South African star grass or Harzol®, *Hypoxis rooperi* contains beta-sitosterol and other sterols, which, in vitro, elevate levels of transforming growth factor beta-1 and induce apoptosis.[42] Although these effects have not been shown in vivo, the results of some of the clinical trials are impressive. In a double-blind, placebo-controlled trial of 200 patients,[43] later extended to an open label study,[44] Harzol® improved symptom score and maximum urinary flow rates very significantly. The I-PSS improved by 7.4 points in the test arm compared with 2.3 points in the control arm and the maximum flow rate by 5.2 ml/sec in the test versus 1.1 ml/sec in the placebo group.[43] In the follow-up open label study, men who continued on Harzol® maintained their symptom and flow rate improvements, but interestingly the 14 men who stopped all BPH therapy maintained similar improvements over the following 12 months, suggesting a possible use of Harzol® in intermittent therapy.[44]

Another compound that contains beta-sitosterol – Azuprostat, derived from *Hypoxis rooperi* as well as *Pinus* (pine) and *Picea* (spruce) – was evaluated in a 6-month randomized placebo-controlled trial involving 177 men.[45] The I-PSS improvements were 8.2 units in the treated arm and 2.8 units in the placebo arm. The flow rate improved by 8.9 ml/sec in the treatment arm and by 4.4 ml/sec in the control group. The size of these improvements is far greater than any other medical treatment and if reproducible would challenge figures achieved by surgical intervention. However, this study raises several issues. The placebo group achieved a mean flow rate improvement of 4.4 ml/sec – greater than most reported flow rate improvements seen in the medical treatment arm of most published series, let alone the placebo arm. Furthermore, although the patients had a mean age of 65 years the mean flow rate in the treatment group was 19.4 ml/sec. This is a value well in excess of the normal for this age

of man and raises serious questions about the study's validity.

These studies, together with two other trials, led Wilt et al[46] in a recent meta-analysis to conclude that beta-sitosterol does improve the symptom score and flow rate of men with BPH. However, its long-term effectiveness, safety and ability to prevent the complications of BPH remain to be established.[46]

There are over 30 phytotherapeutic treatments for symptomatic BPH but the remainder have been evaluated even less than those described above. While there is undoubtedly a role for these agents in the medicinal armamentarium, too little is known about their efficacy and safety at the present time for them to be recommended.

Conclusions

Medical agents are currently not as effective at treating BPH as surgery. This, together with the demands of the aging population, will drive further research to find newer, more effective treatments. A better understanding of the mechanisms of action of the phytotherapies may aid the development of conventional treatments and perhaps standardize alternative treatments. This work will be enhanced by the vast tissue bank accrued from the MTOPS trial. Our understanding of the efficacy of alpha-blockers and 5 alpha-reductase inhibitors is becoming established, although important questions, such as the place of combination therapy and the role of 5ARISs in the prevention of BPH related complications in asymptomatic men, still need to be answered.

References

1. Holtgrewe HL, Bay-Nielsen H, Carlesson P, et al. Proceedings of the 4th International Consultation on Benign Prostatic Hyperplasia (BPH). Plymouth: Plymbridge Distributors; 1998.
2. US Bureau of the Census. http://www.census.gov/ 5-10-2000.
3. Madersbacher S, Haidinger G, Temml C, Schmidbauer CP. Prevalence of lower urinary tract symptoms in Austria as assessed by an open survey of 2,096 men. Eur Urol 1998; 34(2):136–141.
4. Trueman P, Hood SC, Nayak US, Mrazek MF. Prevalence of lower urinary tract symptoms and self-reported diagnosed 'benign prostatic hyperplasia', and their effect on quality of life in a community-based survey of men in the UK. BJU Int 1999; 83(4):410–415.
5. McNicholas TA. Lower urinary tract symptoms

suggestive of benign prostatic obstruction: what are the current practice patterns? Eur Urol 1 A.D.; 39(suppl 3):26–30.

6. McConnell JD, Barry MJ, Bruskewitz R. Clinical practice guideline for benign prostatic hyperplasia: diagnosis and treatment. Department of Health and Human Services. AHCPR publication no. 94–0582; 1994.

7. Denis L, McConnell JD, Yoshida O, et al. Proceedings of the 4th International Consulation on Benign Prostatic Hyperplasia (BPH). Plymouth: Plymouth Health Publication Ltd.; 1997: 669–683.

8. Rhodes T, Jacobson DJ, Jacobson SJ, et al. Longitudinal prostate volume in a community-based sample: long-term follow up in the Olmsted county study of urinary symptoms and health status among men. American Urological Association Annual Meeting. 2002:1059 [Abstract].

8a. Rosen R, O'Leary M, Altwein J et al. Lower urinary tract symptoms and male sexual dysfunction: The multi-national survery of the aging male (MSAM-7). Lancet 2003 (Submitted).

9. Anderson JB, Roehrborn CG, Schalken JA, Emberton M. The progression of benign prostatic hyperplasia: examining the evidence and determining the risk. Eur Urol 2001; 39(4):390–399.

10. Chapple CR, Aubry ML, James S, et al. Characterisation of human prostatic adrenoceptors using pharmacology receptor binding and localisation. Br J Urol 1989; 63(5):487–496.

11. Caine M, Perlberg S, Meretyk S. A placebo-controlled double-blind study of the effect of phenoxybenzamine in benign prostatic obstruction. Br J Urol 1978; 50(7):551–554.

12. Michel MC, Schafers RF, Goepel M. Alpha-blockers and lower urinary tract function: more than smooth muscle relaxation? BJU Int 2000; 86(suppl 2):23–28.

13. Broten T, Scott A, Siegl PKS, Forray C. Alpha-1 adrenoceptor blockade inhibits detrusor instability in rats with bladder outlet obstruction. FASEB J 1998; 12:A445.

14. Heimbach D, Muller SC. Treatment of benign prostatic hyperplasia with alpha 1-adrenoreceptor antagonists. Urologe A 1997; 36(1):18–34.

15. Chapple CR. Pharmacotherapy for benign prostatic hyperplasia – the potential for alpha 1-adrenoceptor subtype-specific blockade. Br J Urol 1998; 81(suppl 1):34–47.

16. Djavan B, Marberger M. A meta-analysis on the efficacy and tolerability of alpha 1-adrenoceptor antagonists in patients with lower urinary tract symptoms suggestive of benign prostatic obstruction. Eur Urol 1999; 36(1):1–13.

17. Kirby RS. Doxazosin in benign prostatic hyperplasia: effects on blood pressure and urinary flow in normotensive and hypertensive men. Urology 1995; 46(2):182–186.

18. McConnell JD, Bruskewitz R, Walsh P, et al. The effect of finasteride on the risk of acute urinary retention and the need for surgical treatment among men with benign prostatic hyperplasia. Finasteride Long-Term Efficacy and Safety Study Group. N Engl J Med 1998; 338(9):557–563.

19. Nickel JC, Fradet Y, Boake RC, et al. Efficacy and safety of finasteride therapy for benign prostatic hyperplasia:

results of a 2-year randomized controlled trial (the PROSPECT study). PROscar Safety Plus Efficacy Canadian Two Year Study. CMAJ 1996; 155(9):1251–1259.

20. Andersen JT, Ekman P, Wolf H, et al. Can finasteride reverse the progress of benign prostatic hyperplasia? A two-year placebo-controlled study. The Scandinavian BPH Study Group. Urology 1995; 46(5):631–637.

21. Boyle P, Gould AL, Roehrborn CG. Prostate volume predicts outcome of treatment of benign prostatic hyperplasia with finasteride: meta-analysis of randomized clinical trials. Urology 1996; 48(3):398–405.

22. Roehrborn CG, Boyle P, Nickel JC, et al. Efficacy and safety of a dual inhibitor of 5-alpha-reductase types 1 and 2 (Dutasteride) in men with benign prostatic hyperplasia. Urology 2002; 60(3):434–441.

23. Lepor H, Williford WO, Barry MJ, et al. The efficacy of terazosin, finasteride, or both in benign prostatic hyperplasia. Veterans Affairs Cooperative Studies Benign Prostatic Hyperplasia Study Group. N Engl J Med 1996; 335(8):533–539.

24. Roehrborn CG. A double-blind comparison of doxazosin and finasteride in symptomatic benign prostatic hyperplasia: a multinational European trial. Eur Urol 2000; 37(suppl 2):1–18.

24a. McConnell JD. The long term effects of medical therapy on the progression of BPH: results from the MTOPS trial. J Urol, 167:265A.

25. Diamond SM, Ismail M, Hubosky S, El–Gabry E. Placebo controlled trial of alpha blockers and finasteride in men with enlarged prostates and LUTS: subjective and objective results after discontinuation of alpha blockers. American Urological Association; 2002 [Abstract].

26. Baldwin KC, Ginsberg PC, Roehrborn CG, Harkaway RC. Discontinuation of alpha-blockade after initial treatment with finasteride and doxazosin in men with lower urinary tract symptoms and clinical evidence of benign prostatic hyperplasia. Urology 2001; 58(2):203–209.

27. Barkin J, Guimaraes M, Do Castelo V, et al. Dutasteride provides sustained symptom relief following short term combination treatment with tamsulosin. American Urological Association; 2002 [Abstract].

28. Sarma AV, Jacobsen SJ, Girman CJ, et al. Concomitant longitudinal changes in frequency of and bother from lower urinary tract symptoms in community dwelling men. J Urol 2002; 168(4 Pt 1):1446–1452.

29. Lowe FC, Fagelman E. Phytotherapy in the treatment of benign prostatic hyperplasia: an update. Urology 1999; 53(4):671–678.

30. ConsumerLab.com. Independent tests of herbal, vitamin and mineral supplements. http://www.ConsumerLab.com

31. Lowe FC. Phytotherapy in the management of benign prostatic hyperplasia. Urology 2001; 58(6 suppl 1):71–76.

32. Plosker GL, Brogden RN. *Serenoa repens* (Permixon). A review of its pharmacology and therapeutic efficacy in benign prostatic hyperplasia. Drugs Aging 1996; 9(5):379–395.

33. Paubert-Braquet M, Momboisse JC, Boichot-Lagente JC. *Pygeum africanum* extract inhibits bFGF and EFG induced proliferation of 3T3 fibroblasts. Biomed Pharmacother 1994; 48:43–47.

34. Marwick C. Growing use of medicinal botanicals forces assessment by drug regulators. JAMA 1995; 273(8):607–609.

35. Debruyne F, Koch G, Boyle P, et al. Comparison of a phytotherapeutic agent (Permixon) with an alpha-blocker (Tamsulosin) in the treatment of benign prostatic hyperplasia: a 1-year randomized international study. Eur Urol 2002; 41(5):497–506.

36. Carraro JC, Raynaud JP, Koch G, et al. Comparison of phytotherapy (Permixon) with finasteride in the treatment of benign prostate hyperplasia: a randomized international study of 1,098 patients. Prostate 1996; 29(4):231–240.

37. Roehrborn CG. BPH clinical research criteria. In: Denis L, Griffiths K, Khoury S, eds. Proceedings of the 4th International Consultation on BPH. Plymouth: Plymouth Health Publications; 1997:437–514.

38. Wilt T, Ishani A, MacDonald R. *Serenoa repens* for benign prostatic hyperplasia (Cochrane Review). The Cochrane Library Issue 3. Oxford: Update Software; 2002.

39. Boyle P, Robertson C, Lowe F, Roehrborn C. Meta-analysis of clinical trials of permixon in the treatment of symptomatic benign prostatic hyperplasia. Urology 2000; 55(4):533–539.

40. Glémain P, Coulange C, Grapin FN, Muszynski RC. No benefit in combining tamsulosin with *Serenoa repens* versus tamsulosin alone on storage/filling and voiding lower urinary tract symptoms. American Urological Association Annual Meeting; 2002 [Abstract].

41. Levin RM, Riffaud JP, Bellamy F, et al. Effects of tadenan pretreatment on bladder physiology and biochemistry following partial outlet obstruction. J Urol 1996; 156(6):2084–2088.

42. Kassen A, Berges R, Senge T. Effect of B-sistosterol (Harzol®) on the expression and secretion of growth factors in primary human prostate stromal cell cultures in vitro. Fourth International Consultation on BPH. 1997:Abstract 31.

43. Berges RR, Windeler J, Trampisch HJ, Senge T. Randomised, placebo-controlled, double-blind clinical trial of beta-sitosterol in patients with benign prostatic hyperplasia. Beta-sitosterol Study Group. Lancet 1995; 345(8964):1529–1532.

44. Berges RR, Kassen A, Senge T. Treatment of symptomatic benign prostatic hyperplasia with beta-sitosterol: an 18-month follow-up. BJU Int 2000; 85(7):842–846.

45. Klippel KF, Hiltl DM, Schipp B. A multicentric, placebo-controlled, double-blind clinical trial of beta-sitosterol (phytosterol) for the treatment of benign prostatic hyperplasia. German BPH-Phyto Study Group. Br J Urol 1997; 80(3):427–432.

46. Wilt TJ, MacDonald R, Ishani A. Beta-sitosterol for the treatment of benign prostatic hyperplasia: a systematic review. BJU Int 1999; 83(9):976–983.

16

The overactive bladder

Gregory S Adey and Graeme S Steele

Introduction

Urinary incontinence (UI) and voiding dysfunction related to overactive bladder (OAB) represent important clinical problems in the United States. Appropriate management of OAB depends on the physician's ability to recognize this entity, perform appropriate investigations and institute therapy accordingly.

Due to improved recognition and better treatment options, OAB has recently come to the fore in urologic surgery. In addition, increased awareness of OAB among the public has prompted physicians to familiarize themselves with this clinical entity. While not life threatening, the social implications associated with UI and OAB are important. With continued advances in technology, the future for treatment of OAB shines bright.

Definition

OAB is a topic relatively new to the field of urology. For the first time OAB is defined and described in the most recent, eighth edition of *Cambell's Urology*.[1] While there is no precise definition for OAB, the Second Consensus Conference on OAB has described it as 'a medical condition referring to the symptoms of frequency and urgency, with or without urge incontinence, when appearing in the absence of local pathologic or metabolic factors that would account for these symptoms'.[2] Symptom severity varies widely and usually correlates with significant changes in quality of life (QL).

Previously, the International Continence Society (ICS) had recommended a classification system modeled after bladder function as seen on urodynamic studies. The ICS definition used the term 'detrusor overactivity' for bladder related incontinence, and then further subdivided this group into detrusor hyperreflexia (neurologic disease present) and detrusor instability (no evidence of neurologic disease).[3] Involuntary bladder contractions were formerly described as any contraction during the filling (cystometry) phase of the urodynamic study that generates greater than 15 cm H_2O pressure. This definition was recently modified to encompass any unstable contraction, regardless of the amount of pressure it generates.

There were many limitations to the earlier definitions of the ICS. Complex terminology in the classifications hindered urologists from discussing results with patients and primary care physicians alike. In addition, only a minority of patients with OAB undergo urodynamic studies, thus the majority of patients with OAB are not correctly categorized. Furthermore, detrusor overactivity was not seen in up to 50% of patients presumed to have OAB.[4] The broader definition supplied by the Consensus Conference appears to have solved many of these conflicts; however, it is not intended to replace those terms supplied by the ICS. The language of the ICS remains the standard for discussion among urologists and other experts on OAB.

Epidemiology

OAB affects both male and female patients; approximately two-thirds of all those affected are women.[5] A large population based survey using trained interviewers in a face-to-face setting, evaluated 1955 individuals within the community, all of whom were older than 60 years. They found the prevalence of UI to be 37.3% in women, 18.9% in men, and 30.0% overall.[6] Almost 40% of the women and 12% of the men were using pads on a regular basis.

Basing the prevalence of OAB on the prevalence of UI may be a gross underestimate of this problem, because 60% of patients with OAB have frequency and urgency, without urge incontinence.[3] Regardless of the magnitude of this problem, UI and OAB impose a significant economic burden on our country. The cost of UI reached $26.6 billion in 1995.[7] Ouslander et al[7] found that half of all nursing home residents were incontinent and, for many of these residents, UI is the problem preventing them from living in the community.

While the incidence of UI increases with increasing patient age, UI is quite common in younger individuals and cannot be thought of as a consequence of aging. In a survey of a general medical practice including over 20 000 patients older than 5 years of age, Thomas et al[8] found that more than 15% of women and 3% of men from each decade of life reported UI. Most current studies show increasing risk of UI associated with childbearing, obesity, hysterectomy and other pelvic surgery, or cognitive impairment.

Much of the ambiguity of the data is a result of poor survey design and overlapping definitions of the types of incontinence. Hampel et al[10] attempted to classify UI by type from a meta-analysis of 48 epidemiologic studies. Among patients with UI, they determined the relative incidence of stress incontinence, urge incontinence and mixed incontinence to be 49%, 22% and 29% in women, and 8%, 73% and 19% in men, respectively. In women, these numbers are similar to a study done by Sand et al,[11] which found 16% to have urge incontinence and 38% to have mixed incontinence. OAB is clearly associated with bladder outlet obstruction, most commonly from benign prostatic enlargement in men, and this explains the very high prevalence of urge and mixed incontinence among men with benign prostatic hypertrophy (BPH).

Clearly more information regarding OAB is required. In this regard, prospective and longitudinal studies using validated evaluative means in order to better qualify and quantify the role played by OAB, are required.

Pathophysiology

A complex combination of local, spinal and central nervous system centers help regulate bladder function. Since the exact cause of OAB is unknown, the complete explanation of the pathophysiology of OAB is impossible.

The physiology involved in the formation, storage and evacuation of urine from the bladder is well described. Normally, afferent activity such as cystometric volume is signaled to the central nervous system via small, myelinated afferent fibers (A-delta fibers). These A-delta fibers pass through the spinal tracts to the brainstem and then on to the periaqueductal gray matter; from there afferent fibers travel to the pontine micturition center.[12] The efferent activity is modulated by voluntary inhibition and the desire to void, if wanted, is then conveyed back to the bladder via the autonomic nervous system. The desire to void results in a relative decrease in sympathetic activity causing relaxation of the urinary sphincter, and a relative increase in the parasympathetic activity causing detrusor muscle contraction. The inhibition of voiding has the opposite effect within the autonomic nervous system. The majority of the time, the central nervous system acts to inhibit the voiding reflex.

All of these neuronal pathways coexist in a delicate balance. Any interruption to this balance may cause UI and the symptoms associated with OAB. In the case of OAB, it is not known if a disruption occurs at the level of detrusor muscle or at the level of the neuron; hence, two competing theories exist.

Neurogenic causes of OAB

Researchers have long known about the voiding dysfunction associated with neurologic injuries. The physiology of such injuries and conditions has been thoroughly investigated. In the case of spinal cord injuries, the afferent pathway is disrupted. A new pathway for afferent signaling is used, and the afferent activity is now carried by unmyelinated C fibers.[13] It is possible that the C fibers act as a short circuit and activate the voiding reflex at the level of the sacral spinal cord, causing the detrusor–external sphincter dyssynergia so often seen in patients with spinal cord injuries.

Blok and Holstege[14] performed positron emission tomography (PET) scanning of patients in their study. They found changes in blood flow to the right prefrontal cortex with voiding, and decreased activity within this same area during voluntary suppression of voiding. If this is the case, cortical neurologic input may play a larger role in micturition than once thought. Sakakibara et al[15] found that 49% of patients with acute brainstem stroke had irritative and obstructive voiding symptoms, and urodynamic studies on this group revealed 73% had detrusor hyperreflexia. This study reinforces what is known about the critical role played by the brainstem in the control of micturition.

The role played by the cerebral cortex requires further study. Voiding dysfunction following stroke is common and, in addition, cerebral cortical changes with aging may lead to OAB.

Myogenic causes of OAB

Some researchers have used light and electron microscopy to examine muscle samples from those patients affected by OAB. Elbadawi et al[16] found there were increased cell-to-cell connections among bladder smooth muscle cells. German et al[17] noted spontaneous muscle activity and associated tetany, also supporting the idea of increased cell coupling. These groups hypothesized that the detrusor overactivity may be the result of facilitated cell-to-cell communication. A prospective study of 23 patients with previously normal bladder function that had developed detrusor overactivity, revealed that the abnormal cell-to-cell conductions correlated directly with degree of bladder overactivity in all 23 cases.[18]

Both of these theories are quite interesting, and they are not altogether separate entities. It is possible that the true answer to the puzzle of OAB lies somewhere in the middle of the neurogenic and myogenic theories, with significant roles played by many factors. Whatever the cause, this area remains a hotbed of research and we are sure to know much more in the coming years.

Diagnostic evaluation

The most important part of the evaluation of those patients presenting with the symptoms of OAB, is proper classification. Initially the distinction between those patients with neurologic disease, and those patients without neurologic disease, must be determined. Secondly, in those patients with incontinence, the type of incontinence needs to be classified.

History

Patient history is the single most important part of the office visit. The practitioner should obtain a complete voiding history from the patient, as well as precipitating causes of the patient's symptoms. It is important in men to determine if there is coincident bladder outlet obstruction along with symptoms of OAB. Efforts should be made to elucidate the cause of any UI as stress, urge or mixed in nature. During the patient interview, the practitioner should attempt to determine the cognitive function of the patient. If the patient has not completed a voiding diary, then one should be encouraged prior to the next visit. Necessary components include total number of voids in 24 hours, voided volume in 24 hours, maximum voided volume and average voided volume.[19] The patient should also note the specific times when symptoms or incontinence occurs. The diary should include data from a minimum of 3 consecutive days. The voiding diary will establish a baseline for evaluating future therapies, and provide validation of patient symptoms, the importance of which cannot be stressed enough.

The practitioner should also include specific questioning regarding symptoms of related conditions. Diabetes mellitus, multiple sclerosis, Parkinson's disease and irritable bowel syndrome will sometimes manifest first with the symptoms of OAB. Bowel and sexual function need to be addressed, including the frequency of bowel movements and possibility of fecal incontinence. Dyspareunia or anorgasmia can be clues to abnormal function of pelvic muscles and nerves. In women, a complete obstetrical and gynecologic history is imperative, including prior pelvic therapies or surgery. Finally, the practitioner needs to determine the patient's family, social and environmental histories.

Physical examination

The primary goals of physical examination of the patient with symptoms of OAB should be pelvic anatomy, pelvic floor function and a complete neurologic examination. The patient should be examined with a moderately full bladder if possible, and in the standing position first.

The neurologic examination should include a thorough inspection of the upper torso and lower back, making note of any surgical scars or possible spinal abnormalities. The patient's gait should be assessed and a full cranial nerve examination undertaken. Peripheral muscle tone, strength and reflexes should be noted. Peripheral sensation should be examined in all four extremities, as well as coordination tests such as finger-to-nose and heel–shin tests. With the female patient in the lithotomy position, sensation within the second, third, and fourth sacral dermatomes may be assessed by light touch.

Ahlberg et al[20] performed a detailed neurologic examination on 45 patients without pre-existing neurologic conditions referred for evaluation of urgency and/or urge incontinence. They found that 82% had abnormal neurologic examinations and upon further work-up, 21% of this group were diagnosed with a neurologic disease, such as multiple sclerosis or dorsal column neuropathy. Abnormalities in the neurologic examination need to be taken seriously and appropriate referral to a specialist when indicated is a necessity.

Female patient

In the female patient, pelvic examination begins in the lithotomy position with observation of the external genitalia, looking for overt evidence of cystocele, prolapse, infection or other lesions. The examination continues with the lower half of the separated vaginal speculum creating traction on the posterior vaginal wall. This allows visualization of the anterior vaginal wall, bladder base and urethra. Movement of the speculum blade to provide traction on the anterior vaginal wall will reveal the remainder of the vaginal vault for inspection. The examination is performed at rest and with Valsalva maneuvers, permitting more thorough inspection for cystocele, rectocele, enterocele and uterine or vaginal prolapse. The urethral meatus should be observed for leakage during Valsalva and afterwards, as delayed urine loss may be the result of unstable detrusor contraction and not true stress incontinence. Urethral palpation and massage can sometimes alert the physician to the possibility of a urethral diverticulum.

Following the speculum examination, a manual pelvic examination should be performed. The patient should be instructed to contract and relax the pelvic floor without the assistance of the gluteus or any other muscles, and at this time the levator musculature can be examined. Note should

be made of pain, spasm or laxity of these muscles. Digital rectal examination should assess the anal sphincter tone and completeness. If it is incontinence or prolapse of which the patient complains, and this finding cannot be reproduced in the lithotomy position, the examination should be repeated in a standing position.

Male patient

Examination of the male patient should include visual inspection of the penis and urethral meatus, ensuring there is no phimosis or distal urethral stricture present. Similar to the female patient, the meatus should also be inspected for leak of urine during and following Valsalva maneuver, especially in those patients having had prior pelvic surgery. Digital rectal examination should note the presence and quality of the anal sphincter muscular tone, presence or absence of the bulbocavernosal reflex, as well as an evaluation of the prostate gland.

Urine examination

The symptoms of OAB may be mimicked by acute urinary infection; therefore, urinalysis and culture is necessary upon initial office visit. Evidence of infection should be treated appropriately and symptoms should be re-evaluated following completion of antibiotic therapy. Recurrent urinary infection should undergo cystoscopic evaluation to exclude the existence of bladder calculi. The presence of microscopic hematuria needs to be evaluated in accordance with the current guidelines set forth by the American Urological Association, as the suspicion for malignancy becomes higher. Urine cytology should also be performed as transitional cell carcinoma-in-situ of the bladder often presents with symptoms of urgency and frequency.

Radiographic studies

Screening radiographic imaging of the majority of patients with symptoms of OAB is probably not necessary. However, those patients with neurogenic bladder disease have a high likelihood of detrusor–external sphincter dyssynergia and do require routine renal ultrasonography, in addition to video urodynamics to more completely define their degree of bladder dysfunction and potential risk for upper tract damage.

Urodynamic studies

The role of urodynamics in the evaluation of patients with the symptoms of OAB is continually debated. Holtedahl et al[21] recently performed a population-based, randomized controlled study of incontinent women. They found that a quarter of the patients who had not had a previous urodynamic evaluation had a revision of their initial diagnosis and subsequent change in therapy after urodynamic study was performed. Despite these changes, the outcome of treatment was no different, suggesting there is not a need for routine use of urodynamics. However, the authors did find that urodynamics were beneficial in complex bladder dysfunction and in those patients who were refractory to conservative therapy.

Opponents of routine urodynamic testing in patients with symptoms of OAB cite poor sensitivity and specificity of urodynamic studies. Detrusor instability defined by urodynamic bladder instability may be seen in 10–40% of asymptomatic patients.[19] Proponents of the use of urodynamic studies are trying to develop good ambulatory monitoring devices that would improve the studies' sensitivity, but there is still dispute over the use of such instruments. The debate regarding potential benefit for routine use of urodynamic studies in patients with OAB will continue for some time to come. In our practice at Brigham and Women's Hospital in Boston, urodynamic studies are routinely used in patients with neurologic pathology and voiding dysfunction, as well as in those patients with OAB who have failed medical therapy.

Therapy

Behavioral therapy

Behavioral therapy for the treatment of the OAB has been in use for many years. This therapy relies on the retraining and re-education of the patient in proper voiding behavior. The mechanism of action remains unknown for behavioral therapy, but it is hypothesized that cortical control is re-established over the hyperexcitable micturition reflex.

In behavioral therapy, the patient is informed as to what constitutes normal voiding patterns. The patient and therapist then compare the normal patterns with the abnormal pattern suffered by the patient as obtained from the patient's voiding diary. The patient is then shown how to contract pelvic floor musculature in response to frequency and urgency and to prevent incontinence. A second strategy employed is the use of timed voiding, also known as bladder drill. Urgency will sometimes exhibit a volume-dependent phenomenon and these patients benefit the most from timed voiding to gradually prolong the voiding interval.

Much of behavioral therapy also uses pelvic floor muscle exercises, or Kegel exercises, in conjunction with the previously defined techniques. These exercises, first reported by Kegel in 1948, involve a repeated series of conscious contractions of the levator musculature with the goal of overall improved strength.[22] Kegel initially described this treatment for stress urinary incontinence, and he reported cure rates of over 80%; however, his outstanding results have never been duplicated. Patients should be instructed to contract and hold the pelvic floor muscles for 10 seconds at a time, and repeat this exercise 10 times in a set. The patient should complete three sets each day, with the knowledge that significant improvement cannot be expected for 6–8 weeks.

Nygaard et al[23] used a 3-month course of pelvic floor muscle exercises to treat 71 women with stress, urge or mixed incontinence. These authors found 56% of the women had greater than 50% reduction in incontinent episodes per day, and the greatest reduction of episodes was seen in the group with urge incontinence. At 6 months, approximately one-third of the women noted good or excellent improvement in their incontinence and desired no further treatment.

It is necessary to note the importance of proper instruction when using verbal techniques to teach patients pelvic floor muscle exercises. Bump et al[24] gave brief verbal instructions for pelvic floor exercises to 47 women, and then studied them with video urodynamics while the women performed these exercises. They found that 25% of the women actually increased intravesical pressure more than 15 cmH$_2$O during attempted contraction of the levator musculature, perhaps worsening their UI.

While there may be perceived benefit from behavioral therapy as measured in outcomes, it does not appear that behavioral therapy improves urodynamic parameters. Elser et al[25] evaluated 204 women with UI treated with behavioral therapy and/or pelvic floor muscle exercises for a period of 12 weeks. Post-treatment urodynamics were available for 181 of the patients, and the authors did not find significant changes in urethral pressure profiles, urethral pressure at the time of Kegel exercises, or cystometric capacities.

Despite minimal improvements found on clinical study, behavioral therapy should remain a first line therapy for practitioners treating OAB. There is minimal cost to the health care practitioner, other than the time and effort invested into proper instruction and technique, and there are few side effects for the patient.

Biofeedback

Similar to behavioral therapy, biofeedback relies on the retraining of the patient in the proper micturition reflex. With biofeedback, the patient receives information (feedback) in the form of visual, auditory or tactile signals, regarding the proper techniques necessary to achieve the goal of therapy.

Vaginal cones

Vaginal cones are a type of biofeedback used for female patients with OAB. The cones are a set of tapered devices designed for insertion into the upper vagina at the time pelvic floor muscle exercises are to be performed. With proper contraction of the levator musculature, the cone should move upward within the vaginal vault. If the patient were to incorrectly use her abdominal muscles instead of the levators, the cone would be pushed downward toward the introitus. The patient is then able to differentiate between these sensations and exercise the proper muscles. The vaginal cones come in a series of sequentially heavier models to assist in the strength training of the pelvic muscles. They are readily available and may be purchased for between $40 and $100.

There are however some problems with vaginal cones. A patient may incorrectly use her leg adductor muscles to keep the cone in place and not actually strengthen the pelvic floor muscles. There is a high cumulative dropout rate of almost 30%, and some patients will simply not use a vaginal device.[3] Vaginal cones obviously have no role in the treatment of men with OAB. However, in women compliant with vaginal cones, satisfaction rates range between 40 and 70%, with a distinct advantage of being used in the privacy of one's home.

Pressure recording (perineometry)

Home biofeedback can also be performed with a pressure monitoring device. These instruments make use of anal or vaginal probes to record the squeeze of these muscles during levator contraction. The device provides both auditory and visual signals to the patient regarding strength of contraction, so the proper musculature may be identified by the patient. The first application of pressure recording, or perineometry, was carried out in the 1950s by Kegel, in an effort to reduce postpartum UI.[22] The main disadvantage to perineometry is that increases in abdominal pressure are transmitted to the probe. Valsalva maneuvers may then be interpreted by the patient as the proper exercise, when in fact they are incorrect. The cost of pressure recording devices is similar to that of vaginal cones. Despite the advantage of home-based use, many patients have the same problems of acceptance for pressure-based devices as with vaginal cones.

Electric stimulation and magnetic therapy

Vaginal cones and pressure recording devices have been gradually replaced by newer technology in recent years, namely electric stimulation and magnetic therapy.

Electric stimulation   Electric stimulation relies on the use of high frequency (50 Hz) stimulation of the pelvic floor muscles to produce contraction. Lower frequencies (2–20 Hz) are also used to inhibit the detrusor muscle and may help control overactivity. There is a wide range of devices available, from inexpensive models to be used at home to high-end sophisticated office-based equipment with electromyelograph (EMG) monitoring. Office-based models require a high degree of patient motivation, as well as specialists trained to use the equipment. Patients often become dissatisfied with the time and effort required for office-based therapy, and use of home electric stimulator biofeedback has therefore become more popular.

The electric stimulation is administered through either anal or vaginal electrodes. Some devices have the ability to use patch electrodes for peripheral stimulation, in either the perianal or posterior tibial distributions.[3] Sand et al[26] used a home-based transvaginal electric stimulator in 35 women, compared to a sham device used in 17 control subjects. After

12 weeks of home therapy, the authors found significant decrease in episodes of urinary leakage per day and per week, and also in pad use. Interestingly, there was significant improvement in vaginal muscle strength in the treatment group when compared to placebo.

Magnetic therapy In 1998, another treatment option emerged for patients apprehensive about using internal probes to treat their OAB. At this time, the Food and Drug Administration (FDA) approved the commercial use of devices using electromagnetic fields to treat UI in the United States. The use of magnetic therapy to treat UI in Europe and Asia preceded that in the US.

The magnetic field is applied in the form of pulses while the patient sits clothed in the treatment chair. The magnetic waves pass through clothing so there is no need for the patient to undress. A typical treatment lasts approximately 20 min. Low frequency stimulation is applied to provoke pulsatile contraction of the pelvic floor muscles, while high frequency stimuli will produce sustained contraction.[3] A standard program usually combines a mixture of high and low frequency stimuli, with adjustments made based on patient comfort. The magnet has a wide field and therefore the patient will also experience contractions of the gluteal and hamstring muscles during therapy. There are few side effects and the treatments are usually well tolerated.

Galloway et al[27] studied 83 women with stress urinary incontinence using magnetic field therapy. The women had 20 min of magnetic therapy, two times per week for 6 weeks. At least 12 weeks of follow-up data were available on 50 patients, and showed reduction in incontinent episodes from 3.3 to 1.7, reduction in pads per day from 2.5 to 1.3, and reduction in mean pad weight from 20 g to 15 g. Seventeen (34%) patients were completely dry. Despite impressive results, limitations of this study include lack of a control group and small study size.

Industry has recently developed cooling systems for the magnetic coils so the device can provide a continuous magnetic stimulus, compared to the pulsed technology currently in use. Previously, continuous magnetic therapy was limited because the coils would overheat if each pulse was more than a few hundred microseconds in length.[28] A small study using continuous magnetic therapy

in 10 15-minute sessions over 5 weeks, comprised of 1 min on/30 seconds off cycles, found urge incontinence was cured or improved in six out of eight patients.[28] It will be interesting to see how larger studies compare between these two types of magnetic therapy.

Magnetic therapy seems to be the biggest challenge to electric stimulation in the treatment of patients with OAB and UI. Magnetic therapy is currently more expensive, but as the technology becomes more commonplace, the cost should become more reasonable. Similar to electric stimulation, many of the studies using electromagnetic fields involve only the population with stress incontinence. Further work needs to be done involving the population with urge and mixed urinary incontinence. It will be difficult to design good control groups in the study of these modalities, but outcome data will have to be interpreted as such.

Pharmacotherapy

The detrusor muscle is comprised mainly of muscarinic receptors under the control of the neurotransmitter acetylcholine, but the micturition response itself is a delicate balance of several neurotransmitter systems.[29] Many areas of the central nervous system are known to have a part in the control of voiding, but there are few drugs acting on these areas that are clinically useful. Antimuscarinic agents remain first line therapy for pharmacologic treatment of the OAB, despite their well-known side effect profile. Without complete knowledge of the pathophysiology of OAB, development of efficacious drugs as a treatment is quite difficult. Nonetheless, an intense amount of research continues to find more successful medicines.

Drugs blocking muscarinic receptors have been in clinical use since the 1960s for the treatment of OAB.[19] There are five well-described subtypes of muscarinic receptors, and their locations may be found throughout the body.[30] Subtypes M_2 and M_3 are the main subtypes found within human detrusor cells, with a respective ratio of 3:1. M_3 receptors are also found in the salivary glands and within the smooth muscle of the intestine. It is the stimulation of these extravesical muscarinic receptors that accounts for the side effects of antimuscarinic agents, such as dry mouth, dry eyes and gastrointestinal effects.

Oxybutynin

The original agent found to have success in the treatment of OAB, oxybutynin chloride remains widely used. Its properties in controlling bladder overactivity were discovered during studies of its uses as an antispasmodic in the colon.[19] Its primary mechanism of action seems to be blockage of the M_3 subtype receptor, also accounting for the large percentage of side effects noted in patients. Oxybutynin is typically dosed in adults as 2.5–5 mg, two to three times daily. Total daily dosage should not exceed 20 mg. In a randomized, controlled, double-blind study, oxybutynin was shown to be effective for symptom improvement, and also showed significant increases in the bladder volume at first unstable contraction and maximum cystometric capacity.[31]

After oral administration, oxybutynin chloride undergoes extensive hepatic and presystemic gastrointestinal metabolism. Oxybutynin is converted to its primary active metabolite, N-desethyloxybutynin, which can appear in the circulation in concentrations 4 to 10 times higher than the parent compound.[32] N-desethyloxybutynin binds more effectively to the muscarinic receptors, and is responsible for the therapeutic as well as the adverse effects of oxybutynin.

Adverse effects were reported in 63% of the patients taking oxybutynin in this study, of which dry mouth was the most common, representing approximately 50% of the complaints.[31] Efforts directed at reducing the side effect profile for oxybutynin have resulted in the development of long-acting and transdermal delivery forms of the drug. The long-acting form of oxybutynin uses an osmotic drug delivery system allowing once daily dosing.[33] The sustained release form of oxybutynin maintains steady plasma concentrations over 24 hours,[34] and lower peak levels of N-desethyloxybutynin are created.[35] The peak active metabolite level after sustained release oxybutynin is less than four times that of the original parent drug dose; this is primarily due to drug metabolism within the colon compared to within the small intestine for the immediate release form. A randomized, double-blind study comparing the sustained release form of oxybutynin to immediate release oxybutynin did not show additional efficacy for the sustained release form.[36] The study did show a significant decrease in moderate to severe dry mouth in the sustained release group as compared to the immediate release group (25% vs 46%). A similar decreased incidence of dry mouth (23%) has been reported by other authors.[33] Once daily dosing of oxybutynin avoids the peaks in blood levels seen with immediate release oxybutynin and prevents some of the concentration-dependent side effects, such as dry mouth. Sustained released oxybutynin is usually dosed as 5–15 mg, once daily, with a maximum daily dosage of 30 mg.

The use of transdermal drug delivery systems aims to increase patient compliance, as well as decrease concentration-dependent side effects of the medication. A randomized, double-blind study comparing transdermal delivery of oxybutynin to immediate release oxybutynin did not show a significant difference between the two forms of the drug.[37] There was, however, significant reduction in dry mouth reported by the transdermal group (38% vs 94%), and none described this as intolerable. Randomized double-blind studies have also been conducted comparing different dosages of the transdermal patches.[32] The transdermal delivery form for oxybutynin has not yet been released to the public but the preliminary studies hold promise as effective therapy.

In an effort to improve side effect profiles, some research has examined the stereogenic properties of oxybutynin.[38] The D-isomer appears to be the more active of the isomers, but it appears that the antispasmodic effects of oxybutynin are not stereoselective. Current compounds are composed of a racemic mixture of the two isomers. Efforts are being made to construct purified compounds of the S-isomer, which potentially may have fewer adverse effects. As new drugs are developed to treat overactive bladder, efforts continue to improve the formulation of oxybutynin.

Tolterodine

In the mid 1990s, researchers developed a new antimuscarinic agent with much promise in treating overactive bladder. Tolterodine, the new agent, has been shown to be equally potent at blocking bladder muscarinic receptors, but has a much smaller effect on receptors within the salivary glands.[39] Binding studies using radioligands show tolterodine has eight times less potency at blocking muscarinic receptors within the parotid gland when compared to oxybutynin.[40] Unlike oxybutynin, tolterodine lacks the specificity for certain muscarinic subtypes.[40]

The development of this new drug was driven by the large number of adverse events reported by those patients taking oxybutynin, particularly dry mouth. Many head-to-head studies between oxybutynin and tolterodine have been performed and conclude that the effects on treating bladder symptoms are similar.[41] Appell[39] compared the results from four phase III clinical trials of tolterodine and found both tolterodine and oxybutynin significantly decreased incontinent episodes, significantly improved voided volumes, and significantly improved patient perception of their bladder condition when compared to placebo. There were no significant differences in efficacy when tolterodine was compared to oxybutynin. The main differences between the drugs were found in the side effect profiles. Appel found dry mouth to be the most frequently reported adverse event, occurring in 40% of those taking 2 mg tolterodine twice per day compared to 78% in the oxybutynin group (5 mg three times daily).[39] The degree of severity of dry mouth was also significantly different, with 60% in the oxybutynin group citing moderate or severe conditions, compared to 17% in the tolterodine group. In the oxybutynin group, 20% actually withdrew from the studies because of symptoms, compared to only 8% taking tolterodine.

Some consider the high incidence of side effects with oxybutynin is a result of study dosage, claiming many clinicians actually use dose escalation with oxybutynin to help lessen the incidence of side effects such as dry mouth. A randomized, double-blind, placebo-controlled study from the UK and Ireland used dose escalation in the group taking oxybutynin and still found significantly lower adverse events reported by the tolterodine group.[42] Dry mouth was seen in 37% of those taking tolterodine compared to 61% taking oxybutynin.

Tolterodine is normally prescribed as 1–2 mg twice daily. Recent efforts to further improve the drug have yielded an extended release form of tolterodine. In a large, randomized, prospective, placebo-controlled study, van Kerrebroeck et al[43] found that the rate of dry mouth was 23% lower with the extended release form of tolterodine compared to the immediate release. The investigators found that urge incontinence episodes were reduced by 71% from baseline in those taking the extended release form, compared with 60% reduction seen in those taking immediate release tolterodine. Onset of action of tolterodine is estimated to occur within 1 week of starting therapy.[44] However Appell found maximum efficacy is not reached until 5–8 weeks after treatment initiation.[39] The recommended dosage for extended release tolterodine is 4 mg once daily.

Capsaicin and resiniferatoxin

The majority of drug therapy for OAB is by oral administration; however, some research has investigated the use of intravesical agents in the treatment of OAB. Intravesical administration is certainly more involved than oral medications, but scientists aim for high clinical efficacy without the observation of systemic side effects. Currently, their use is limited to those hyperreflexive bladders from spinal cord injuries or neurodegenerative disease.

Capsaicin has been identified as a possible intravesical agent to treat OAB. Capsaicin is the active ingredient found within the hot peppers of the genus Capsicum. Capsaicin is also a specific neurotoxin for afferent C fiber neurons. In 1878, Hogyes was the first to note that the irritation from capsicol, an extract from Capsicum, was mediated by sensory nerves.[45] Resiniferatoxin is the ultrapotent analog of capsaicin, and comes from the cactus-like plants of *Euphorbia resinifera*. Resiniferatoxin is 1000 times more potent than capsaicin. These agents are collectively referred to as vanilloids, named for the specific membrane receptor to which capsaicin and resiniferatoxin bind in primary sensory neurons.

The ion channel that vanilloids activate was recently discovered and named vanilloid receptor subtype 1.[46] After vanilloid binding, the channel opens allowing an influx of sodium and calcium ions and causing depolarization of the neuron. These receptors are non-selective and increases in temperature will cause similar depolarization. C fibers are found throughout the body and serve to detect noxious stimuli. The C fibers in our fingertips contain vanilloid receptor subtype 1 and serve to warn us about hot temperatures. The C fibers within the bladder also contain vanilloid receptor subtype 1, and serve to warn us of irritative conditions within the bladder. These C fibers are very sensitive to vanilloids. Capsaicin and resiniferatoxin act first by stimulating, and then by desensitizing the C fibers that may be responsible for the detrusor overactivity.[45] The desensitizing properties of vanilloids have been used to treat other conditions. Capsaicin is now available as a topical preparation to treat the neuropathic pain associated with conditions such as herpes zoster.

Neither capsaicin nor resiniferatoxin has been approved by the FDA for routine intravesical use in patients with OAB. The largest series with long-term follow up using intravesical capsaicin comes from two centers in Belgium and England.[47] De Ridder et al used repeat intravesical instillation of 100 ml of 1–2 mM capsaicin in 30% ethanol in saline solution for 79 patients with refractory OAB. The solution was left in place for 30 min and then the bladder was drained completely. The majority of their patients had neurological disease, with multiple sclerosis being the most common. The authors found that 44% of patients achieved complete continence and another 36% claimed satisfactory improvement in their incontinence. Clinical benefit persisted for 3–6 months following a single instillation of the capsaicin solution. Interestingly, of all of the patients who had poor compliance on bladder cystometry pretreatment, none had clinical or urodynamic improvement from capsaicin.[47]

The irritant properties of capsaicin that account for its actions are also at the center of some of its limitations. The majority of the patients in the previous study[47] noted the occurrence of irritative voiding symptoms and/or suprapubic pain that developed after capsaicin administration. Incontinence typically worsened during this period, lasting 2–10 days. Symptoms then disappeared and the patients' incontinence clinically improved or returned to baseline. Many believe that resiniferatoxin will be more efficacious than capsaicin to treat OAB, in part because of its increased potency. Studies using resiniferatoxin have used concentrations as small as 100 nM. It is possible that these small concentrations may be able to desensitize C fibers without causing other noxious effects.[45]

Preliminary data suggest that there may be some benefit to intravesical therapy for patients suffering from OAB. Unfortunately, the long-term safety of intravesical vanilloids is unknown, and will have to be elucidated before their use will become approved. If intravesical agents prove to be safe, they may redefine current therapy for OAB. Oral therapy remains the first line choice of pharmacotherapy, but the use of these medications is limited by their side effect profile. In-office, intravesical treatment for 30 min at a time, two to three times yearly, without the troubling side effects, may sound very appealing to those patients with OAB.

Implantable neurostimulator

Success at treating urinary incontinence with pelvic floor electric stimulation developed the interest in implantable devices. This interest was fueled as Tanagho and Schmidt showed that stimulation of sacral spinal nerves at S3 and S4 could reduce bladder hyperactivity and incontinent episodes.[48] An implantable sacral neuromodulator (InterStim, Medtronic Inc, Minneapolis, MN) is currently in use in the United States. It is indicated for treatment of urinary urgency and frequency, as well as for the treatment of urge incontinence.

In order to be eligible for implantation of the neuromodulator, a patient must first undergo a percutaneous trial electric stimulation. Under local anesthesia, a hollow 20-gauge needle is inserted into the S3 or S4 foramen.[19] The needle will deliver a charge to the nerves within the foramen and the responses are measured externally. The wave forms are used to guide a small temporary electrode through the hollow needle and into the sacral nerve. Following this, the electrode is attached to an external stimulator and therapy is commenced for a period of between 3 and 7 days. If at least a 50% clinical improvement occurs during the trial stimulation period, the patient is typically eligible for the implantable device. The implantable system consists of an implantable pulse generator, a unilateral, transforaminally-placed electrode, and extension wiring between these two items.[49] The exact mechanism of action in neurostimulation has not been elucidated.

Studies from both the United States and Europe report promising results from implantable neuromodulators. Schmidt et al[50] implanted stimulators in 34 patients and at 6 months 47% were completely dry, and an additional 29% had greater than 50% reduction in incontinent episodes. Bosch and Groen[51] studied 45 patients with implantable neurostimulators for refractory urgency and urge incontinence. At a mean follow up of 47 months,

THE OVERACTIVE BLADDER **205**

40% were cured of their incontinence, and 20% had at least 50% reduction in the number of incontinent episodes. The studies involve smaller numbers of male patients, but for unknown reasons, the results are better when implanted in female patients.[51] Adverse effects from the implantable neuromodulators include pain from the impulses, pain from the generator implant site, electrode migration, and changes in bowel habits. The reoperation rate is between 32 and 37%, the majority being for electrode repositioning.[50,51] When electric stimulation is discontinued, patients have been shown to return to their baseline incontinence.[50] There have been no instances of permanent nerve damage from the implantable neuromodulators.[51]

Most of the studies with implantable devices are in patients with symptoms refractory to behavioral and medical therapy, and the success rates are encouraging. The procedure is minimally invasive, but the reoperation rate remains fairly high. When therapy is effective, it must be continued throughout life. With continued application of this technology, the complication rate will lessen and this modality may become attractive to more patients.

Surgical therapy

Many attempts at developing surgical therapy for the OAB have failed, and augmentation cystoplasty remains the mainstay of surgery for those refractory cases. Augmentation cystoplasty involves using an isolated segment of bowel to increase the capacity of the urinary bladder. The goal of the procedure is the development of a larger volume, lower pressure reservoir. It engages the principles of the myogenic theory of OAB, in hopes of disrupting the contractility of the detrusor muscle.

Augmentation cystoplasty has excellent results in over 70%, and another 20% will have significant improvement, but the procedure is often fraught with complications.[52] The use of bowel in the urinary system often leads to metabolic abnormalities and calculus formation. A retrospective review of 122 augmentation cystoplasties using primarily detubularized ileum at mean follow up of 3 years, found 16% required surgical revision at some point, 21% developed bladder stones, and 13% were incontinent of urine.[52]

The future of surgical therapy for OAB may change dramatically with the introduction of tissue engineered products for in vivo use. Many other agents, such as pericardium and dura mater, have been tried but lack of a muscular layer has led to inevitable graft failure at various points with each.[19] A tissue engineered bladder has been constructed by Atala et al in dogs, which proved to be capacious and did show some evidence of neurogenicity.[53] The ability to use autologous tissue for augmentation cystoplasty would potentially significantly improve the number of adverse events and the appeal for this modality of treatment.

Conclusion

The overactive bladder is a significant problem to people of both sexes and all age groups. It represents a significant economic burden in the US alone. It is a complex of symptoms, ranging from urinary urgency and frequency to urge incontinence, in patients without a neurologic explanation. An estimated 13 million Americans[54] are affected by OAB, at a cost of over $26 billion.[6] These figures are a few years out of date and, because of underreporting, they are probably significant underestimates of the true magnitude of OAB.

Only recently has OAB been described as a separate entity within the realm of voiding dysfunction. Not much is known about the pathophysiology of OAB. Two theories, myogenic and neurogenic, exist as possible explanations. Efforts to define the dysfunction occurring in patients with OAB will aid the development of novel ways to treat this condition.

Currently, the mainstay of treatment for OAB is primarily behavioral and pharmacologic. Bladder training and biofeedback have been used to obtain substantial results in certain patients, but their success is not predictable. Magnetic therapy holds promise as a non-invasive and simple means to treat OAB, but long-term results are needed. Anticholinergic therapy has been in use for a few decades, but patient compliance is often limited by troublesome side effects, such as dry mouth and constipation. Recent advancements within the pharmaceutical industry have led to the development of longer acting agents and new, bladder specific medications with fewer side effects. The potential development of intravesical agents that are both effective and safe may eliminate side effects such as dry mouth altogether.

Those patients with refractory symptoms of OAB despite multiple modalities often find themselves exploring surgical options for treatment. Newer technology has brought implantable neurostimulators that can be placed minimally invasively. Augmentation cystoplasty remains a final option for some patients with OAB. Hopefully, tissue engineering technology with autologous bladder tissue will improve the complication rate for augmentation cystoplasty by eliminating the use of bowel for reconstruction.

As the awareness of overactive bladder continues to increase, the research into its causes and solution continues to expand. What just a few years ago was not even recognized in the field of urology, now sits at the fore. The algorithm of treatment of OAB promises to be redefined in the next few years. The practicing urologist needs to pay special attention to this in order to provide his or her patients with the best possible solution to a very troublesome problem.

References

1. Wein AJ. Pathophysiology and categorization of voiding dysfunction. In: Walsh PC, Retik AB, Vaughan EJ, et al (eds). Campbell's Urology, 8th edn. New York: Saunders; 2002:898.
2. Abrams P, Wein A. Introduction. Overactive bladder and its treatments. Urology 2000; 55(suppl 5A):1.
3. Payne CK. Advances in nonsurgical treatment of urinary incontinence and overactive bladder. Campbell's Urology – Update 1999; 1:1.
4. Griffiths D. Clinical aspect of detrusor instability and the value of urodynamics: a review of the evidence. Eur Urol 1998; 34(suppl 1):13–15.
5. Payne CK. Epidemiology, pathophysiology, and evaluation of urinary incontinence and overactive bladder. Urology 1998; 51(suppl 2A):3.
6. Diokno AC, Brock BM, Brown MB, Herzog AR. Prevalence of urinary incontinence and other urological symptoms in the noninstitutionalized elderly. J Urol 1986; 136:1022–1025.
7. Wagner TH, Hu T-W. Economic costs of urinary incontinence in 1995. Urology 1998; 51:355–361.
8. Ouslander JG, Kane RL, Abrass IB. Urinary incontinence in elderly nursing home patients. JAMA 1982; 248:1194–1198.
9. Thomas TM, Plymat KR, Blannin J, Meade TW. Prevalence of urinary incontinence. Br Med J 1980; 281:1243–1245.
10. Hampel C, Wienhold D, Benken N, et al. Definition of overactive bladder and epidemiology of urinary incontinence. Urology 1997; 50(suppl 6A):4–14; discussion 15–17.
11. Sand PK, Hill RC, Ostegard DO. Supine urethroscopic and standing cystometry as screening methods for detection of detrusor instability. Obstet Gynecol 1987; 70:57–60.
12. Fowler CJ. Bladder afferents and their role in the overactive bladder. Urology 2002; 59(suppl 5A):37–42.
13. de Groat WC, Kawatani M, Hisamitsu T, et al. Mechanisms underlying the recovery of urinary bladder function following spinal cord injury. J Auton Nerv Syst 1990; 30:S71–S77.
14. Blok BFM, Holstege G. The central control of micturition and continence: implications for urology. BJU Int 1999; 83(suppl 2):1–6.
15. Sakakibara R, Hattori T, Yasuda K, Yamanishi T. Micturitional disturbance and the pontine tegmental lesion: urodynamic and MRI analyses of vascular cases. J Neurol Sci 1996; 141(1–2):105–110.
16. Elbadawi A, Yalla SV, Resnick NM. Structural basis of geriatric voiding dysfunction. III. J Urol 1993; 150:1681–1695.
17. German K, Dedwani J, Davies J, et al. Physiologic and morphometric studies into the pathophysiology of detrusor hyperreflexia in neuropathic patients. J Urol 1995; 153:1678–1683.
18. Elbadawi E, Hailemariam S, Yalla SV, Resnick NM. Structural basis of geriatric voiding dysfunction. VII. Prospective ultrastructural/urodynamic evaluation of its natural evolution. J Urol 1997; 157:1814–1822.
19. Wright EJ. From backwater to headwater: evolving concepts in understanding and treating the overactive bladder. Campbell's Urology – Update 2001; 2:1.
20. Ahlberg J, Edlund C, Wikkelso C, et al. Neurological signs are common in patients with urodynamically verified "idiopathic" bladder overactivity. Neurourol Urodyn 2002; 21:65–70.
21. Holtedahl K, Verelst M, Schiefloe A, Hunskaar S. Usefulness of urodynamic evaluation in female urinary incontinence – lessons from a population-based, randomized, controlled study of conservative treatment. Scand J Urol Nephrol 2000; 34:169–174.
22. Kegel AH. The functional restoration of the perineal muscles. Am J Obstet Gynecol 1948; 56:238.
23. Nygaard IE, Kreder KJ, Lepic MM, et al. Efficacy of pelvic floor muscle exercises in women with stress, urge, and mixed urinary incontinence. Am J Obstet Gynecol 1996; 174:120–125.
24. Bump RC, Hurt WG, Fantl JA, Wyman JF. Assessment of Kegel pelvic muscle exercise after brief verbal instruction. Am J Obstet Gynecol 1991; 165:322–327; discussion 327–329.
25. Elser DM, Wyman JF, McClish DK, et al. The effect of bladder training, pelvic floor muscle training, or combination training on urodynamic parameters in women with urinary incontinence. Neurourol Urodyn 1999; 18:427–436.
26. Sand PK, Richardson DA, Staskin DR, et al. Pelvic floor electrical stimulation in the treatment of genuine stress incontinence: a multicenter, placebo-controlled trial. Am J Obstet Gynecol 1995; 173:72–79.
27. Galloway NT, El-Galley RES, Sand PK, et al. Extracorporeal magnetic innervation therapy for stress urinary incontinence. Urology 1999; 53:1108–1111.
28. Yamanishi T, Yasuda K, Suda S, et al. Effect of functional continuous magnetic stimulation for urinary incontinence. J Urol 2000; 163:456–459.

29. Andersson K-E. Treatment of overactive bladder: other drug mechanisms. Urology 2000; 55(suppl 5A):51–57; discussion 59.

30. Andersson K-E. The overactive bladder: pharmacologic basis of drug treatment. Urology 1997; 50(suppl 6A):74–84; discussion 85–89.

31. Thuroff JW, Bunke B, Ebner A, et al. Randomized, double-blind, multicenter trial on treatment of frequency, urgency, and incontinence related to detrusor hyperactivity: oxybutynin versus propantheline versus placebo. J Urol 1991; 145:813–816; discussion 816–817.

32. Dmochowski RR, Davila GW, Zinner NR, et al. Efficacy and safety of transdermal oxybutynin in patients with urge and mixed urinary incontinence. J Urol 2002; 168:580–586.

33. Gleason DM, Susset J, White C, et al. Evaluation of a new once-daily formulation of oxybutynin for the treatment of urinary urge incontinence. Urology 1999; 54:420–423.

34. Gupta SK, Shah J, Sathyan G. Evidence for site specific presystemic metabolism of oxybutynin following oral administration. Clin Pharmacol Ther 1997; 61:227.

35. Gupta SK, Sathyan G. Pharmacokinetics of an oral once-a-day controlled-release oxybutynin formulation compared with immediate-release oxybutynin. J Clin Pharmacol 1999; 39:289–296.

36. Anderson RU, Mobley D, Blank B, et al. Once daily controlled versus immediate release oxybutynin chloride for urge urinary incontinence. J Urol 1999; 161:1809–1812.

37. Davila GW, Daugherty CA, Sanders SW. A short-term, multicenter, randomized double-blind dose titration study of the efficacy and anticholinergic side effects of transdermal compared to immediate release oral oxybutynin treatment of patients with urge urinary incontinence. J Urol 2001; 166:140–145.

38. Koch P, McCullough JR, Blum PS, et al. Pharmacokinetics and safety of (S)-oxybutynin in normal healthy volunteers. FASEB J 1998; 12:A142.

39. Appell R. Clinical efficacy and safety of tolterodine in the treatment of overactive bladder: a pooled analysis. Urology 1997; 50(suppl 6A):90–96.

40. Nilvebrant L, Hallen B, Larsson G. Tolterodine: a new bladder selective, muscarinic receptor antagonist: pre-clinical pharmacological and clinical data. Life Sci 1997; 60:1129–1136.

41. Abrams P, Freeman R, Anderstrom C, Mattiasson A. Tolterodine, a new antimuscarinic agent: as effective but better tolerated than oxybutynin in patients with an overactive bladder. BJU Int 1998; 81:801–810.

42. Malone-Lee J, Shaffu B, Anand C, Powell C. Tolterodine: superior tolerability than and comparable efficacy to oxybutynin in individuals 50 years old or older with overactive bladder: a randomized controlled trial. J Urol 2001; 165:1452–1456.

43. Van Kerrebroeck P, Kreder K, Jonas U, et al. Tolterodine once-daily: superior efficacy and tolerability in the treatment of overactive bladder. Urology 2001; 57:414–421.

44. Atan A, Konety BR, Erickson JR, et al. Tolterodine for overactive bladder: time to onset of action, preferred dosage, and 9-month follow-up. Tech Urol 1999; 5:67–70.

45. Chancellor MB, de Groat WC. Intravesical capsaicin and resiniferatoxin therapy: spicing up the ways to treat the overactive bladder. J Urol 1999; 162:3–11.

46. Caterina MJ, Schumacher MA, Tominaga M, et al. The capsaicin receptor: a heat-activated ion channel in the pain pathway. Nature 1997; 389:816–824.

47. De Ridder D, Chandiramani V, Dasgupta P, et al. Intravesical capsaicin as a treatment for refractory detrusor hyperreflexia: study with long-term follow-up. J Urol 1997; 158:2087–2092.

48. Schmidt RA. Application of neurostimulation in urology. Neurourol Urodyn 1988; 7:585.

49. Janknegt RA, Hassouna MM, Siegel SW, et al. Long-term effectiveness of sacral nerve stimulation for refractory urge incontinence. Eur Urol 2001; 39:101–106.

50. Schmidt RA, Jonas U, Oleson KA, et al. Sacral nerve stimulation for treatment of refractory urinary urge incontinence. J Urol 1999; 162:352–357.

51. Bosch JLHR, Groen J. Sacral nerve modulation in the treatment of patients with refractory motor urge incontinence: long-term results of a prospective longitudinal study. J Urol 2000; 163:1219–1222.

52. Flood HD, Malhotra SJ, O'Connell HE, et al. Long-term results and complications using augmentation cystoplasty in reconstructive urology. Neurourol Urodyn 1995; 14:297–309.

53. Oberpenning FO, Meng J, Yoo J, et al. De novo reconstitution of a functional urinary bladder by tissue engineering. Nature Biotech 1999; 17:149–155.

54. Fantl JA, Newman DK, Colling J, et al. Urinary incontinence in adults: acute and chronic management. Clinical Practice Guideline, No. 2, 1996 Update. Rockville, Maryland: US Department of Health and Human Services, Public Health Service, Agency for Health Care Policy and Research. AHCPR Publication No. 96-0682; March 1996.

17

Three-dimensional imaging of the upper urinary tract

Shirley Mak, Uday Patel and Ken Anson

Historical development of 3-dimensional imaging

With the advent of CT imaging, it became possible to extract the 3-dimensional information from a volume composed of a stack of sectional slices[1,2] resulting in computer-synthesized display of underlying spatial relationships.[3] In 1977, 5 years after the introduction of CT by Sir Godfrey Newbold Hounsfield, Herman published his first clinical 3-dimensional reconstructions of the lung and heart of a dead dog.[3] Herman and his co-workers further developed the technique to identify and *render* bone surface in a CT data set[4] and started to use this technique for patients with unusual spine disorders. Hemmy, a co-investigator of Herman, subsequently pursued the application of 3-dimensional imaging of craniofacial surgery.[5] In 1990, this pioneering work involving several international collaborations resulted in an atlas of craniofacial deformities illustrated with 3-dimensional images[6] and the modern era of 3-dimensional imaging was born.

Technical aspects

To understand the clinical value of 3-dimensional imaging, it is necessary to discuss the general principles of data acquisition, reconstruction techniques and image display methods.

Data acquisition

One basic principle of radiographic data acquisition techniques underpins all areas of 3-dimensional imaging, i.e. the acquisition of digitized 3-dimensional volume datasets.

Modern computed tomography utilizes ionizing radiation to generate a series of individual axial scans in suspended respiration during continuous rotation of an X-ray tube–detector assembly in a spiral fashion. Raw data from the detectors are computer processed and a gray-scale image is constructed from the *digital* data and displayed on a monitor.

Magnetic resonance imaging does not employ ionizing radiation. It is an application of an external magnetic field generated by a powerful cryogenic electromagnet which causes alignment of the spinning proton within each hydrogen atom. Subsequent emissions of absorbed radio signals by the protons are detected by suitably placed receiver coils. Computer analysis of the radio signals detected allows the spatial distribution of hydrogen atoms to be established and the data are displayed as a 2-dimensional gray-scale image on the monitor.

Ultrasound imaging is an application that uses pulses of high-frequency sound waves and the detection of *echoes* returning from various tissue interfaces. The time interval between transmission and detection of each pulse is measured. Since the speed of sound is known, the depth of each tissue interface can be calculated. The spatial relationships between the various interfaces encountered by the beam can thus be determined and displayed in a visual form on the image monitor.

Table 17.1 outlines applications of the commonly recognized 3-dimensional imaging modalities to the upper urinary tract.

It must be emphasized that the position of the data (or signal) in relation to its 3-dimensional space in all three modalities must be precisely known. With further manipulation, a variety of volume models can be synthesized.

Reconstruction techniques and display methods

Reconstruction processes allow the generation of a 3-dimensional image from a set of digitized 2-

Table 17.1 Applications of the commonly recognized 3-dimensional imaging modalities to the upper urinary tract

3-Dimensional modalities	Advantages	Disadvantages	Proven applications
CT	Fast acquisition Readily available Accurate 3-dimensional reconstruction Good definition of anatomy and radiodense/radiolucent calculi	Ionizing radiation Radiation dosage required to generate narrowly collimated axial slices suitable for reconstruction Inferior soft tissue definition to MR Viewing dependent on attenuation gradient (difficult in poorly opacified urinary tract)	3-Dimensional reconstruction of pelvicalyceal system and renal calculi Preoperative planning and simulation of radical nephrectomy and nephron sparing surgery Evaluation of donor and recipients in renal transplant surgery 3-Dimensional CT reconstruction and CT angiography in PUJ obstruction CT ureterorenoscopy to assess strictures, tumors and stones
MRI	Readily available Non-ionizing radiation Good soft tissue definition Integration of different techniques to represent an all-in-one investigation MR urography provides anatomical, pathological and physiological information Potential real-time interactivity	Long acquisition time Poor representation of radiodense calculi and other calcifications Patient factors and preference	MR urography of the obstructed and non-obstructed upper urinary tract Feasible though limited assessment of MR urography in urolithiasis Utility of MR urography ± MR angiography in the assessment of tumor disease, renal anomalies and renal transplantation MR ureterorenoscopy in the assessment of neoplastic lesions, PUJ stenosis, strictures and extrinsic compression
US	Non-invasive Real-time interactivity Newer contrast agents allowing optimal viewing	Operator dependent Limited availability	Research phase

PUJ, pelviureteric junction.

dimensional images (Fig. 17.1). The 3-dimensional model commonly demonstrates either a specific area on the surface of the object or an inner structural area within the object. Furthermore, software-based measuring tools allow the generation of linear and volumetric measurements of the structure of interest.

The different types of *rendering* technique assume that the basis is a volumetric data set composed of consecutive images of thin cross-sectional slices while the patient remains immobile throughout *data acquisition*. These axial images are then combined within computer memory and then resolved by the computer as a 3-dimensional matrix composed of *voxels* with various *attenuation* values (Table 17.2).

Surface rendering

Surface rendering is a process which determines apparent surfaces of the organ within the volume of data and an image representing the surface of the object of interest is displayed. *Thresholding* technique is used to select the structures of interest. In this technique, each voxel intensity

within the volume is determined to be within a specific range of attenuation values. The fidelity of the rendered image to actual anatomy is dependent in part on the value range selected. Current display systems offer a variety of options for rendering parameters and features. The operator can control the color, shading, texture and transparency; as well as the rendering *algorithm* used: shaded, texture mapped, wire-frame, hidden line, etc. This rendering technique offers optimum visualization of small structures with well-differentiated surfaces. In contrast to volume rendering, this method greatly reduces the amount of 3-dimensional data manipulation and hence leads to a faster and more efficient reconstruction. However, a common criticism is that the surface is derived from only a small percentage of the available data and subtle image features may be distorted or misrepresented.

Volume rendering

Volume rendering uses the information from all voxels within a given volume of radiological data set to reconstruct images. The computer builds a

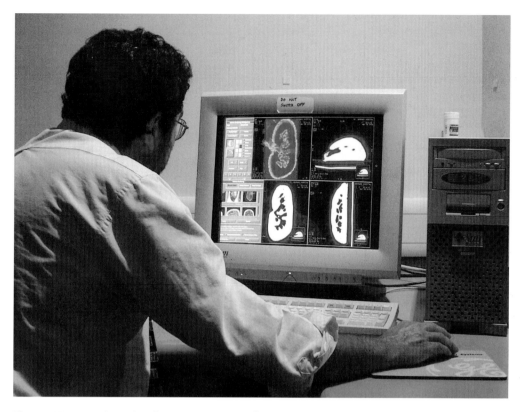

Figure 17.1 3-Dimensional CT reconstruction from digitized 2-dimensional radiographic data of porcine pelvicalyceal system using Advantage workstation 3.1, GE Medical Systems and Advantage Navigator AW 2.0 software.

Table 17.2 Computer software programs used in 3-dimensional reconstruction common to all imaging modalities

Advantages	Disadvantages	Future expectations
Unlimited viewing perspectives	Operator dependent	Reduction in cost of memory and processor
Interactive viewing	Moderately steep learning curve	power
Provides consistent, accurate information	Difficult to detect small lesions (< 5 mm)	Wider availability
Relatively short reconstruction time	Limited textural and surface characterization	Advance in computer software to generate
Linear and volumetric measurements	Does not allow biopsy of lesions for diagnosis	user-friendly programs with improved
of pathological lesions	Visualization during virtual endoscopy	object definition
Allows assessment of system proximal	dependent on degree of dilatation	Real-time interactivity with integration into
to stenotic lesions	of the ureter	intraoperative surgical planning and
Allow assessment of position		education through simulation
(in relation to other anatomical		
structures) and extension of lesions		

3-dimensional grid as it places each digitized 2-dimensional image into its correct location within the cuboid volume. It casts 'rays' through this volume and projects the results onto a 2-dimensional plane (Fig. 17.2). By assigning different optical transparencies or colors to different tissues, certain attenuations can be rendered transparent and others opaque. Images can be rendered in gray scale or color. As this technique incorporates all the available data, it leads to optimum fidelity of resultant images (Fig. 17.3). However, much more computer power is required to perform volume rendering at a reasonable speed. Surface shading can be added to the tissues classified as opaque to generate more detail as a hybrid form of surface and volume rendering.

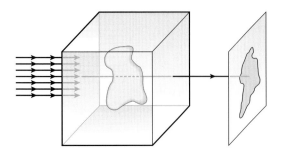

Figure 17.2 Volume rendering. Diagram shows how a ray interacts with a 3-dimensional volume image. The voxel values along each ray can be multiplied by selected factors and summed to produce different effects. (Reproduced with permission from Downey et al 2000.[85])

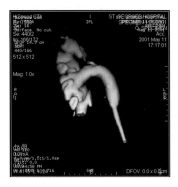

Figure 17.3 3-Dimensional CT volume-rendered reconstruction of contrast-enhanced porcine pelvicalyceal system. This is a volume-rendered image with depth information. The 3-dimensional complexity and relationship of the collecting system can be appreciated by rotating the image on the monitor.

Maximum intensity projection (MIP)
This technique generates images derived from the most 'intense' voxel along each 'ray'. MIP has proved to be particularly useful in creating angiographic images from CT and MRI data sets. However, this display method will obscure information with lower intensities. The resultant images are typically not displayed with surface shading or other depth cues making the appreciation of 3-dimensional relationships difficult.

Multiplanar reformatting
This method enables the viewer to assess the volume of radiographic data in multiple planes. This information can be viewed in three *orthogonal* planes. Computer-based interface tools allow the

planes to be rotated and repositioned for analysis. Alternatively, the 3-dimensional image can be displayed as a *polyhedron*. The appropriate imaging plane can be 'painted' on each face of the polyhedron, which can be rotated to obtain the desired image orientation. Any of the faces can be moved in and out in sections to be viewed in context with the rest of the anatomy.

Fly-through and fly-around
'*Fly-through*' and '*fly-around*' functions were developed from computer technologies used in the entertainment industry. The computations guide a virtual camera over the volume of interest for dynamic viewing, applied clinically to hollow structures as virtual endoscopy. The journey of the virtual camera can be determined by manual interaction or semi-automatic point placement. A curve fit to these points permits the calculation of intermediate points and can be saved for future playback of the 'fly-through' sequence. The 'fly-around' enables the viewer to isolate a structure within the volumetric data for protracted viewing. The image projected on display represents a view from the surface of a sphere that has the region of interest at its centre. The sphere can be rotated by the use of the mouse to visualize the structure from different perspectives (Fig. 17.4, Table 17.3).

Current clinical capabilities of 3-dimensional imaging

3-Dimensional computed tomography
Spiral CT allows *helicoidal* acquisition of data by using a continuous X-ray tube rotation with table feed. This compiles a data set of continuous anatomic information without the establishment of arbitrary boundaries at section interfaces that occurs in conventional CT imaging.[7,8] The acquisition time of helical CT is very short and is getting shorter still. Studies can be completed within one apnea with resulting narrowly *collimated* high quality images that are well suited for processing into 3-dimensional figures.

Renal calculi
Recent work has shown the value of spiral CT for renal calculus disease. Stones are easily detected on non-contrast CT scans as high-density foci in the kidney, ureter or bladder; even those that are

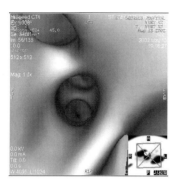

Figure 17.4 Fly-through sequence demonstrating the upper urinary tract of porcine model. Using the mouse, the operator can 'fly-through' the collecting system and assess areas of mucosal abnormalities. This interactive 'road map' can also provide valuable anatomical and pathological information to help preoperative planning.

Table 17.3 3-Dimensional image display formats

Type of display	Features
Surface rendering	Reconstructs images of the surface of the organ
Volume rendering	Reconstructs images of the internal structures of the organ
Maximum intensity projection	Images derived from the most intense voxels. No depth cues
Multiplanar reformatting	Analysis of a volume of radiographic data in multiple planes
Fly-through	Dynamic viewing of internal hollow structure through a virtual camera
Fly-around	Protracted viewing of structure of interest from different perspectives

radiolucent on plain film radiography. Density values for stones can be selected and 3-dimensional images created. The reconstructed images can accurately show the size and the spatial location of intrarenal calculi, both of which have a bearing on clinical management.

The accuracy of traditional methods of estimating linear measurements of urinary calculi may generate considerable variability. Lam and colleagues have suggested that the inconsistencies in the success rates reported for lithotripsy of certain calculi may reflect 'the inaccuracy and non-reproducibility' of conventional 2-dimensional imaging methods.[9] Olcott and colleagues conducted 3-dimensional CT studies on the linear measurements of a variety

of calculi within simulated kidneys inside an abdominal phantom and found that this modality of imaging produced a mean collective error of less than 1% along all three axes (x, y and z) while plain radiography and linear nephrotomography, the modalities traditionally used for measuring the size of calculi, produced corresponding mean measurement errors of approximately 17%.[10]

Due to the difficulty in the accurate measurement of stones with irregular contours, Yamaguchi suggested that it would be more appropriate to measure the total volume of residual stone burden rather than the length in postlithotripsy patients with staghorn calculi.[11] Fortunately, 3-dimensional CT is capable of providing direct volumetric analyses that are accurate to a mean error of 5%.[10] Hubert and colleagues have successfully applied 3-dimensional CT reconstruction in the assessment of staghorn calculi and the follow-up of radiolucent stones[12] and have found that it contributes significantly to the choice of the most appropriate ports for percutaneous stone surgery as well as facilitating perioperative pelvicalyceal exploration. Conversely, Liberman et al[13] found that the application of 3-dimensional spiral CT reconstruction in 10 patients with complex staghorn calculi added minimal additional information over that obtained from careful interpretation of standard radiographic studies for guiding nephrolithotomy. They concluded that this modality cannot be recommended as a routine preoperative study for such patients.[13]

Buchholz[14] reported a successful case of percutaneous nephrolithotomy in a morbidly obese woman with a large renal staghorn calculus, further complicated by malrotation and hypermobility of the kidney. As conventional 2-dimensional imaging failed to provide sufficient information for safe percutaneous approach, 3-dimensional CT reconstruction was used in this instance which exerted significant influence in the pretreatment decision making process.[14]

Renal masses

The role of CT in the evaluation of renal lesions is well established[15] and is the preferred imaging technique for suspected renal tumors, tumor staging and detection of metastatic disease. Benign renal lesions that mimic tumors including cystic disease, infection and benign tumors can also be defined by CT.[16] With improvements in CT imaging and the increased availability of ultrasound, the detection of small or indeterminate renal masses occurs with greater frequency – as many as 33% of renal masses are 'incidental tumors'. These smaller, often low grade lesions are more amenable to nephron sparing surgery with favorable results.[17] The 5-year survival after nephron sparing surgery for small stage I tumors may be up to 100%.[18]

As early as 1994, it was also recognized that 3-dimensional CT could aid in the evaluation of patients undergoing nephron sparing surgery.[19] In a study of 17 consecutive patients with suspected renal masses, Smith et al[20] performed helical CT with subsequent generation of volume-rendered 3-dimensional images. This study concluded that 3-dimensional imaging coupled with CT angiography provided a thorough and accurate assessment of these malignant lesions and it was felt that such imaging modalities assisted the planning of operative management of these patients.[20]

In a separate study, triphasic spiral CT scans were performed in 60 consecutive patients undergoing nephron sparing surgery for renal neoplasms during which a videotape was prepared using volume-rendering software, which demonstrated the position of the kidney, the location and depth of the tumor, the renal arteries and veins as well as the relationship of the tumor to the collecting system. These tapes were viewed by the radiologists and urologists in the operating room at the time of surgery and immediately correlated with pathologic findings. This imaging modality accurately identified all tumor locations and 96% of renal arteries. Only three small accessory arteries and two short veins were missed.[21]

Recently, Wunderlich and colleagues published similar results. They examined the value of 3-dimensional CT in the preoperative simulation of nephron sparing surgery in 36 patients undergoing transperitoneal radical nephrectomy. They compared preoperative and intraoperative findings and found that 3-dimensional CT consistently and accurately demonstrated anatomical information relevant to surgical planning. They also successfully simulated partial nephrectomy as part of their study (Fig. 17.5).[22]

Pelvic ureteric junction obstruction
Traditional treatment of pelviureteric junction (PUJ) obstruction has been by open pyeloplasty

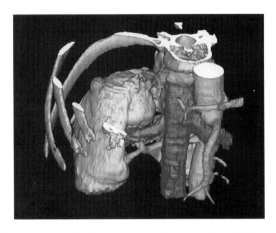

Figure 17.5 3-Dimensional volume-rendered CT showing a right kidney with two small renal cell carcinomas and vascular system. (Reproduced with permission from Wunderlich et al 2000.[22])

with successful long term results.[23] Recently, minimally invasive modalities such as antegrade or retrograde endopyelotomy,[24–26] Acusise endopyelotomy[27] and laparoscopic pyeloplasty[28,29] have been developed as attractive alternative therapeutic options.

For endopyelotomy procedures, the presence of major vessels close to the PUJ is potentially hazardous. Attention has been paid recently to the imaging of such vessels. Although endoluminal sonography provides considerable information on the location and nature of these obstructing vessels,[30] 3-dimensional spiral CT angiography generated a more informative spatial image, less invasively. The 3-dimensional images are far more intelligible for the urologist in identifying the obstructing vessels. Moreover, ureterovascular hydronephrosis characterized by the spatial relationship between the malrotated renal pelvis and the anterior crossing vessels can be visualized more definitively and hence influence the choice of therapeutic management.[31]

In a study conducted by Quillin and colleagues, good correlation was found between 3-dimensional CT angiograms and laparoscopic or open surgical findings in all patients undergoing such surgery. Uncomplicated endopyelotomies were performed in patients in whom no significant vessels were seen posterior or posterolateral to the PUJ.[32]

Hemorrhagic or vascular complications of endopyelotomy occur in 10% of cases, with 3–4% necessitating blood transfusion. Such a serious complication may be a result of blind incision made to a crossing vessel. The standard recommendation is for posterolateral incision though crossing vessels are as frequently situated posteriorly as anteriorly. Spiral CT and reconstruction may help to guide the direction of incision, thereby avoiding hemorrhagic complications.[33]

Renal transplantation

Potential live renal donors undergo extensive preoperative evaluation, which includes medical history, laboratory testing and radiological imaging.[34–36] Traditionally, imaging has included excretory urography (IVU) and conventional renal arteriography.[37–39] IVU is used to confirm two normally functioning kidneys and ureters and identify parenchymal lesions, renal calculi and congenital anomalies; renal arteriography is performed to delineate the vascular anatomy and any existing vascular disease.

The traditional role of these 2-dimensional imaging modalities has been challenged by helical CT angiography which provides a fast, minimally invasive mode of arteriogram-like evaluation of vascular anatomy in these patients. Recently, a few studies have indicated that this new modality of imaging may have an accuracy rate sufficient to replace intravenous pyelogram (IVP) and renal arteriography. Cochran and associates reported that CT arteriography is as accurate as conventional arteriography in revealing the number of renal vessels and can replace catheter angiography.[40]

In a report published by Del Pizzo et al,[41] helical 3-dimensional CT is deemed highly accurate in the assessment of renal arterial anatomy with results correlated with laparoscopic findings of sensitivity, specificity and accuracy of 91%, 98% and 96%, respectively. However, high level of contrast enhancement was not achieved in venous structures on CT arteriograms generating less impressive results of sensitivity, specificity and accuracy of 65%, 100% and 97%. Misdiagnoses were documented as cases of early venous bifurcations and supernumerary tributary veins.[41] Lerner and colleagues generated visually pleasing, highly accurate 3-dimensional reformatted images from CT angiography in their series of potential renal donors. In addition, they found that total preoperative imaging costs were decreased by 50% compared to IVP and renal arteriography. The procedure-related patient discomfort and potential morbidity were also significantly reduced.[42]

However, there seems to be a learning curve in the performance and interpretation of these 3-dimensional studies. A study conducted by Kaynan and colleagues evaluated the findings in 'early' and 'late' groups of patients and found that the ability to detect early renal arterial division improved throughout the study. They concluded that given the relative convenience of CT angiography compared to conventional methods, the cost savings and the comparable results, this 3-dimensional imaging modality is a good alternative in the assessment of live renal donors.[43]

Hofmann et al[44] also recognized an adjunctive use of 3-dimensional helical CT in renal transplant recipients. Real-time, volume-rendered 3-dimensional angiography can be performed on both the allografts as well as the native renal artery. In a recent report, they suggested that stenotic lesions were identified in transplant renal arteries, findings were confirmed by CT angiography and the lesions were relieved by angioplasty (Fig. 17.6).

It is clear that postprocessing of CT datasets can integrate information from a large number of axial sections into 3-dimensional images depicting the genitourinary tract in a variety of new types of presentation. The often compelling representations of normal and diseased structures and the ability to represent important anatomical relationships in easily comprehensible ways appears to give this new technology much promise for future applications.

CT virtual endoscopy

The rapid pace of technological advance in the last decade has made it possible to simulate virtual endoscopies based on various imaging modalities. Processing of such volumetric data is based on two computer techniques: *perspective projection* and *real-time 3-dimensional surface and volume rendering*. Flying through the anatomy can be produced by a freehand approach or by application of a mathematically model-generated path (central pathway navigation). The lumen wall can be made transparent to view adjacent structures. A specific point can be targeted and the axial, sagittal and coronal plane images displayed to provide better

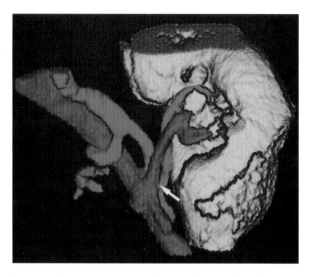

Figure 17.6   3-Dimensional CT surface rendered image of transplanted kidney with arrowed end-to-side anastomosis between renal vein and external iliac vein. (Reproduced with permission from Sebastia et al 2001.[45])

anatomical definition. Moreover, computer algorithms have been developed that calculate luminal wall thickness and integrate this with information about the curvature and convexity of the organ. This technique allows the identification and scrutinization of pathologic 'hot spot' areas (Fig. 17.7).

A high 'visual gradient' is required between the visceral lumen and wall to allow differentiation of structures. Predominantly air-filled spaces such as the paranasal sinuses,[46] larynx[47] and the tracheobronchial tree[46,48,49] offer optimal conditions for CT due to high attenuation gradient between air and mucosa. Similarly, datasets for virtual colonoscopy are acquired following transrectal air insufflation. This imaging modality has been extensively studied in the diagnosis and screening of patients at risk of colorectal cancers with encouraging results.[50,51]

Virtual ureterorenoscopy

Endoscopic procedures to evaluate the renal collecting system represent the gold standard for investigation of the urothelium. Diagnostic indications include filling defects, unilateral hematuria, positive urine cytology and surveillance after tumor resection.[52] However, these procedures are invasive and general anesthesia is usually required.

Virtual reality imaging has not been extensively applied to the upper urinary tract although the implications of its clinical usefulness are readily apparent. Takebayashi et al[53] examined surface rendering CT nephroscopy in 23 patients with suspected renal pelvic carcinoma and correlated findings with pathologic specimens retrospectively. Results showed that CT nephroscopy revealed 92% of carcinomas whereas axial CT images demonstrated only 83%. However, CT nephroscopy failed to detect one sessile and one polypoid tumor. Overall, CT nephroscopic images gave a good representation of pathological findings. They concluded that this technology is superior to axial CT for the detection of infiltrating and pedunculated carcinomas.[53]

In a more recent study, the same authors assessed the usefulness of CT ureteroscopic imaging for diagnosing ureteral tumors.[54] They conducted surface rendering CT ureteroscopy in 16 patients with ureteral stenosis and suspected ureteral tumors. Results were correlated with surgical and pathologic findings. CT ureteroscopy correctly detected all 22 lesions except one carcinoma in situ, one polypoid carcinoma and one hyperplastic polyp. The sensitivity and specificity of this technique for detecting ureteral tumors and carcinomas

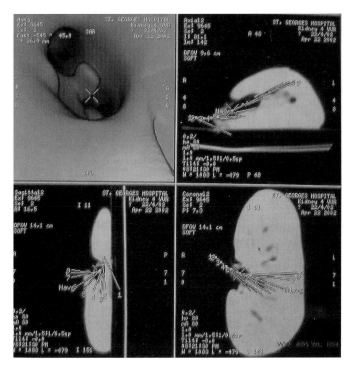

Figure 17.7   Axial, sagittal and coronal sections representing the location of the pelvicalyceal calculus. Numbered lines depict pathway navigation.

were 81% and 100%, and 80% and 75% respectively when tumors without stalks were considered carcinoma. They suggested that CT ureteroscopy is apparently useful to evaluate the complex morphology of ureteral tumors. Its advantages include the ability of proximal visualization in ureteral stenosis and enabling the evaluation of extraluminal extension of ureteral lesions and extrinsic compression from other sources.

However, CT ureterorenoscopy does have its inherent limitations, particularly a lack of information about flat urothelial abnormalities; unlike optical endoscopy, virtual endoscopy cannot evaluate the color, texture and the fine surface characteristics of these lesions. This technique is also limited as biopsy is unobtainable. Furthermore, these images cannot be achieved in patients in whom excretion of contrast into the upper urinary tract is impeded by renal dysfunction or high-grade tumor obstruction[54] and with current technology, depressed pelvicalyceal system and ureter are difficult to analyze.

The feasibility and accuracy of 3-dimensional reconstruction of the upper urinary tract and applied virtual ureterorenoscopy have been studied recently in several series of in vitro experiments. Mak and colleagues performed 3-dimensional CT reconstruction of porcine kidneys with subsequent comparative assessment of their pelvicalyceal parameters with those measured from their respective resin casts representing the true pelvicalyceal anatomy. They found significant correlations between the two sets of measurements affirming the accuracy of this 3-dimensional imaging modality (Fig. 17.8). Following on from this preliminary work, they applied such technology in the generation of virtual ureterorenoscopy with the aim of assessing its feasibility and value in the preoperative planning of endourological procedures of the upper urinary tract. These studies have demonstrated that virtual ureterorenoscopy is not only feasible but is also an accurate technique in the assessment of the locations of simulated pathologies (Fig. 17.9).[55,56]

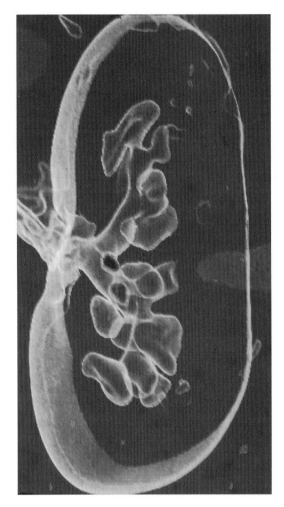

Figure 17.8 Volume-rendered CT image of air-contrasted porcine kidney demonstrating two radiodense lower infundibular calculi.

Allan and colleagues have also conducted a study on the feasibility and sensitivity of upper tract virtual endoscopy. They compared this imaging modality with flexible ureteroscopy in the context of adequacy of procedure, cost, sensitivity and specificity in 10 patients with upper tract pathologies which included transitional cell carcinoma (TCC), stone and strictures. They concluded that virtual ureteroscopy is feasible, safer, and cheaper and causes less morbidity than conventional ureteroscopy.[57]

Although virtual ureterorenoscopy has its inherent disadvantages in the management of malignant lesions in the upper tract, with improve-ment in technology it may play an important role in selected cases of upper tract urothelial tumors[58] and for planning endoscopic stone surgery. It is clear that the application of virtual ureterorenoscopy to the management of upper tract pathologies holds great value.

3-Dimensional magnetic resonance imaging

Magnetic resonance imaging has several intrinsic strengths that make it an attractive modality for 3-dimensional imaging. Multiplanar image acquisition with unique soft tissue definition is achievable with this technology. The use of gadolinium chelates as dynamic contrast agents avoids the need for nephrotoxic, allergenic iodinated contrast media.[59,60] Its utilization of non-ionizing radiation also makes it ideal for children and pregnant women. Furthermore, with the advent of 'open magnets', interactive magnetic resonance is already feasible.

However, magnetic resonance imaging of the upper urinary tract has suffered from greater technical limitations as it has a much slower acquisition time, with at times, disabling respiratory misregistration. However, the availability of faster and stronger gradient magnetic coils promises the reduction of ventilatory motion *artifact*. Furthermore, surface imaging coils are being developed to enable a more sensitive reception of the MR signal (higher *signal-to-noise* ratio, SNR).

Advances in computer software have generated new pulse sequences such as *2- and 3-dimensional gradient echo sequences*, which can provide high-resolution images within a single breath-hold. These sequences also allow the generation of MR angiography, dynamically enhanced renal and upper tract mass lesion images and contrast-enhanced MR urography (Fig. 17.10). *Fast 2-dimensional heavily T2-weighted sequences* (which can also be applied within a single breath-hold) and *high-resolution respiratory-triggered T2-weighted sequences* both give excellent contrast as well as eliminating ventilatory motion artifact, and are the result of modern technological advances which play an important part in making this imaging modality more clinically applicable.

As with other imaging modalities, MRI has its own intrinsic limitations. They include cost and availability. Patient factors such as those with MR-

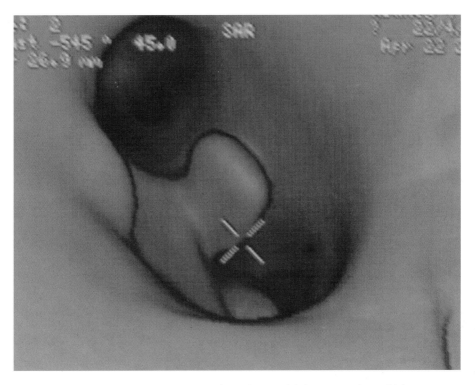

Figure 17.9 Virtual ureterorenoscopy of porcine model demonstrating calculus.

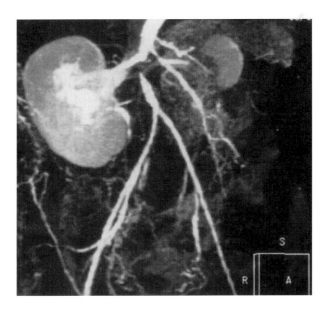

Figure 17.10 Magnetic resonance derived maximum intensity projection of kidney and renal vasculature. Note that there is no depth or 'surface' information. (Reproduced from Davis et al 1997.[61])

incompatible implanted devices and those with claustrophobia may influence the ultimate choice of investigation in favor of other imaging modalities. Whether T1 or T2 weighted, MR information can be digitized and presented in any 3-dimensional format as with CT.

MR urography

MR urography can be performed unenhanced or after intravenous gadolinium. The unenhanced study utilizes *T2-weighted static-fluid sequences* to provide excellent visualization of the obstructed and dilated urinary tract.[62] The gadolinium-enhanced study, performed using *T1-weighted gradient-echo excretory sequences*, provides morphological and functional information of the obstructed and non-obstructed urinary tract in patients with normal or moderately impaired renal function.[63] The MR urographical data are manipulated using *maximum intensity projection* to provide a 3-dimensional view of the entire excretory system.

Renal calculi

Calcification is better represented by other imaging modalities such as CT and 2-dimensional X-ray studies than MR, but MR urography has been used to demonstrate calculi as round or branched signal voids with the application of static-fluid MR urography[64–66] and excretory MR urography.[62]

However, it is recommended that one should include a single plain film radiograph in the analysis of MR urography for confident detection of calcifications[62] as filling defects are somewhat non-specific and other lesions such as blood clot, debris, small tumor and surgical clips can give rise to similar MR urographic appearances.[62,65,67,68]

Although this imaging modality has limited application in acute urolithiasis except in the pregnant woman, it may still play a potential role in patients with chronic stone disease affecting the urinary tract. Valuable information about the true location of renal calculi and the anatomical configuration of the pelvicalyceal system may be obtained which serves to predict therapeutic success.[69]

Intrinsic tumors of the upper urinary tract

Retrograde pyelography is commonly regarded as the mainstay in the range of diagnostic investigations available for ureteral TCC. CT has also proved to be of great value in the representation of these

lesions.[70] However, initial results suggest that MR urography may also have a role in reducing the need for invasive retrograde pyelography in this clinical context.[62]

Several studies have documented that advanced intrinsic tumor growths can be diagnosed with both static-fluid and excretory MR urography.[62,66,71–73] The signs of endoluminal tumor growth described for standard IVU and retrograde pyelography[70] also applies to the morphological features found in MR urography and maximum intensity projection.[62,72,74] MR urography can be combined with conventional MR imaging and contrast-enhanced MR angiography to establish an all-in-one imaging modality to examine bilateral kidneys, renal vascular supply and perfusion, and the urinary tract, thus removing the need for separate investigations with other modalities such as ultrasonography, intravenous urography and CT for both intrinsic and extrinsic lesions.[75]

Anomalies of the urinary tract

Static-fluid and excretory MR urography are complementary techniques in the early detection of pediatric anomalies.[76–78] Urological anomalies are also common findings in MR urography of adult patients.[62,66,72,73]

T2-weighted static-fluid MR urography has proved useful for the visualization of ureteroceles,[78] bladder diverticula,[73] megaureters,[76,78] markedly obstructed duplex systems,[66,72,73,78] pelviureteric obstruction[66,73,76] and cystic kidney diseases.[72,73,76,78]

T1-weighted dynamic contrast enhanced excretory MR urography has great potential in the representation of small variations and anomalies that occur in the non-dilated urinary tract such as ectopic ureters[77] and non-dilated duplex systems.[77] Both static-fluid and excretory MR urography are also able to demonstrate dystrophic and horseshoe kidneys.[62,77,78]

Magnetic resonance virtual ureterorenoscopy

Magnetic resonance virtual endoscopy has been successfully applied to the study of vessels, biliary tract, colon and cerebral ventricles.[79–82] In urology, virtual magnetic resonance ureterorenoscopy can be generated from MR urographic data using thresholding and reconstruction techniques common to other imaging modalities. Several studies using various magnetic sequences have been performed to assess the feasibility and diagnostic performance of virtual ureterorenoscopy in the morphological representation of upper urinary tract.

Nolte-Ernsting and co-workers conducted 28 contrast-enhanced MR urographic examinations with subsequent postprocessing of such data to generate virtual ureterorenoscopy. They reported that all the filling defects diagnosed by MR urography could be evaluated from the endoluminal view using virtual ureterorenoscopy. However, the exact characterization of upper tract lesions based only on the assessment of surface detail endoluminally was difficult.[83]

Neri et al[63] conducted a feasibility study on unenhanced surface rendering MR virtual ureteroscopy applied to 26 patients with various upper tract pathologies including neoplastic lesions, PUJ stenosis, postoperative fibrotic strictures and extrinsic compression of the ureter. They found that virtual ureteroscopy was feasible in patients with ureteric diameters greater than 5 mm and that the non-dilated contralateral side could only be partially explored in 11 (43%) of patients. MR ureteroscopy depicted the endoluminal appearance, position and extension of the lesions with respect to the collecting system.[63]

Beer and colleagues conducted a study to assess the diagnostic performance of both enhanced and unenhanced MR urographic data with subsequent combined analysis of *maximum intensity projection* and virtual endoscopy in 36 patients with urological pathologies. They concluded that maximum intensity projection is comparable to virtual endoscopy in the evaluation of the upper urinary tract.[84]

Although still in the early stages of development, MR ureterorenoscopy is certainly feasible. It allows observers to visualize the pelvicalyceal system and to see the effects of abnormalities on the urinary tract lumen. Whether it will evolve as a useful clinical tool remains to be seen. In theory, it is more promising than CT ureterorenoscopy because of its better tissue characterization and the promise of real-time interactivity. However, in practice, current magnetic resonance imaging is limited by imaging artifact and background noise.

3-Dimensional ultrasonography

3-Dimensional ultrasonography offers noninvasive real-time interactivity and flexibility in contrast to other tomographic imaging techniques. 3-Dimensional images can be reconstructed from data obtained with a single sweep of the ultrasound beam across the targeted organ with the accurate recording of the exact relationship between anatomical structures allowing unrestricted access to an infinite number of viewing planes. This imaging modality has theoretical advantages over conventional 2-dimensional ultrasound because it may decrease interobserver variability and the limited viewing perspective.[85]

In urology, intraluminal 3-dimensional ultrasound is applicable for the evaluation of anterior urethral strictures[86] and, when combined with urodynamics, in the assessment of voiding in patients with posterior urethral strictures.[87]

3-Dimensional transrectal ultrasonography has a fully established role in the evaluation, cryoablation and radiotherapy (in combination with CT-based radiation planning therapy (RPT) and transperineal prostate implantation (TPI) systems) of prostate cancer (Fig. 17.11).[88–91]

However, as far as imaging of the upper urinary tract is concerned, this modality remains very much in the research phase. There are several reasons for this:

- It is difficult to obliterate acoustic barriers (e.g. air) to generate an artifact-free 3-dimensional database.
- A translational stage has also to be realized in order to determine *transducer* position and orientation, i.e. accurate 3-dimensional spatial information.[92,93]
- There is an associated learning curve attached to data manipulation and postprocessing techniques with variable reconstruction times according to the speed of the computer algorithms.[85]

Applications of 3-dimensional ultrasound

Recently, technological advances have enabled the acquisition and visualization of 3-dimensional ultrasonographic images (either in gray scale or Doppler) using a sophisticated position sensor and a conventional 2-dimensional ultrasound machine. New computer software can now facilitate the visualization of voxel data in any plane with

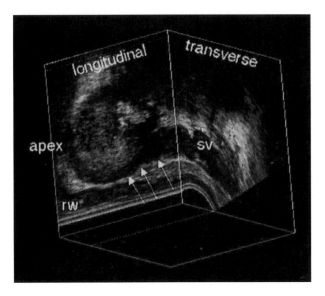

Figure 17.11 3-Dimensional ultrasound reconstruction of the prostate showing arrowed hypoechoic tumor invading seminal vesicles (SV). This is an example of a multiplanar reformatted reconstruction. rw, rectal wall (Reproduced from Downey et al 2000.[85])

additional postprocessing modality which allows for effects of varying probe pressure and correction of small errors in the position sensor readings. There is also provision for the calculation of volume and a special tool to deal with large structures that cannot be scanned with a single sweep of the ultrasound probe.[94]

With these recent advances, increased research in 3-dimensional ultrasound imaging is anticipated. If fruitful, this will be a major advance as the real-time interactivity may make intraoperative surgical planning possible, a feature that is impossible with 3-dimensional CT or MRI.

Conclusion

In the past decade, 3-dimensional imaging has become increasingly feasible in clinical practice and may make a huge impact in urological surgery in the near future. Currently, its clinical value is limited to surgical management for calculi, renal masses and PUJ obstruction, using 3-dimensional CT and image analysis of 3-dimensional CT or MR angiography. Areas of active research are virtual ureterorenoscopy and the development

of real-time, interactive 3-dimensional studies, particularly on interactive magnetic resonance and ultrasound.

The present limitations of this modality are related to object definition and validation. The inevitable future technologic advances will be in the areas of improved resolution and rapid acquisition. In display and data analysis, computer hardware advances with reduction of cost in memory and processor power will lead to more sophisticated software development.

The next generation of surgical systems will permit the implementation of surgical procedures beyond the current limitations of human performance. 3-Dimensional reconstructions generated by computed tomography, magnetic resonance imaging, ultrasound or other scanning techniques will act to integrate the entire spectrum of surgical care from diagnosis to preoperative planning through to intraoperative navigation and education through simulation. By working through the computer-generated image, first with preoperative planning and then during telepresence or image-guided procedures, new approaches to surgery will be possible.

Glossary

Algorithm – the mathematical process used in image reconstruction.

Artifact – an error induced by the incorrect processing of the image by the array processor or attenuation measurements from within the object being scanned.

Attenuation – the absorption of transmitted energy by various components of the object.

Collimate – to make parallel.

Data acquisition – collection and transformation of ionizing or non-ionizing radiation into digital signal.

Digital – electronic technology that generates, stores and processes data in terms of state digits referred to as a bit (a string of bits that a computer can address as a group is a byte).

Echoes – reflected sound waves.

Helicoidal – forming or arranged in a spiral.

Orthogona – 'involving right angles' Greek *ortho* = right, *gon* = angled.

Perspective projection – perception that near objects appear larger than objects that are located further than view point.

Polyhedron – a solid formed by planed faces.

Rendering – data manipulating technique used in 3-dimensional imaging.

Resolution – sharpness of an image represented by the number of pixels (basic 2-dimensional units of radiographic data) contained in a display monitor.

Signal-to-noise ratio – a measure of the electromagnetic field strength relative to background interference in decibels (dB).

Thresholding – technique used to segment structures of interest based attenuation gradient in Hounsfield units between different tissues at the interface.

Transducer – electronic device that converts energy from one form to another.

Voxel – a 3-dimensional volume element of radiographical data (a 3-dimensional pixel [2-dimensional picture element]).

References

1. Glenn WVJ, Johnston RJ, Morton PE, Dwyer SJ. Image generation and display techniques for CT scan data: thin transverse and reconstructed coronal and sagittal planes. Invest Radiol 1975; 10:403–416.

2. Mazziotta JC, Huang HK. THREAD (three-dimensional reconstruction and display) with biomedical applications in neuron ultrastructure and computerized tomography. National Computer Conference, New York. 1976.

3. Herman GT, Liu HK. Display of three-dimensional information in computed tomography. J Comput Assist Tomogr 1977; 1:155–160.

4. Herman GT, Liu HK. Three-dimensional display of human organs from computed tomograms. Comput Graph Image Process 1979; 9:1–21.

5. Hemmy DC, David DJ, Herman GT. Three-dimensional reconstruction of craniofacial deformity using computed tomography. Neurosurgery 1983; 13:534–541.

6. David DJ, Hemmy DC, Cooter RD. Craniofacial deformities: atlas of three-dimensional reconstruction from computed tomography. New York: Springer-Verlag; 1990.

7. Kalender WA, Seissler W, Klotz E, Vock P. Spiral volumetric CT with single-breath-hold period technique, continuous transport and continuous scanner rotation. Radiology 1990; 176:181–183.

8. Rubin GD, Dake MD, Napel SA, et al. Three-dimensional spiral CT angiography of the abdomen: initial clinical experience. Radiology 1993; 186:147–152.

9. Lam HS, Lingeman JE, Russo R, Chua GT. Stone surface area determination techniques: a unifying concept of staghorn stone burden assessment. J Urol 1992; 148(3 Pt 2):1026–1029.

10. Olcott EW, Sommer FG, Napel S. Accuracy of detection and measurement of renal calculi: in vitro comparison of three-dimensional spiral CT, radiography, and nephrotomography. Radiology 1997; 204(1):19–25.

11. Yamaguchi A. Extracorporeal shock wave lithotripsy monotherapy for staghorn calculi. Eur Urol 1994; 25(2):110–115.

12. Hubert J, Blum A, Cormier L, et al. Three-dimensional CT-scan reconstruction of renal calculi. A new tool for mapping-out staghorn calculi and follow-up of radiolucent stones. Eur Urol 1997; 31(3):297–301.

13. Liberman SN, Halpern EJ, Sullivan K, Bagley DH. Spiral computed tomography for staghorn calculi. Urology 1997; 50(4):519–524.

14. Buchholz N-P. Three-dimensional CT scan stone reconstruction for the planning of percutaneous surgery in a morbidly obese patient. Urologia Int 2000; 65:46–48.

15. Bluemke DA, Fishman EK. Spiral CT of the abdomen: clinical applications. Crit Rev Diagn Imaging 1993; 34103–34157.

16. Bosniak MA. The small (< 3.0 cm) renal parenchymal tumor. Radiology 1991; 179:307–317.

17. Polascik TJ, Meng MV, Epstein JI, Marshall FF. Intraoperative sonography for the evaluation and management of renal tumors: experience with 100 patients. J Urol 1995; 154:1676–1680.

18. Licht MR, Novick AC, Goormastic M. Nephron sparing surgery in incidental versus suspected renal cell carcinoma. J Urol 1994; 152:39–42.

19. Chernoff DM, Silverman SG, Kikinis R, et al. Three-dimensional imaging and display of renal tumors using spiral CT: potential aid to partial nephrectomy. Urology 1994; 43:125–129.

20. Smith PA, Marshall FF, Corl FM, Fishman EK. Planning nephron-sparing renal surgery using 3D helical CT angiography. J Comput Assist Tomogr 1999; 23(5):649–654.

21. Coll DM, Uzzo RG, Herts BR, et al. 3-dimensional volume rendered computerized tomography for preoperative evaluation and intraoperative treatment of patients undergoing nephron sparing surgery. J Urol 1999; 161(4):1097–1102.

22. Wunderlich H, Reichelt O, Schubert R, et al. Preoperative simulation of partial nephrectomy with three-dimensional computed tomography. BJU Int 2000; 86(7):777–781.

23. O'Reilly P, Brooman PB, Mak S, et al. Long term results of Anderson-Hynes pyeloplasty for ureteropelvic junction obstruction. BJU Int 2001; 87(4):287–289.

24. Kuenkel M, Korth K. Endopyelotomy: long-term follow-up of 143 patients. Endourology 1990; 4:109.

25. Motola JA, Fried R, Badlani GH, Smith AD. Failed endopyelotomy: implications for future surgery on the ureteropelvic junction. J Urol 1993; 150(3):821–823.

26. Meretyk I, Meretyk S, Clayman RV. Endopyelotomy: comparison of ureteroscopic retrograde and antegrade percutaneous techniques. J Urol 1992; 148(3):775–782; discussion 782–783.

27. Chandhoke PS, Clayman RV, Stone AM, et al Endopyelotomy and endoureterotomy with the acucise ureteral cutting balloon device: preliminary experience. J Endourol 1993; 7(1):45–51.

28. Janetschek G, Peschel R, Frauscher F, Franscher F. Laparoscopic pyeloplasty. Urol Clin North Am 2000; 27(4):695–704.

29. Brooks JD, Kavoussi LR, Preminger GM, et al. Comparison of open and endourologic approaches to the obstructed ureteropelvic junction. Urology 1995; 46(6):791–795.

30. Bagley DH, Liu JB, Goldberg BB, Grasso M. Endopyelotomy: importance of crossing vessels demonstrated by endoluminal ultrasonography. J Endourol 1995; 9(6):465–467.

31. Kumon H, Tsugawa M, Hashimoto H, et al. Impact of 3-dimensional helical computerized tomography on selection of operative methods for ureteropelvic junction obstruction. J Urol 1997; 158(5):1696–1700.

32. Quillin SP, Brink JA, Heiken JP, et al. Helical (spiral) CT angiography for identification of crossing vessels at the ureteropelvic junction. AJR Am J Roentgenol 1996; 166(5):1125–1130.

33. Farres MT, Pedron P, Gattegno B, et al. Helical CT and 3D reconstruction of ureteropelvic junction obstruction: accuracy in detection of crossing vessels. J Comput Assist Tomogr 1998; 22:300–303.

34. Lowell JA, Taylor RJ. The evaluation of the living renal donor, surgical techniques and results. Semin Urol 1994; 12:102–107.

35. Riehle RAJ, Steckler R, Naslund EB, et al. Selection criteria for the evaluation of living related renal donors. J Urol 1990; 144:845–848.

36. Spanos PK, Simmons RL, Kjellstrand CM, et al. Screening potential related transplant donors for renal disease. Lancet 1974; 1:645–649.

37. Derauf B, Goldberg ME. Angiographic assessment of potential renal transplant donors. Radiol Clin North Am 1987; 25:261–265.

38. Walker TG, Geller SC, Delmonico FL, et al. Donor renal angiography: its influence and the decision to use the right or left kidney. AJR Am J Roentgenol 1988; 151:1149–1151.

39. Kjellevand TO, Kolmannskog F, Pfeffer P, et al. Influence of renal angiography in living potential renal donors. Acta Radiol 1991; 32:368–370.

40. Cochran ST, Krasny RM, Danovitch GM, et al. Helical CT angiography for examination of living renal donors. AJR Am J Roentgenol 1997; 168(6):1569–1573.

41. Del Pizzo JJ, Sklar GN, You-Cheong JW, et al. Helical computerized tomography arteriography for evaluation of live renal donors undergoing laparoscopic nephrectomy. J Urol 1999; 162(1):31–34.

42. Lerner LB, Henriques HF, Harris RD. Interactive 3-dimensional computerized tomography reconstruction in evaluation of the living renal donor. J Urol 1999; 161(2):403–407.

43. Kaynan AM, Rozenblit AM, Figueroa KI, et al. Use of spiral computerized tomography in lieu of angiography for the preoperative assessment of living renal donors. J Urol 1999; 161:1769–1775.

44. Hofmann LV, Smith PA, Kuszyk BS, et al. Three-dimensional helical CT angiography in renal transplant recipients: a new problem-solving tool. AJR Am J Roentgenol 1999; 173:1085–1089.

45. Sebastia C, Quiroga S, Boye R, et al. Helical CT in renal transplantation: normal findings and early and late complications. Radiographics 2001; 21:1103–1117.

46. Rubin GD, Beaulieu CF, Argiro V, et al. Perspective volume rendering of CT and MRI images; applications for endoscopic imaging. Radiology 1996; 199:321–330.

47. Rodenwaldt J, Kopka L, Roedel R, Grabbe R. Three-dimensional surface imaging of the larynx and trachea by spiral CT: virtual endoscopy. Rofo Fortschr Geb Rontgenstr Neuen Bildgeb Verfahr, 1996; 165(1):80–83.

48. Vining DJ, Liu K, Choplin RH, Haponik EF. Virtual bronchoscopy. Relationships of virtual reality endobronchial simulations to actual bronchoscopic findings. Chest 1996; 109(2):549–553.

49. Feretti G, Knoplioch J, Coulomb M. Virtual bronchoscopy: multiplanar reformation and 3D shaded surface displays of tracheobronchial tree. Radiology 1995; 197(P):201 (suppl).

50. Fenlon HM, Barish MA, Ferrucci JT. Virtual colonoscopy – technique and applications. Ital J Gastroenterol Hepatol 1999; 31(8):713–720.

51. Morrin MM, Farrell RJ, Kruskal JB. Virtual colonoscopy. N Engl J Med 2000; 342(10):738; discussion 738–739.

52. Rowbotham C, Anson KM. Benign lateralizing haematuria: the impact of upper tract endoscopy. BJU Int 2001; 88(9):841–849.

53. Takebayashi S, Hosaka M, Takase K, et al. Computerized tomography nephroscopic images of renal pelvic carcinoma. J Urol 1999; 162(2):315–318.

54. Takebayashi S, Hosaka M, Kubota Y, et al. Computerized tomographic ureteroscopy for diagnosing ureteral tumors. J Urol 2000; 163(1):42–46.

55. Mak S, Cattini G, Patel U, Anson K. The evaluation of 3-dimensional CT pelvicalyceal reconstruction as a guide to endoscopic navigation for intrarenal surgery. In: BAUS Section of EndoUrology 1st Annual Meeting. Medical Education Centre, Northern General Hospital, Sheffield. 2001.

56. Mak S, Cattini G, Patel U, Anson K. Virtual ureterorenoscopy and 3-dimensional pelvicalyceal anatomical reconstructions as a guide to endoscopic navigation – feasibility studies in a pig kidney model. J Urol 2002; 167(4):75.

57. Allan JD, Moussa SA, Connell M, Tolley DA. A comparison of virtual and flexible ureteroscopy in the assessment of upper tract pathology. J Endourol 2000; 14(suppl 1):A8.

58. Elliott DS, Segura JW, Lightner D, et al. Is nephroureterectomy necessary in all cases of upper tract transitional cell carcinoma? Long-term results of conservative endourologic management of upper tract transitional cell carcinoma in individuals with a normal contralateral kidney. Urology 2001; 58(2):174–178.

59. Prince MR, Arnoldus C, Frisoli JK. Nephrotoxicity of high-dose gadolinium compared with iodinated contrast. J Magn Reson Imaging 1996; 6:162–166.

60. Niendorf HP, Dinger JC, HausteinJ, et al. Tolerance data of Gd-DTPA: a review. Eur J Radiol 1991; 13:15–20.

61. Davis CP, Hany TF, Wildermuth S, et al. Postprocessing techniques for gadolinium-enhanced three-dimensional MR angiography. Radiographics 1997; 17:1061–1077.

62. Nolte-Ernsting CC, Bucker A, Adam GB, et al. Gadolinium-enhanced excretory MR urography after low-dose diuretic injection: comparison with conventional excretory urography. Radiology 1998; 209(1):147–157.

63. Neri E, Boraschi P, Carmella D, et al. MR virtual endoscopy of the upper urinary tract. AJR Am J Roentgenol 2000; 175(6):1697–1702.

64. Roy C, Saussine C, LeBras Y, et al. Assessment of painful ureterohydronephrosis during pregnancy by MR urography. Eur Radiol 1996; 6(3):334–338.

65. Regan F, Petronis J, Bohlman M, et al. Perirenal MR high signal – a new and sensitive indicator of acute ureteric obstruction. Clin Radiol 1997; 52(6):445–450.

66. Tang Y, Yamashita Y, Namimoto T, et al. The value of MR urography that uses HASTE sequences to reveal urinary tract disorders. AJR Am J Roentgenol 1996; 167(6):1497–1502.

67. Roy C, Saussine C, Jahn, C, et al. Evaluation of RARE-MR urography in the assessment of ureterohydronephrosis. J Comput Assist Tomogr 1994; 18(4):601–608.

68. O'Malley ME, Soto JA, Yucel EK, Hussain S. MR urography: evaluation of a three-dimensional fast spin-echo technique in patients with hydronephrosis. AJR Am J Roentgenol 1997; 168(2):387–392.

69. Nolte-Ernsting C, Tacke J, Adam GB, et al. Diuretic-enhanced gadolinium excretory MR urography: comparison of conventional gradient-echo sequences and echo-planar imaging. Eur Radiol 2001; 11:18–27.

70. Goldman SM, Bohlman ME, Gatewood OM. Neoplasms of the renal collecting system. Semin Roentgenol 1987; 22(4):284–291.

71. Catalano C, Pavone P, Laghi A, et al. MR pyelography and conventional MR imaging in urinary tract obstruction. Acta Radiol 1999; 40(2):198–202.

72. Rothpearl A, Frager D, Subramanian A, et al. MR urography: technique and application. Radiology 1995; 194(1):125–130.

73. Klein LT, Frager D, Subramanian A, Lowe FC. Use of magnetic resonance urography. Urology 1998; 52(4):602–608.

74. Reuther G, Kiefer B, Wandl E. Visualization of urinary tract dilatation: value of single-shot MR urography. Eur Radiol 1997; 7(8):1276–1281.

75. Verswijvel GA, Oyen RH, Van Poppel HP, et al. Magnetic resonance imaging in the assessment of urologic disease: an all-in-one approach. Eur Radiol 2000; 10(10):1614–1619.

76. Borthne A, Nordshus T, Reiseter T, et al. MR urography: the future gold standard in paediatric urogenital imaging? Pediatr Radiol 1999; 29(9):694–701.

77. Staatz G, Nolte-Ernsting CC, Adam GB, et al. Feasibility and utility of respiratory-gated, gadolinium-enhanced T1-weighted magnetic resonance urography in children. Invest Radiol 2000; 35(8):504–512.

78. Sigmund G, Stoever B, Zimmerhackl LB, et al. RARE-MR-urography in the diagnosis of upper urinary tract abnormalities in children. Pediatr Radiol 1991; 21(6):416–420.

79. Davis CP, Ladd CP, Romanowski BJ, et al. Human aorta: preliminary results with virtual endoscopy based on three-dimensional MR imaging data sets. Radiology 1996; 199(1):37–40.

80. Luboldt W, Debatin JF. Virtual endoscopic colonography based on 3D MRI. Abdom Imaging, 1998; 23(6):568–572.

81. Shigematsu Y, Korogi Y, Hirai T, et al. Virtual MRI endoscopy of the intracranial cerebrospinal fluid spaces. Neuroradiology 1998; 40(10):644–650.

82. Neri E, Boraschi P, Braccini G, et al. MR virtual endoscopy of the pancreaticobiliary tract. Magn Reson Imaging 1999; 17(1):59–67.

83. Nolte-Ernsting CC, Krombach G, Staatz G, et al. Virtual endoscopy of the upper urinary tract based on contrast-enhanced MR urography data sets. Rofo Fortschr Geb Rontgenstr Neuen Bildgeb Verfahr 1999; 170(6):550–556.

84. Beer A, Saar B, Link TM, et al. Virtual endoscopy of the urinary tract from T2-weighted and gadolinium-enhanced T1-weighted MR urographic images. Rofo Fortschr Geb Rontgenstr Neuen Bildgeb Verfahr 2001; 173(11):997–1005.

85. Downey DB, Fenster A, Williams JC. Clinical utility of three-dimensional US. Radiographics 2000; 20(2):559–571.

86. McAninch JW, Laing FC, Jeffrey RB Jr. Sonourethrography in the evaluation of urethral strictures: a preliminary report. J Urol 1988; 139(2):294–297.

87. Nerstrom H, Holm HH, Christensen NE, et al. 3-dimensional ultrasound based demonstration of the posterior urethra during voiding combined with urodynamics. Scand J Urol Nephrol 1991; 137(suppl):125–129.

88. Garg S, Fortling B, Chadwick D, et al. Staging of prostate cancer using 3-dimensional transrectal ultrasound images: a pilot study. J Urol 1999; 162(4):1318–1321.

89. Chin JL, Downey DB, Onik G, Fenster A. Three-dimensional prostate ultrasound and its application to cryosurgery. Tech Urol 1996; 2(4):187–193.

90. Kini VR, Edmundson VK, Vicini FA, et al. Use of three-dimensional radiation therapy planning tools and intraoperative ultrasound to evaluate high dose rate prostate brachytherapy implants. Int J Radiat Oncol Biol Phys 1999; 43(3):571–578.

91. Zelefsky MJ, Yamada Y, Cohen G, et al. Postimplantation dosimetric analysis of permanent transperineal prostate implantation: improved dose distributions with an intraoperative computer-optimized conformal planning technique. Int J Radiat Oncol Biol Phys 2000; 48(2):601–608.

92. Hell B. 3D sonography. Int J Oral Maxillofac Surg 1995; 24(1 Pt 2):84–89.

93. Sohn C, Grotepass J. 3-dimensional organ image using ultrasound. Ultraschall Med 1990; 11(6):295–301.

94. Prager R, Gee A, Treece G. The Stradx 3D Ultrasound Acquisition and Visualisation System. 3D ultrasound research in the SVR Group at Cambridge University Engineering Department. 2002.

18

Future prospects for nephron conservation in renal cell carcinoma

Erik Havranek and Chris Anderson

Introduction

Renal cancer is now the sixth most common cancer in men and women in the UK. It comprises about 8% of all solid cancers and is a heterogeneous group of tumors. The majority (i.e. over 85%) are renal cell adenocarcinomas. There are 4800 new cases of renal cancer diagnosed annually in England and Wales (181 000 worldwide). This corresponds to an approximate incidence of 9.6 per 100 000. Unlike many other cancers, the incidence has been rising over the last 20 years at a faster rate than can be explained by better and earlier diagnosis alone.

Surgery remains the only reliable cure for (early stage) renal cell cancer. Spontaneous regressions have been reported but are very rare. Immunotherapy, chemotherapy and radiotherapy are all disappointing compared with surgery. As the size of newly diagnosed tumors decreases with the increased proportion of incidentally diagnosed early cancers, the potential scope for nephron conservation is obvious. The number of small incidentally discovered tumors has risen over the last 25 years by at least 50%.[1] In a recent series of 180 partial nephrectomies, 85% of tumors were discovered incidentally, usually by ultrasound or CT and only 14% were symptomatic.[2] Asymptomatic incidentally discovered tumors are often small and hence more amenable to partial nephrectomy.

Nephron sparing surgery for renal cancer was first pioneered by Czerny in 1887.[3] In 1950, Vermooten suggested indications for partial nephrectomies.[4] However a study in 1969 by Robson et al[5] showed that radical nephrectomy was superior at limiting hematological cancer spread compared with the partial and simple nephrectomies carried out in the 1950s and 1960s. They described radical nephrectomy as early ligation of the renal vessels, removal of the kidney, perinephric fat, ipsilateral

adrenal gland and all regional lymph nodes. This led to radical nephrectomy becoming the gold standard of renal cancer surgery as the logical belief was that this approach would maximize potential for cure. This significantly delayed the acceptance of partial nephrectomy as a feasible treatment.

In 1980, Jacobs et al[6] reported better survival in partial nephrectomy patients with synchronous cancers compared to bilateral radical nephrectomy followed by dialysis. Many other reports have since shown promising results for partial nephrectomies. An improved understanding of cancer physiology, better imaging as well as improved surgical methods have led to a slow replacement of radical nephrectomy by partial nephrectomy in selected cases of renal cancer.

Nephron sparing surgery or partial nephrectomy is becoming increasingly widely accepted, as indications to operate and surgical techniques are refined and more follow-up data are available. The main issues of contention have been adequate clearance margins in cancer surgery, appropriate follow up to detect possible recurrence and cancer specific survival rates. The aim of the operation is to conserve physiological units of the kidney, while removing the pathological lesion without compromising cure.

Long-term follow-up data have now shown that partial nephrectomy in selected cases of renal cell carcinoma (RCC) can be performed with low morbidity, preservation of renal function, low local recurrence rate and high patient satisfaction.[7] Concern regarding local recurrence is still the major factor slowing wide acceptance of partial nephrectomy. As emerging evidence is showing that survival of partial and radical nephrectomy patients is comparable, it would seem reasonable to preserve as much renal parenchyma as possible.

Advances in renal imaging, improved surgical techniques, methods to prevent ischemic renal injury and better postoperative management (including improvements in renal replacement therapy) have made nephron sparing surgery a serious alternative to radical nephrectomy. The dedication of several specialists to revisiting partial nephrectomy, which fell into disrepute in the 1960s, has contributed to the availability of long-term, prospective cancer-free survival data. Over 1800 patients who underwent partial nephrectomy have been reported in the literature since 1980. Overall cancer specific survival appears to be 72–100% with more recent reports consistently > 90%. The mean follow up ranged from 24 to 75 months.[8] Furthermore, hospital costs and the rate of complications have been shown to be similar for partial and radical nephrectomies.[9] The evidence base supporting partial nephrectomy is steadily increasing and progressively less invasive methods of achieving nephron sparing are being studied.

Indications for partial nephrectomy

Indications are commonly subdivided into three categories: imperative (or absolute), relative and elective (Table 18.1). In current practice imperative indications for nephron sparing surgery comprise situations where more extensive surgery would render the patient anephric or with limited renal function with subsequent need for renal replacement therapy. This includes patients with a lesion in a solitary kidney, patients with bilateral renal tumors and patients with impaired renal function. Partial nephrectomy should be considered even for tumors greater than 4 cm in imperative situations.

Relative indications need to be considered for selected patients in whom local, systemic or

Table 18.1 Indications for nephron sparing surgery[8]

Imperative
Tumors in single kidneys
Impaired function of contralateral kidney
Bilateral synchronous tumors
Relative
Von Hippel–Lindau disease (VHLD) and other forms of hereditary renal cell carcinoma
Elective
Consider patients with tumors 4 cm or less
Indeterminate cystic lesions with malignant potential[10]

genetic conditions threaten the contralateral kidney's future in terms of function or by risk of developing a subsequent contralateral tumor.[8] Von Hippel–Lindau disease is one such example, which in contrast to non-hereditary RCC, develops at a younger age and is usually multicentric and bilateral. The decision whether to offer partial nephrectomy should be based on the age of the patient, comorbidities, the risk of disease progression and the likelihood of remaining renal function being affected by these conditions.

While imperative indications are relatively undisputed, elective indications for patients with normal contralateral kidneys are still approached with caution by many surgeons, who are reluctant to consider offering partial nephrectomy for cancer. The risk of developing a metachronous tumor or renal impairment in the contralateral kidney of an otherwise healthy patient is small. Whether the potential benefit of nephron sparing outweighs the potential risk of local recurrence is still to be conclusively decided. Currently advocated indications for elective partial nephrectomies include tumors of 4 cm and smaller. Until recently lesions with a polar location have been favored but current evidence shows that centrally located tumors have similar outcomes. The evidence broadly shows that there is no statistical differences in 5-year survival of radical nephrectomy compared with partial nephrectomy patients for tumors of 4 cm or less. However, few prospective studies are available and further refinement of indications is still necessary. A multicenter trial to determine the benefits of partial nephrectomy for small incidental RCCs would be useful in future.[11]

The largest series of partial nephrectomies so far has been published by Hafez and colleagues.[12,13] Five hundred patients treated before 1997 were reviewed with overall 5-year survival rates of 81% and cancer specific 5-year survival rates of 93%, with outcome much better in patients with tumor sizes of 4 cm or less. Only 2.7% developed local recurrence in the remnant kidney. Negative predictive factors for survival included high grade, high stage, bilateral disease and a tumor size of greater than 4 cm. Subsequent data from the same institution showed that there was no difference in 5-year cancer specific survival, tumor recurrence or renal function in centrally versus peripherally located tumors.

A 10-year follow-up study was published by Fergany et al in 2000.[14] All 107 patients treated in

Table 18.2 Published series of partial nephrectomies

Study	Year	No of patients	Local recurrence (%)
Marberger et al[15]	1981	72	8
Morgan & Zincke[16]	1990	104	6
Steinbach et al[17]	1992	121	4
Moll et al[18]	1993	142	1
Van Poppel et al[19]	1998	76	0
Hafez et al[11]	1999	485	3
Belldegrun et al[20]	1999	146	3
Lee et al[21]	2000	79	0

a single institution prior to 1989 were reviewed. Nephron sparing surgery was carried out in 90% of patients for imperative indications such as the presence of only one kidney. Cancer specific survival was 88% at 5 years and 73% at 10 years; 26% died of metastatic disease. For tumors smaller than 4 cm survival was 98% at 5 years and 92% at 10 years. Table 18.2 shows a list of several published partial nephrectomy series.

A Mayo Clinic study has shown that the incidence of postoperative chronic renal impairment 10 years after surgery is 11% after partial nephrectomy compared to 22% after radical nephrectomy.[22] Fergany et al, in a 10-year follow-up study, showed that 6.5% of partial nephrectomies carried out for mainly imperative indications progressed to end-stage renal failure.[14] Uzzo and Novick[8] argue that elective partial nephrectomies are at lower risk than imperative ones due to the nature of their disease. In view of the good results of nephron sparing surgery in patients with tumours 4 cm or less,[17,18,21,23–26] and because it is impossible to calculate the risk to contralateral renal function in each patient, it seems reasonable that partial nephrectomy is offered to such individuals.

Nephron sparing surgery in Von Hippel–Lindau disease

Von Hippel–Lindau disease (VHLD) is the most frequent cause of familial renal cancer. It is an autosomal dominant disorder with variable penetrance characterized by retinal angiomas, hemangioblastomas of the central nervous system, pheochromocytomas, epididymal cystadenomas, pancreatic and renal cysts and carcinomas. Renal cell cancer will develop in 45% of these patients, often with

bilateral synchronous or metachronous renal tumors.[27–29] In order to avoid a lifelong need for dialysis or renal transplantation, bilateral nephrectomy can be delayed by close monitoring and carrying out nephron sparing surgery as and when lesions arise.

During surgery, careful inspection of the whole kidney is crucial with removal of any coexistent suspicious lesions. Intraoperative ultrasound is particularly useful in excluding these synchronous lesions. Histopathologically, RCC in these patients is characterized by both solid tumors and renal cysts that contain either frank RCC or a lining of hyperplastic clear cells representing incipient RCC.[13] Several studies now support partial nephrectomy in VHLD.[30–33] In a study of 52 patients with VHLD, Walther et al[34] suggest that in partial nephrectomies for lesions below 3 cm, metastases did not occur during a medium follow up of 5 years.

Steinbach et al[31] reported cancer specific survival rates at 5 and 10 years of 100% and 81%, respectively. However survival free of local recurrence was 71% at 5 years and only 15% at 10 years, with further partial nephrectomy or removal of renal remnant being performed in these cases. It is likely that most of these local recurrences were a manifestation of residual microscopic RCC that was not removed at the original surgery.

Partial nephrectomy can therefore provide effective initial treatment for patients with RCC and VHLD. These patients must however be followed closely with a lifelong protocol, because most will eventually develop locally recurrent RCC with concomitant need for repeat renal surgery.

Preoperative preparation

In general terms, preoperative work-up for partial nephrectomies is the same as for radical nephrectomies. History, physical examination and routine preoperative investigations such as full blood count, cross-match, clotting screen, serum electrolytes, creatinine, serum liver function tests and electrocardiogram are carried out. If the preoperative serum creatinine is abnormal, a measure of the glomerular filtration rate should be obtained. Additional tests include urinalysis or urine dipstick to screen for proteinuria. Radiological tests to rule out locally advanced or metastatic disease include chest X-ray, and abdominal and pelvic CT. Bone scan, chest or head CT are done if considered relevant. MRI has not been shown to be better than CT[35] but can be used in patients in whom CT contrast is contraindicated.

Because partial nephrectomy is technically more difficult than radical nephrectomy, more precise information about the anatomy is desirable preoperatively. Arteriography can be useful to delineate intrarenal vasculature, which can help in tumor excision and minimizing blood loss and injury to surrounding parenchyma. This is particularly helpful if two or more renal arterial segments are involved.

Three-dimensional images of renal vasculature and soft tissue anatomy have much improved preoperative imaging and provide topographic roadmaps for surgery and multiplanar views of intrarenal anatomy.[36,37] This has been confirmed by studies in several centers.[36,38–40] CT reformatting or MRI can accurately delineate the tumor itself and establish its relationship to the pelvicalyceal system and vasculature. Knowledge of vessel anatomy can minimize perioperative blood loss and maximize the chances of a well-perfused remnant. The 3-dimensionally reconstructed images can be viewed during surgery.

This technology is superseding more invasive investigations and therefore limiting the necessity for arteriography, venography and excretion urography.

Operative techniques: open partial nephrectomy

Basic principles of open partial nephrectomy include:

- early vascular control
- minimizing renal ischemia
- complete tumor excision with negative margins
- careful closure of the collecting system
- closure of renal defect.[41]

Several different techniques exist and are described in detail in other publications.[41–43] The most commonly used techniques include polar segmental nephrectomy, wedge resection for peripheral tumors[2,44] and major transverse resection with removal of a healthy margin.[1,2] Simple tumor enucleation risks leaving tumor behind[45,46] if the pseudocapsule is invaded. Central tumors are removed by transparenchymal incision or exploration from renal hilum.[35] Extracorporeal partial nephrectomy with autotransplantation is only

rarely needed in exceptionally large and anatomically challenging cases.[41,47,48]

Transperitoneal and retroperitoneal routes of access vary according to the surgeon's preference or anatomical factors. In the retroperitoneal approach, an incision in the flank through 11th rib can be used to achieve maximal exposure. Gerota's fascia is mobilized and opened, and all perirenal fat except that overlying the tumor is excised. The cortex of the whole kidney is thoroughly inspected to exclude any synchronous lesions not seen on preoperative imaging.

For small peripheral renal tumors it may not be necessary to control the renal artery. In most cases however, partial nephrectomy is most effectively performed after temporary renal artery occlusion. This measure not only limits intraoperative bleeding but by reducing renal tissue turgor, also improves access to intrarenal structures. Temporary occlusion of the renal vein is debatable as there are advantages in leaving it patent. This measure would decrease intraoperative renal ischemia and by allowing venous backbleeding, facilitates hemostasis by enabling identification of small transsected renal veins. These advantages need to be balanced against the obvious benefit of operating in a bloodless field if the renal vein is temporarily occluded. However, temporary occlusion of the renal veins is widely accepted as routine practice with centrally located tumors.[13]

If ischemic time is likely to be longer than 30 min, renal hypothermia is used to protect against postischemic renal injury. Surface cooling with ice slush for 10–15 min to decrease the core temperature to approximately 15–20°C will prolong safe ischemic time to up to 3 hours[49] by reducing oxygen need. Clamping and unclamping the artery should be avoided as this may cause reperfusion injury. Renal injury can be reduced by vigorous pre- and intraoperative hydration, together with mannitol 5–10 min before arterial clamping to reduce intracellular swelling. Mannitol is readministered after unclamping to induce diuresis.[8]

Intraoperative ultrasound can be used to delineate surface markings of completely intrarenal tumor as well as to check for presence of undiscovered multifocal lesions.[8,35,50,51] Resection itself is carried out with a scalpel; although an ultrasonic scalpel, waterjet dissectors, laser beam, microwave tissue coagulator and other tools have been tried, none has shown any advantage over conventional methods. Watertight closure of the collecting system with absorbable suture material is advocated to prevent urinary fistula formation.[8] Stents are placed prophylactically only if major reconstruction is anticipated. Methylene blue may be used to identify entry into the collecting system. It can also be injected directly into the collecting system later to help visualize leaks.[50] Bleeding vessels should be ligated with absorbable sutures when encountered before they retract into parenchyma. Larger vessels are located medially within or near the renal sinus. After venous clamp removal manual hyperventilation increases venous pressure and may reveal additional bleeding points.

Diathermy or lasers can be used, but damage to the collecting system and to sutures should be avoided. An argon beam coagulator may be used giving an additional cautery depth of 2–3 mm for increased safety.[8] Renal remnants can be reconstructed over hemostatic agent (e.g. oxidized cellulose). The effectiveness of fibrin sealants to facilitate hemostasis and closure is being investigated in clinical trials and their application is at this stage largely experimental. Intraoperative frozen section to demonstrate adequacy of resection margins can be considered but is not necessary in all cases.[35,44,51] The kidney can be fixed to psoas to prevent ureteric kinking.[50] A tubed drain is left in the perinephric space before flank closure. It is advisable to keep this in position for at least 7 days due to the usual delayed presentation of ischemic urinary fistulae. Patients can be admitted to a high dependency unit overnight postoperatively for close fluid balance monitoring.

Complications

Comparable rates of morbidity and mortality after partial and radical nephrectomies have been reported, for example in the US National Veterans Administration trial.[52] Table 18.3 shows a summary of reported complications of partial nephrectomies.

Reversible postoperative acute vascular necrosis may occur but should not cause renal failure where a normal contralateral kidney is present.[11] Hemorrhage is the commonest early postoperative complication. Usually hemorrhage occurs from the operated renal bed and is revealed in the drains. Re-exploration often results in nephrectomy and therefore super-selective radiological remobilization may be preferable.[8,11] Delayed formation of

arteriocalyceal fistulae can result in gross hematuria and requires urgent selective embolization.[11] Renal artery thrombosis resulting from renal artery clamping is often not recognized until patient follow up.[53] If recognized early, the patient should be taken back to theater immediately. The rate of postoperative complications is decreasing as more experience and better case selection is achieved.

Results and long-term follow up

Evidence is accumulating from partial nephrectomies on substantial numbers of patients, showing good results for tumors of 4 cm or less.[1,2,8,20,21,35,54,55] The results of the European Organization of Research and Treatment of Cancer (EORTC) trial (protocol 30904) in partnership with North American collaborative groups, are still awaited to determine the outcomes of elective partial versus radical nephrectomy for tumors smaller than 5 cm. Risk of recurrence seems to be related to tumor stage rather than tumor size,[56] grade or histologic pattern.[57]

Debate surrounds the issue of whether or not local recurrence is due to incomplete resection of tumor or undetected multifocality, which is present synchronously or develops later (i.e. metachronously). Local recurrence is more common after imperative surgery as margins tend to be smaller.[11] Multifocality appears to be related to tumor size. Tumors < 4 cm are associated with a multifocal incidence of less than 5%, compared to 15% in tumors of all sizes (Table 5 in Uzzo & Novick[8]). Overall recurrence after partial nephrectomy is reported in 0–10% of cases (Table 4 in Uzzo

Table 18.3 Complications reported* after partial nephrectomy[8]

Complication	Percentage
Deaths	1.6
Urinary fistulae	7.4
Renal impairment	6.3
Dialysis	4.9
Infection/abscess	3.2
Bleeding	2.8
Reoperation	1.9
Spleen injury	0.6

* 1129 patients, reported in nine studies with overall complication rates between 4 and 30%.

& Novick[8]). Risk of recurrence in the remnant is nearly the same as developing secondary clinical renal tumors in the contralateral kidney.[2,58,59]

Renal intraepithelial neoplasia (RIN) may be an explanation for local recurrence but its natural history is unknown.[60] The incidence of local recurrence is lower than might be predicted and it is possible that immunologically mediated spontaneous regression of secondary foci, possibly caused by cytotoxic lymphocytes,[44] is the reason for this.

Follow-up protocol

In properly selected patients, nephron-sparing surgery yields excellent long-term patient survival, free of cancer, particularly for low stage RCC. To date however, there has been no consensus on a standard surveillance protocol following these operations in patients with localized RCC.

The literature reports that surveillance for recurrent malignancy after partial nephrectomy can be tailored according to the initial pathological tumor stage.[13] All patients should be evaluated with medical history, physical examination and selected urine and serum studies at appropriate intervals (Table 18.4). Studies should include serum creatinine measurement and urine dipstick to detect proteinuria. In cases where renal impairment is suspected confirmation with 24-hour creatinine clearance or EDTA (ethylene diamine tetraacetic acid) glomerular filtration rate is recommended. The frequency for radiographic investigations is also stage dependent with little evidence supporting rigorous investigation for early stage disease.

Laparoscopic techniques[61–63]

Clayman et al[64] were the first to report a laparoscopic nephrectomy in 1991. Since then, laparoscopic partial nephrectomies have also gained considerable popularity. Studies have shown that while technically demanding, laparoscopy is a feasible alternative to open resection with comparable follow-up results over up to 35 months.[65–69] Operating time remains longer with laparoscopic surgery, while hospital stay is shorter, less analgesia is necessary and convalescence is faster.[70,71] However long-term data are awaited to determine whether or not the risk of recurrence is higher than with open techniques.

Particular areas of concern are the potential for direct cancer spread during resection, and the risk of hemorrhage and urinary extravasation despite the use of instruments such as an ultrasonic scalpel, argon beam coagulation or surgical glues. Laparoscopic partial nephrectomy is probably most suitable for small superficial, preferably exophytic lesions as other tumors can be difficult to locate even with laparoscopic ultrasound.[72] It should be noted that the technique of cold ischemia has not yet been perfected and most cases reported in the literature employ warm ischemia. However several centers are actively developing the technology to cool kidneys laparoscopically, which will hopefully soon extend the ischemic time available.

Operative procedure

The operative technique is still undergoing refinement at various centres but common features are described as follows: Preoperatively a description of the renal vasculature is obtained by either arteriograpy or 3-dimensional CT. Bowel preparation is usually given. A ureteral catheter is usually placed to enable retrograde infusion of a colored liquid (e.g. methylene blue) to identify breaches of the collecting system. A transperitoneal approach is chosen for central or anterior renal lesions, while peripheral lateral or posterior lesions are best approached retroperitoneally.

Table 18.4 St George's Hospital, London: follow-up protocol* for partial nephrectomies

Pathological tumor stage	History, physical exam, urine dipstick, bloods	Chest X-ray, abdominal CT scan
T1	At 6 months then annual for 5 years	Annual for 3 years and at 5 years
T2 (imperative cases only)	6 monthly for 3 years then annual until year 5	Annual
T3	6 monthly for 3 years then annual	Chest X-ray 6 monthly for 3 years then annual. CT scan annual

* All patients at 6 weeks postop: physical examination, full blood count, creatinine, urine dipstick; alkaline phosphatase if abnormal preop, repeat EDTA glomerular filtration rate prior to 6 month visit.

Three or four laparoscopic ports are used. Intra-operative ultrasound is used to check the position of the lesion and exclude any further lesions. The retroperitoneal space is entered via Petit's triangle and space is created by balloon dilatation. If the transperitoneal approach is used, the colon is mobilized medially. The liver or spleen is mobilized superiorly if necessary. Perirenal fat is removed. The vascular pedicle is isolated by careful hilar dissection. (Various devices are available for temporary vascular occlusion of arterial and venous pedicle vessels.) The tumor is excised with sharp dissection including a 0.5–1 cm margin of normal parenchyma. Hemostasis at the resection site may be achieved with a variety of methods including bipolar electrocautery, harmonic scalpel, argon beam coagulation or gelatin sponge soaked in fibrin glue. The renal bed should be biopsied and sent for frozen section to ensure clear resection margins. The collecting system is repaired with sutures once identified with the retrograde perfusion. A tubed drain is placed. The lesion is removed using a bag and extending one of the port site incisions if necessary.

Laparoscopic partial nephrectomy

In the largest study published to date, Gill et al[69] report the Cleveland Clinic experience of 50 patients undergoing laparoscopic partial nephrectomy since 1999. Mean warm ischemic time was 23 min (range 9–40 min), mean tumor size 3 cm (1.4–7 cm), mean surgical time 3 hours (0.75–5.8 hours) and mean blood loss 270 ml (40–1500 ml). The collecting system was entered in 18 cases (36%) and suture repaired in all cases. All procedures were successfully completed without the need for conversion to open repair. Thirty-four (68%) patients had renal cell cancer. All margins were clear and after a mean follow up of 7 months (range 1–17 months), no patient had local recurrence, portsite disease or metastatic disease. Three major complications (6%) were reported: one intra-operative hemorrhage, one delayed hemorrhage requiring nephrectomy and one urinary leak.

Laparoscopic partial nephrectomy is a relatively novel technique requiring considerable surgical expertise. Small studies have shown excellent outcomes and appear comparable to open partial nephrectomy series. It is likely that refinements in instrumentation facilitating hemostasis and collecting system closure as well as improved techniques

of renal cooling will help promote this minimally invasive technique.

Other types of minimally invasive partial nephrectomy

Many have questioned whether small renal tumors could be managed by means other than extirpative surgery. With the diagnosis of ever smaller incidental renal cell cancers in often high risk or very elderly patients, less invasive forms of tumor ablation are being explored. The goal of any such technique is destruction of the renal lesion with preservation of the normal renal parenchyma. Many of these techniques are being employed in the treatment of other tumors or benign conditions in or outside urology.[73] A common factor to most techniques is that one or more probes is placed directly into the tumor via open surgery, laparoscopy or percutaneously. Monitoring is carried out using ultrasound or magnetic resonance imaging.

All these techniques need much more investigation with improvement in technology before they will be accepted into routine clinical practice for highly selected patients. Techniques will need to be standardized and long-term outcome data obtained.

Cryotherapy

Freezing damages cells irreversibly by disrupting cell membranes and organelles via ice crystal formation. It also disrupts the microvasculature and causes a hyperosmolar insult.[74] This results in coagulative necrosis beyond the boundaries of the lesion.[75] Necrosis is later resorbed and replaced by fibrosis and scarring.

Cryoprobes are inserted directly into the lesion and cooled by liquid nitrogen[73] or by expanding argon-gas[75] according to the Joule Thompson principle to $-180°C$ or $-135°C$ respectively. Renal pedicle clamping is not necessary.[76] Open, laparoscopic or MRI guided percutaneous probe insertion has been reported. A variety of probe sizes (1.5 to 8 mm) have been used, with the smallest producing adequate freezing with least bleeding[76a]. The formation of the ice ball is monitored during the procedure by intra-operative ultrasound although MRI may be used in future for monitoring percutaneous procedures. Ultrasound shows a characteristic hyperechoic advancing crescent with posterior acoustic shadow as the ice ball advances.[77] An ideal rim of death of 1 cm beyond the tumor edge has been described to achieve temperatures in the target tissue of –40°C and 100% cellular death.[78,79] Most investigators advocate repeating the freeze/thaw cycle to ensure adequate cell death although no direct comparison of single versus repeat freeze/thaw cycles in RCC have been published. The rationale is based on evidence for increased cyto-toxicity in prostate and hepato-cellular carcinoma.

In the largest series published so far, Sung et al[79a] describes 50 patients undergoing laparoscopic cryoablation. Posterior and posterolateral tumors were approached retroperitoneally and anterior as well as anterolateral tumors were approached transperitoneally. Significantly the lesions were biopsied to obtain a tissue diagnosis. The cryoprobe was inserted directly via laparoscopy and ultrasound was used to determine the extent of the ice ball. The procedure was well tolerated. Serial follow-up MRIs over 12 months demonstrated progressive resorption of the well-demarcated, non-enhancing cryolesions. Biopsies were performed in 21 patients at a mean follow-up of 11.2 months with no evidence of residual or recurrent disease. However subsequently one patient had a positive biopsy and underwent laparoscopic radical nephrectomy.[73]

Shingleton and Sewell[80] studied percutaneous cryoablation with MRI control on 20 patients with mean diameter lesions of 3 cm. At a mean follow-up of 9.1 months only one patient had evidence of persistent tumor The same authors reported four patients with Von Hippel Lindau disease undergoing the same procedure, with two requiring re-treatment for residual disease.[81] No complications were reported and at follow up of between 2 to 23 months, no evidence of recurrence was evident. Long-term data are required, but this technique may avoid the need for multiple surgical procedures in Von Hippel Lindau patients.

Potential although rare complications reported in human or animal studies[73] include injury to adjacent organs, small bowel obstruction, pelvi-ureteric junction obstruction, potential fistula formation, parenchymal haemorrhage and transient rise in creatinine. There is also a theoretical risk of tumor portsite metastasis, although this has not been reported in any series.

Long-term outcome data and refinement of indications for cryotherapy are necessary before its place in the treatment of renal tumors can be decided. Particularly pathological evidence of tumor ablation is needed to support its efficacy.[68]

Radio frequency ablation (RFA)

Radio frequency ablation works by converting radio frequency (RF) waves into heat, resulting in thermal damage to parenchymal tissue. RF electrodes are introduced percutaneously or laparoscopically under visual or radiological guidance (ultrasound, CT or MRI). Frictional heating occurs and when tissue temperature rises above 70°C, direct cytological destruction occurs.

As RF energy can be applied in different forms, several innovations have been possible to enhance the size of the RF lesion. Originally energy was applied though a "dry" electrode causing rapid increase in temperature, tissue desiccation and charring around the tip of the probe. This increased impedance (tissue resistance to energy flow), limiting the size of the radio lesion. By infusing the tissues with a fluid capable of electrical conduction ("wet" RF), the energy can be spread away from the electrode in a centrifugal manner, thereby preventing the increase in impedance caused by "dry" RF and creating larger lesions in a shorter treatment time.[98–100] Bipolar or monopolar electrodes with multiple hooks and retractable insulating shields allowing for a longer electrode tip have also enabled a larger zone of effect. Temperature based systems monitor the size of the lesion created by thermo couples at the electrode tip allowing a more gradual increase in the current delivered to the tissues. Alternative systems employ impedance based monitoring of lesion size by detecting the increased impedance caused by tissue destruction.

Zlotta et al[86] and Walther et al[87] reported that histological analysis of ablated lesions subsequently removed by nephrectomy showed complete tumor destruction. The same technology has been used during open partial nephrectomy to reduce intraoperative bleeding. By achieving coagulation of the tumor before excision beyond the tumor margins, resection along the coagulation borders with minimal bleeding has been demonstrated.[88]

Numerous studies have reported promising preliminary results with the majority of patients showing no enhancement of lesions on post operative CT or MRI scans.[101–103] Particular efficiency was shown in lesions 3 cm or less.

Probably the most significant concerns are the

findings of positive histology in some of the RFA studies. Some studies have shown radiological enhancement on post operative scans and viable cancer cells were confirmed by histology upon lesion resection.[104-106] However the fact that some animal studies have shown complete tumor ablation indicates that the inconsistency of tumor ablation therefore may not be caused by the failure of the technology itself but rather by the inability to accurately monitor the progression of the RFA lesion in real time. Fine bubbles can be seen on ultrasound within the treated area, but their presence is unreliable.

This technique of renal tumor ablation has demonstrated interesting results. However larger studies with long term clinical and radiographic follow up are required to determine the ultimate role and efficacy of this treatment.

High intensity focused ultrasound (HIFU)

HIFU has previously been demonstrated to ablate tissue thermally with cellular destruction by coagulative necrosis. HIFU is commonly delivered through minimally invasive transrectal or trans-cutaneous probes but to enable tissue ablation in the kidney delivery has been achieved either trans-cutaneously or directly to the kidney. The percu-taneous method has caused skin burns, induration and incomplete tumor necrosis in animal studies. The direct application of HIFU energy to renal tissue has avoided the limitations of the transcuta-neous method, but at the cost of an open surgical approach. A recent study using laparoscopy to deliver direct HIFU energy demonstrated complete tissue necrosis of renal lesions with sharp demarca-tion from adjacent normal tissue in porcine models. It was considered feasible and safe with no signi-ficant alteration of the remaining parenchyma.[93]

Microwave thermotherapy

The application of transurethral microwave therapy (TUMT) in benign prostatic hypertrophy has prompted interest in its use in renal tumor ablation. Probes are inserted directly into the tumor and the tumor cells are destroyed by thermal energy. Rabbit tumor models show that without damaging surrounding organs, this technique can be used to ablate tumors both safely and success-fully.[94] Temperatures of 84°C and 55°C were achieved 5 mm and 1 cm respectively away from the probe, with complete coagulative necrosis.

Microwave thermotherapy can also be used as part of the resection procedure to reduce bleeding, obviating the need for renal artery clamping.[95]

At present this method is experimental and has only been tried in animal models. Significantly more data and clinical trials are required.

Laser interstitial thermal therapy

Another means of delivering thermal energy to the tumor is by placement of laser fibers directly into the mass. This form of treatment has been used in other types of cancer outside urology as well as for benign prostatic hypertrophy.[73] Laser interstitial thermal therapy has been reported on three patients with inoperable renal tumors.[96] A YAG laser placed percutaneously was used with real-time thermal monitoring in the interventional MRI scanner. Tumor sizes up to 4.5 cm appeared amenable to this treatment. The short reported follow up seemed encouraging, but further evaluation will be necessary. This technique should however be considered experimental[73] at this stage owing to the lack of laboratory and clinical data evaluating its efficacy.

Interstitial photon radiation ablation

Interstitial photon radiation ablation has been shown to be safe and feasible on a canine model.[97] Probe placement directly into kidney induced 2.5 cm lesions. Histopathology confirmed coagu-lative necrosis and on serial follow-up CT scans the lesions decreased in size at 3 and 6 months. Peri-operative monitoring of the extent of treatment seems to be difficult, in that treatment requires to be achieved by careful adjustment of treatment time and dosage. This form of radiation therapy has been successfully used in the treatment of other tumors and further studies may show it to be useful in the management of renal cell carcinoma.[73]

Conclusion

While EORTC data are awaited for elective indications of partial nephrectomies, existing data support such surgery for tumors of 4 cm or less. With conscientious follow up and good patient cooperation, conserving nephrons can only be beneficial in the long run.

Further improvements in and more widespread use of 3-dimensional contrast-enhanced imaging preoperatively to visualize renal vasculature, parenchyma and collecting system will make planning and surgery more precise. In future more minimally invasive forms of this surgery may well prevail. This will include laparoscopy, energy-based ablation therapies as well as the possibility of operative robotics. Of these, laparoscopy is already in regular use but long-term follow-up data are awaited before it can become the operation of choice.

References

1. Russo P. Renal cell carcinoma: presentation, staging, and surgical treatment. Semin Oncol 2000; 27(2):160–176.
2. Filipas D, Fichtner J, Spix C, et al. Nephron-sparing surgery of renal cell carcinoma with a normal opposite kidney: long-term outcome in 180 patients. Urology 2000; 56(3):387–392.
3. Herczel E. Ueber Nierenextirpation. Beitr Klin Chir 1890; 6:485.
4. Vermooten V. Indications for conservative surgery in certain renal tumours: a study based on the growth patterns of renal cell carcinoma. J Urol 1950; 64:200.
5. Robson CJ, Churchill BM, Anderson W. The results of radical nephrectomy for renal cell carcinoma. J Urol 1969; 163(suppl):157.
6. Jacobs SC, Berg SI, Lawson RK. Synchronous bilateral renal cell carcinoma: total surgical excision. Cancer 1980; 46:2341.
7. Clark PE, Schover LR, Uzzo RG, et al. Quality of life and psychological adaptation after surgical treatment for localized renal cell carcinoma: impact of the amount of remaining renal tissue. Urology 2001; 57(2):252–256.
8. Uzzo RG, Novick AC. Nephron sparing surgery for renal tumors: indications, techniques and outcomes. J Urol 2001; 166(1):6–18.
9. Shekarriz B, Upadhyay J, Shekarriz H, et al. Comparison of costs and complications of radical and partial nephrectomy for treatment of localized renal cell carcinoma. Urology 2002; 59(2):211–215.
10. Bosniak MA. The use of the Bosniak classification system for renal cysts and cystic tumors. J Urol 1997; 157(5):1852–1853.
11. Van Poppel H, Dilen K, Baert L. Incidental renal cell carcinoma and nephron sparing surgery. Curr Opin Urol 2001; 11(3):281–286.
12. Hafez KS, Fergany AF, Novick AC. Nephron sparing surgery for localized renal cell carcinoma: impact of tumor size on patient survival, tumor recurrence and TNM staging. J Urol 1999; 162(6):1930–1933.
13. Novik AC. Radical nephrectomy and nephron-sparing surgery for localized renal cell carcinoma. In: Bukowski RM, Novick A, eds. Renal cell carcinoma. Molecular biology, immunology and clinical management. Totowa, New Jersey: Humana Press; 2000:163–172.
14. Fergany AF, Hafez KS, Novick AC. Long-term results of nephron sparing surgery for localized renal cell carcinoma: 10-year follow up. J Urol 2000; 163(2):442–445.
15. Marberger M, Pugh RC, Auvent J, et al. Conservative surgery for renal cell carcinoma: the EIRSS experience. Br J Urol 1981; 53:528.
16. Morgan WR, Zincke H. Progression and survival after renal-conserving surgery for renal cell carcinoma: experience in 104 patients and extended follow-up. J Urol 1990; 144:852.
17. Steinbach F, Stockle M, Muller SC, et al. Conservative surgery of renal cell tumors in 140 patients: 21 years of experience. J Urol 1992; 148(1):24–29.
18. Moll V, Becht E, Ziegler M. Kidney preserving surgery in renal cell tumors: indications, techniques and results in 152 patients. J Urol 1993; 150(2 Pt 1):319–323.
19. Van Poppel H, Bamelis B, Oyen R, et al. Partial nephrectomy for renal cell carcinoma can achieve long-term tumour control. J Urol 1998; 160:674.
20. Belldegrun A, Tsui KH, Dekernion JB, Smith RB. Efficacy of nephron-sparing surgery for renal cell carcinoma: analysis based on the new 1997 tumor-node-metastasis staging system. J Clin Oncol 1999; 17(9):2868–2875.
21. Lee CT, Katz J, Shi W, et al. Surgical management of renal tumors 4 cm or less in a contemporary cohort. J Urol 2000; 163(3):730–736.
22. Lau WK, Blute ML, Weaver AL, et al. Matched comparison of radical nephrectomy vs nephron-sparing surgery in patients with unilateral renal cell carcinoma and a normal contralateral kidney. Mayo Clin Proc 2000; 75(12):1236–1242.
23. Petritsch PH, Rauchenwald M, Zechner O, et al. Results after organ-preserving surgery for renal cell carcinoma. An Austrian multicenter study. Eur Urol 1990; 18(2):84–87.
24. Provet J, Tessler A, Brown J, et al. Partial nephrectomy for renal cell carcinoma: indications, results and implications. J Urol 1991; 145(3):472–476.
25. Butler BP, Novick AC, Miller DP, et al. Management of small unilateral renal cell carcinomas: radical versus nephron-sparing surgery. Urology 1995; 45(1):34–40.
26. Lerner SE, Hawkins CA, Blute ML, et al. Disease outcome in patients with low stage renal cell carcinoma treated with nephron sparing or radical surgery. J Urol 1996; 155(6):1868–1873.
27. Richards RD, Mebust WK, Schimke RN. A prospective study on Von Hippel–Lindau disease. J Urol 1973; 110(1):27–30.
28. Horton WA, Wong V, Eldridge R. Von Hippel–Lindau disease: clinical and pathological manifestations in nine families with 50 affected members. Arch Intern Med 1976; 136(7):769–777.
29. Loughlin KR, Gittes RF. Urological management of patients with von Hippel–Lindau's disease. J Urol 1986; 136(4):789–791.
30. Novick AC, Streem SB. Long-term followup after nephron sparing surgery for renal cell carcinoma in von Hippel–Lindau disease. J Urol 1992; 147(6):1488–1490.
31. Steinbach F, Novick AC, Zincke H, et al. Treatment of renal cell carcinoma in von Hippel–Lindau disease: a multicenter study. J Urol 1995; 153(6):1812–1816.
32. Walther MM, Choyke PL, Weiss G, et al. Parenchymal sparing surgery in patients with hereditary renal cell carcinoma. J Urol 1995; 153(3 Pt 2):913–916.
33. Persad RA, Probert JL, Sharma SD, Haq A, Doyle PT. Surgical management of the renal manifestations of von Hippel–Lindau disease: a review of a United Kingdom case series. Br J Urol 1997; 80(3):392–396.
34. Walther MM, Choyke PL, Glenn G, et al. Renal cancer in families with hereditary renal cancer: prospective

analysis of a tumor size threshold for renal parenchymal sparing surgery. J Urol 1999; 161(5):1475–1479.

35. Black P, Filipas D, Fichtner J, et al. Nephron sparing surgery for central renal tumors: experience with 33 cases. J Urol 2000; 163(3):737–743.

36. Wyatt SH, Urban BA, Fishman EK. Spiral CT of the kidneys: role in characterization of renal disease. Part II: Neoplastic disease. Crit Rev Diagn Imaging 1995; 36(1):39–72.

37. Smith PA, Marshall FF, Fishman EK. Spiral computed tomography evaluation of the kidneys: state of the art. Urology 1998; 51(1):3–11.

38. Coll DM, Uzzo RG, Herts BR, et al. 3-dimensional volume rendered computerized tomography for preoperative evaluation and intraoperative treatment of patients undergoing nephron sparing surgery. J Urol 1999; 161(4):1097–1102.

39. Chernoff DM, Silverman SG, Kikinis R, et al. Three-dimensional imaging and display of renal tumors using spiral CT: a potential aid to partial nephrectomy. Urology 1994; 43(1):125–129.

40. Uzzo RG, Novick AC. Von Hippel–Lindau disease: clinical and molecular considerations for the urologist. AUA Update Series 1999; 18:137.

41. Novick AC. Partial nephrectomy for renal cell carcinoma. Urol Clin North Am 1987; 14(2):419–433.

42. Polascik TJ, Pound CR, Meng MV, et al. Partial nephrectomy: technique, complications and pathological findings. J Urol 1995; 154(4):1312–1318.

43. Campbell SC, Novick AC. Surgical technique and morbidity of elective partial nephrectomy. Semin Urol Oncol 1995; 13(4):281–287.

44. Van Poppel H. Nephron sparing surgery in renal cell carcinoma. Braz J Urol 2000; 26:342–353.

45. Novick AC, Zincke H, Neves RJ, Topley HM. Surgical enucleation for renal cell carcinoma. J Urol 1986; 135(2):235–238.

46. Marshall FF, Taxy JB, Fishman EK, Chang R. The feasibility of surgical enucleation for renal cell carcinoma. J Urol 1986; 135(2):231–234.

47. Wickham JE. Conservative renal surgery for adenocarcinoma. The place of bench surgery. Br J Urol 1975; 47(1):25–36.

48. Calne RY. Treatment of bilateral hypernephromas by nephrectomy, excision of tumour, and autotransplantation. Report of three cases. Lancet 1973; 2(7839):1164–1167.

49. Novick AC. Renal hypothermia: in vivo and ex vivo. Urol Clin North Am 1983; 10(4):637–644.

50. Chan DY, Marshall FF. Partial nephrectomy for centrally located tumors. Urology 1999; 54(6):1088–1091.

51. Grasso M, Salonia A, Lania C, et al. Conservative surgery in small renal tumors: our experience. Arch Esp Urol 1999; 52(10):1102–1107.

52. Corman JM, Penson DF, Hur K, et al. Comparison of complications after radical and partial nephrectomy: results from the National Veterans Administration Surgical Quality Improvement Program. BJU Int 2000; 86(7):782–789.

53. Inoue Y, Ohtake T, Kameyama S, et al. Increased renal retention of 99mTc-methylene diphosphonate after nephron-sparing surgery. J Nucl Med 1999; 40(3):418–421.

54. Barbalias GA, Liatsikos EN, Tsintavis A, Nikiforidis G.

55. Bilen CY, Mahalati K, Ozen H, et al. Multicentricity in renal cell carcinoma. Int Urol Nephrol 1999; 31(3):295–299.

56. Miller J, Fischer C, Freese R, et al. Nephron-sparing surgery for renal cell carcinoma – is tumor size a suitable parameter for indication? Urology 1999; 54(6):988–993.

57. Baltaci S, Orhan D, Soyupek S, et al. Influence of tumor stage, size, grade, vascular involvement, histological cell type and histological pattern on multifocality of renal cell carcinoma. J Urol 2000; 164(1):36–39.

58. Kinouchi T, Mano M, Saiki S, et al. Incidence rate of satellite tumors in renal cell carcinoma. Cancer 1999; 86(11):2331–2336.

59. Schlichter A, Wunderlich H, Junker K, et al. Where are the limits of elective nephron-sparing surgery in renal cell carcinoma? Eur Urol 2000; 37(5):517–520.

60. Van Poppel H, Nilsson S, Algaba F, et al. Precancerous lesions in the kidney. Scand J Urol Nephrol 2000; 205(suppl):136–165.

61. Kozlowski PM, Winfield HN. Laparoscopic partial nephrectomy and wedge resection for the treatment of renal malignancy. J Endourol 2001; 15(4):369–374.

62. Janetschek G, Jeschke K, Peschel R, et al. Laparoscopic surgery for stage T1 renal cell carcinoma: radical nephrectomy and wedge resection. Eur Urol 2000; 38(2):131–138.

63. van Ophoven A, Tsui KH, Shvarts O, et al. Current status of partial nephrectomy in the management of kidney cancer. Cancer Control 1999; 6(6):560–570.

64. Clayman RV, Kavoussi LR, Soper NJ, et al. Laparoscopic nephrectomy: initial case report. J Urol 1991; 146(2):278–282.

65. Janetschek G, Daffner P, Peschel R, Bartsch G. Laparoscopic nephron sparing surgery for small renal cell carcinoma. J Urol 1998; 159(4):1152–1155.

66. Hoznek A, Salomon L, Antiphon P, et al. Partial nephrectomy with retroperitoneal laparoscopy. J Urol 1999; 162(6):1922–1926.

67. Winfield HN, Donovan JF, Lund GO, et al. Laparoscopic partial nephrectomy: initial experience and comparison to the open surgical approach. J Urol 1995; 153(5):1409–1414.

68. McDougall EM, Elbahnasy AM, Clayman RV. Laparoscopic wedge resection and partial nephrectomy – the Washington University experience and review of the literature. JSLS 1998; 2(1):15–23.

69. Gill IS, Desai MM, Kaouk JH, et al. Laparoscopic partial nephrectomy for renal tumor: duplicating open surgical techniques. J Urol 2002; 167(2 Pt 1):469–474; discussion 475–476.

70. Novick AC. Nephron-sparing surgery for renal cell carcinoma. Br J Urol 1998; 82(3):321–324.

71. Herr HW. Partial nephrectomy for unilateral renal carcinoma and a normal contralateral kidney: 10-year followup. J Urol 1999; 161(1):33–34.

72. Schulam PG, Dekernion JB. Laparoscopic nephrectomy for renal-cell carcinoma: the current situation. J Endourol 2002; 15(4):375–376.

73. Murphy DP, Gill IS. Energy-based renal tumor ablation: a review. Semin Urol Oncol 2001; 19(2):133–140.

74. Breining H, Helpap B, Minderjahn A, Lymberopoulos

S. Histological and autoradiographic findings in cryonecrosis of the liver and kidney. Cryobiology 1974; 11(6):519–525.

75. Edmunds TB Jr, Schulsinger DA, Durand DB, Waltzer WC. Acute histologic changes in human renal tumors after cryoablation. J Endourol 2000; 14(2):139–143.

76. Campbell SC, Krishnamurthi V, Chow G, et al. Renal cryosurgery: experimental evaluation of treatment parameters. Urology 1998; 52(1):29–33.

76a. Pantuck AJ, Zisman A, Cohen J, et al. Cryosurgical ablation of renal tumors using 1.5-millimeter, ultrathin cryoprobes. Urology. 2002; 59:130–133.

77. Onik GM, Reyes G, Cohen JK, Porterfield B. Ultrasound characteristics of renal cryosurgery. Urology 1993; 42(2):212–215.

78. Chosy SG, Nakada SY, Lee FT Jr, Warner TF. Monitoring renal cryosurgery: predictors of tissue necrosis in swine. J Urol 1998; 159(4):1370–1374.

79. Gill IS, Novick AC, Meraney AM, et al. Laparoscopic renal cryoablation in 32 patients. Urology 2000; 56(5):748–753.

79a. Sung G, Meraney AM, Schweizer DK, et al. Laparoscopic renal cryoablation in 50 patients: immediate follow-up. J Urol. 2001; 165:158.

80. Shingleton WB, Sewell PE Jr. Percutaneous renal tumor cryoablation with magnetic resonance imaging guidance. J Urol 2001; 165(3):773–776.

81. Shingleton WB, Sewell PE Jr. Percutaneous renal cryoablation of renal tumors in patients with von Hippel–Lindau disease. J Urol 2002; 167(3):1268–1270.

82. Zlotta AR, Raviv G, Peny MO, et al. Possible mechanisms of action of transurethral needle ablation of the prostate on benign prostatic hyperplasia symptoms: a neurohistochemical study. J Urol 1997; 157(3):894–899.

83. Schulman CC, Zlotta AR. Transurethral needle ablation of the prostate (TUNA). A new treatment of benign prostatic hyperplasia using interstitial radiofrequency energy. J Urol (Paris) 1995; 101(1):33–36.

84. Siperstein AE, Rogers SJ, Hansen PD, Gitomirsky A. Laparoscopic thermal ablation of hepatic neuroendocrine tumor metastases. Surgery 1997; 122(6):1147–1154.

85. Hall WH, McGahan JP, Link DP, deVere White RW. Combined embolization and percutaneous radiofrequency ablation of a solid renal tumor. AJR Am J Roentgenol 2000; 174(6):1592–1594.

86. Zlotta AR, Wildschutz T, Raviv G, et al. Radiofrequency interstitial tumor ablation (RITA) is a possible new modality for treatment of renal cancer: ex vivo and in vivo experience. J Endourol 1997; 11(4):251–258.

87. Walther MC, Shawker TH, Libutti SK, et al. A phase 2 study of radio frequency interstitial tissue ablation of localized renal tumors. J Urol 2000; 163(5):1424–1427.

88. Gettman MT, Bishoff JT, Su LM, et al. Hemostatic laparoscopic partial nephrectomy: initial experience with the radiofrequency coagulation-assisted technique. Urology 2001; 58(1):8–11.

89. Li-Ming S, Jarrett TW, Kavoussi LR, Solomon SB. Percutaneous CT-guided radiofrequency ablation of small renal masses in poor surgical risk patients: preliminary resuts. J Urol 2002; 167(4 suppl):1 [5-25-2002; abstract]

90. Polascik TJ, Hamper U, Lee BR, et al. Ablation of renal tumors in a rabbit model with interstitial saline-augmented radiofrequency energy: preliminary report of a new technology. Urology 1999; 53(3):465–472.

91. Zlotta AR, Schulman CC. Ablation of renal tumors in a rabbit model with interstitial saline-augmented radiofrequency energy. Urology 1999; 54(2):382–383.

92. Rendon RA, Kachura JR, Sweet JM, et al. The uncertainty of radio frequency treatment of renal cell carcinoma: findings at immediate and delayed nephrectomy. J Urol 2002; 167(4):1587–1592.

93. Paterson RF, Shalhav AL, Lingeman JE, et al. AUA 2000 Abstract No. 8. J Urol 2002; 167(4 suppl):2 [5-25-2002; abstract]

94. Kigure T, Harada T, Yuri Y, et al. Laparoscopic microwave thermotherapy on small renal tumors: experimental studies using implanted VX-2 tumors in rabbits. Eur Urol 1996; 30(3):377–382.

95. Naito S, Nakashima M, Kimoto Y, et al. Application of microwave tissue coagulator in partial nephrectomy for renal cell carcinoma. J Urol 1998; 159(3):960–962.

96. de Jode MG, Vale JA, Gedroyc WM. MR-guided laser thermoablation of inoperable renal tumors in an open-configuration interventional MR scanner: preliminary clinical experience in three cases. J Magn Reson Imaging 1999; 10(4):545–549.

97. Chan DY, Koniaris L, Magee C, et al. Feasibility of ablating normal renal parenchyma by interstitial photon radiation energy: study in a canine model. J Endourol 2000; 14(2):111–116.

98. Calkins H, Langberg J, Sousa J, et al. Radiofrequency catheter ablation of accessory atrioventricular connections in 250 patients. Abbreviated therapeutic approach to Wolff- Parkinson-White syndrome. Circulation. 1992 ;85:1337–1346.

99. Hoey MF, Mulier PM, Leveille RJ, et al. Transurethral prostate ablation with saline electrode allows controlled production of larger lesions than conventional methods. J Endourol. 1997; 11:279–284.

100. Leveille RJ, Hoey MF, Hulbert JC, et al. Enhanced radiofrequency ablation of canine prostate utilizing a liquid conductor: the virtual electrode. J Endourol. 1996; 10:5–11.

101. Gervais DA, McGovern FJ, Wood BJ, et al. Radio-frequency ablation of renal cell carcinoma: early clinical experience. Radiology. 2000; 217:665–672.

102. de Baere T, Kuoch V, Smayra T, et al. Radio frequency ablation of renal cell carcinoma: preliminary clinical experience. J Urol. 2002; 167:1961–1964.

103. Li-Ming S, Jarrett TW, Kavoussi LR, Solomon SB. Percutaneous CT-guided radiofrequency ablation of small renal masses in poor surgical risk patients: preliminary resuts. J Urol.suppl. 2002; 167:1.

104. Pavlovich CP, Walther MM, Choyke PL, et al. Percutaneous radio frequency ablation of small renal tumors: initial results. J Urol. 2002; 167:10–15.

105. Rendon RA, Kachura JR, Sweet JM, et al. The uncertainty of radio frequency treatment of renal cell carcinoma: findings at immediate and delayed nephrectomy. J Urol. 2002; 167:1587–1592.

106. Michaels MJ, Silverman M, Libertino JA, Burlington MA. Absence of total tumor necrosis in radiofrequency ablated renal tumors. J Urol.suppl. 2003; 165:21.

19

Urethral stricture surgery: the state of the art

Daniela E Andrich and Anthony R Mundy

Introduction

Urethral strictures are very common. From Hospital Episode Statistics in the United States and in the UK they affect males with an increasing incidence from about one in every 10 000 males aged 25 to about one in every 1000 males aged 65 or more. Traditionally strictures were associated with gonococcal urethritis and with external urethral trauma. In the UK nowdays they are more commonly associated with iatrogenic injury or are otherwise idiopathic. Gonococcal urethritis is now very much less common, although external trauma is more common than it was. Other causes include hypospadias surgery (included in Table 19.1 under iatrogenic) and lichen sclerosus (balanitis xerotica obliterans, BXO) (included in Table 19.1 under inflammatory), both of which are increasingly common.

Urethral dilation has been used for the treatment of urethral strictures for literally thousands of years. By comparison, internal urethrotomy has a comparatively short history of 150 years. The history of open urethroplasty is short indeed, having only been used with any regularity for some 50 years.

This chapter will review current diagnosis and treatment and close with a view as to how the future may develop.

Pathology

The pathology of (non-traumatic) urethral stricture disease has not been widely studied and not for many years. The best explanation was proposed by Chambers and Baitera.[1] They showed, in a series of autopsy studies, that the first change in urethral stricture disease is a change in the urethral epithelium from a pseudostratified columnar epithelium, which is relatively flexible and waterproof, to a squamous epithelium which is less flexible and less waterproof. These two characteristics are important because whereas most epithelia are supported by either a lamina propria or a muscle layer which is substantial, the urethral epithelium lies more or less directly on the spongy tissue of the corpus spongiosum. A less flexible and waterproofing squamous epithelium, poorly supported, is more than usually prone to microscopic tears or ulcers during distension on voiding. These heal with the formation of microscopic plaques which eventually, with increasing number, coalesce to form a stricture. This leads to obstruction which then causes even more distension proximal to the original stricture which extends the pathological problem and therefore the stricture more proximally.

Presentation

Symptoms and signs
The usual presenting symptom is a weak stream and usually there are no physical signs to accompany this in the developed world. Where medical care is less freely available or has not been sought patients may present with very severe voiding

Table 19.1 Etiology of urethral strictures (personal series)

Urethral stricture	Percentage
Congenital	22
Traumatic	
External	29
Iatrogenic	14
Inflammatory	16
Idiopathic	19

difficulty and sometimes with gross hematuria as a consequence of straining to void.[2] Because recurrent urinary tract infection is a frequent complication of obstructed voiding such patients may also have chronic epididymo-orchitis and palpable fibrosis affecting the genital tract.[3] Frank acute retention is uncommon but may occur.

Despite the incidence noted above, most patients with urethral strictures present in their 30s and 40s rather than later but there is some overlap with the 'prostate' age group, thereby confusing the underlying etiology.

Investigation

The first line of outpatient investigation is a urinary flow rate study to look at peak flow and flow pattern, a midstream specimen of urine to look for complicating urinary tract infection and an ultrasound scan to look for a thick walled, poorly emptying bladder or upper tract changes. The mainstays of definitive diagnosis are radiological and endoscopic.

Radiological evaluation

Radiological evaluation should include an ascending urethrogram and micturating cystogram performed together. The ascending urethrogram should be performed in the lateral position with the penis under stretch to observe the full length of the urethra. Unless contrast has been shown to fill all parts of the urethra and the bladder it cannot be regarded as adequate.[4] With a tight stricture it may be difficult to fill the urethra proximal to a stricture and it is for this reason that a micturating cystogram to show the proximal urinary tract during voiding is useful.

Endoscopic evaluation

Endoscopic evaluation may be helpful, although it may only be possible to view the urinary tract downstream of the stricture. In those with an indwelling suprapubic catheter, flexible cystoscopy through the suprapubic catheter tract may be possible and in many instances is valuable in assessing the length of the stricture and the state of the urethra upstream of the stricture.

Treatment

Although it has long been recognized that dilation and urethrotomy are rarely curative it was not until recently that there was objective evidence to support this assertion. In recent years there have been several good studies, particularly from Rome[5] and Cape Town[6,7] to show that this is so. It is also now clear that urethrotomy and dilation are equally effective in most circumstances. It is also clear that the only strictures that respond to either technique are first time strictures, never previously treated, and generally short sharp strictures of the bulbar urethra. If a procedure has to be repeated then it will have to be repeated, albeit in some instances only occasionally, for the rest of the patient's life. Generally speaking, the time to recurrence is less than 1 year. Strictures of the penile urethra rarely respond to either modality.

Most instances of urethrotomy or dilation are palliative rather than curative. There is nothing wrong with palliation, of course, as long as both patient and surgeon realize that this is the case.

Alternatives to instrumentation

There is a common belief that if a surgical instrument costs £60 000 then it must be 60 000 times more effective than an instrument that costs £1. Thus the feeling is that laser urethrotomy must be effective when cold knife urethrotomy (or dilation) have failed. This is not so. Laser urethrotomy is no more effective than visual internal urethrotomy.

Clean intermittent self-catheterization has been advocated by some[8] and indeed is widely used, following urethrotomy. Thus instead of the patient having repeated instrumentation under some form of anesthesia by a doctor, the patient simply dilates the stricture himself (or holds it open), without anesthesia, with a catheter. This is undoubtedly a way of reducing hospital attendance but it is no more a cure of urethral stricture than urethrotomy or dilation performed by a doctor.

A range of urethral stents of varying materials and varying complexity (and varying cost) have been described as an alternative way of holding the urethra open after a visual internal urethrotomy.[9–11] The best known is the Urolume®. This has been used for recurrent bulbar strictures and has proved to be useful in some (generally elderly) patients in whom urethroplasty would be unnecessarily invasive. Younger patients however frequently complain about pooling of urine causing postmicturition dribble and pooling of seminal fluid causing reduced ejaculation.[12] It can also be uncomfortable, particularly in those who ride bicycles. Most surgeons who have ever had to take one out have never put another one in and so the role of stents appears to be restricted simply to the elderly.

Thus for most patients the only realistic alternative to urethrotomy or dilation is urethroplasty. Urethroplasty may be positively indicated as the first line of treatment when there has been urethral disruption and it is simply not possible to perform urethrotomy or dilation. It may be the treatment of choice for a short stricture with spongiofibrosis that looks unlikely to respond to urethrotomy. In most patients however it is the second line of treatment after one instrumentation has failed and when the patient prefers cure by urethroplasty rather than palliation by continuing urethral dilation or clean intermittent self-catheterization.

General principles of urethroplasty

Anastomotic versus substitution urethroplasty

There are essentially two forms of urethroplasty: anastomotic, in which the urethral stricture is excised, the two ends are spatulated and end-to-end anastomosis is performed; and substitution urethroplasty, in which the urethra is reconstructed using some non-urethral material. Both can be very successful. However, as a matter of general principle, excision and end-to-end anastomosis gives a better cure rate and one that is sustained in the long term; it also carries a lower complication rate than substitution (Tables 19.2 and 19.3).[13] Substitution urethroplasty gives almost as good results in the first year or two after surgery but by 5 and 10 years it is clear that there is a steady deterioration with time.

Tables 19.2 and 19.3 report historical data in patients followed up for more than 15 years and there is no doubt that with modern operative techniques (particularly utilizing the whole range of modern techniques that are currently available for substitution urethroplasty) the long-term results are better. Nonetheless, there is the same picture of deterioration with time, for two possible reasons: first because any material other than urethra is not inherently as good as urethra, and secondly because in substitution urethroplasty it appears

Table 19.2 Re-stricture rates after urethroplasty

| Procedure | Length of follow up | | | |
	1 year (%)	5 years (%)	10 years (%)	15 years (%)
Anastomotic urethroplasty	7	12	13	14
Substitution urethroplasty	12	21	30	42

Table 19.3 Complications after urethroplasty

Complication	Anastomotic urethroplasty (%)	Substitution urethroplasty (%)
Urgency*	66	–
Stress incontinence*	37	–
Impotence		
Temporary*	26	10
Permanent	7	2
Palpable/visible pouch	–	12
Postmicturition dribble	–	28
Urinary tract dribble	–	5
Chordee	–	3
Urethrocutaneous fistula	–	3
Total	7	33**

*Complications of the underlying trauma (in the case of anastomotic urethroplasty) or which are only temporary. ** There are a total of 53 complications in 33 patients because some patients had more than one complication.

that the whole urethra is disease prone (possibly for the reasons given above – see Pathology) whereas in anastomotic urethroplasty the urethra is frequently normal up until the episode of (usually) trauma which caused the problem.

Anastomotic urethroplasty

An anastomotic urethroplasty is performed when there is a traumatic defect of the bulbar urethra following a straddle or fall-astride injury, or of the posterior (often called membranous) urethra after a pelvic fracture injury. It can also be used for a short, that is to say less than 2 cm (and preferably less than 1 cm) stricture of the bulbar urethra.[14] It can be used in the bulbar urethra because there is elasticity in this structure that allows the procedure to be performed without compromising erections. Excision and end-to-end anastomosis cannot be performed in the penile urethra without compromising erection and therefore should not be performed at all. Thus the limitations on anastomotic urethroplasty are that it is confined to the bulbar urethra or more proximally and that it can only be used in the bulbar urethra for relatively short strictures. Unfortunately most strictures are longer than excision and end-to-end anastomosis will allow.

Substitution urethroplasty

Substitution urethroplasty could, in theory, be used anywhere but it should be confined to those areas where an anastomotic urethroplasty is not possible. Certainly to use a substitution rather than an anastomotic repair for a pelvic fracture urethral distraction defect or for a fall-astride injury where the urethral lumen has been completely disrupted or obliterated would substantially increase the likelihood of long-term problems, particularly of recurrent stricture.[15]

Clearly there are two possible approaches to substitution urethroplasty for a long stricture: the diseased segment could be excised and replaced with a tube or the strictured segment could be opened and a patch put on to hold it open. Unfortunately tube grafts (or flaps – see below for the difference) have three times the re-stricture rate in the long-term than a stricturotomy and patch procedure and so the latter is to be preferred unless the urethral wall positively should be excised.[16] If this is the case the best practice is to

excise and put in a patch between the two ends of the urethra at the first stage, leaving the patient voiding through a proximal urethrostomy in the interim, and then to roll the patch into a tube at a second stage when the re-stricture rate is no more than with a one-stage stricturotomy and patch.[16] Indications for excision of the urethra and a two-stage circumferential repair include previous surgery for hypospadias where the urethral remnant is severely compromised, lichen sclerosus (BXO)[17] and rarities such as arteriovenous malformations and tumors.

Grafts and flaps

Having decided that most urethral stricture problems are best treated by stricturotomy and patch the next question is: what should be used for the patch? There are two main types of material – grafts and flaps.[18] A graft is a free transfer of tissue without an attached blood supply. A flap is a transfer of tissue with its blood supply attached. Typically, for urethroplasty, local genital skin flaps are used and penile skin in particular. Scrotal skin flaps may be valuable but as a general rule are more prone to problems than flaps of penile shaft skin, away from the hair-bearing area. Materials for grafts include genital skin, the skin from behind the ear (the post-auricular Wolfe graft, PAWG) and buccal mucosal grafts (BMG), all of which are satisfactory because they have a dense subdermal vascular plexus which means that 'take' is good.[19] Skin from other areas of the body has a poor subdermal plexus and so take is poor.

Grafts and flaps are equally good for most circumstances.[20] Flaps are positively indicated when there is infection, ischemia or after previous surgery. They have the disadvantage that they are tedious and time consuming to raise for strictures of the bulbar urethra. Grafts are quick to raise and are perfectly applicable to most stricture circumstances and so are preferred by most reconstructive surgeons for routine stricture repair in the bulbar urethra.[21] In the penile urethra a flap is preferred for a simple stricture because it is quicker and easier to raise. Thus for routine stricturotomy and patch procedures of the bulbar urethra a graft should be used. For complicated cases a flap should be used and in rare circumstances where excision of the urethra is indicated – usually only to excise a Urolume® stent and replace the urethra – a two-stage reconstruction is preferred. In the penile urethra simple strictures should be repaired by a (Orandi) flap technique.[22] Complex strictures, usually due to previous hypospadias surgery or BXO, are best repaired by urethral excision and a two-stage circumferential repair.

Finally, having decided that a stricturotomy and patch using a free graft is preferable for most strictures, where should the stricturotomy be made and the patch put? Traditionally the patch was placed ventrally but this was associated with a relatively high incidence of outpouching of the patch due to lack of support causing pooling of urine, irritative symptoms and even frank recurrent urinary infection.[23] By placing the stricturotomy and subsequent patch dorsally, support is provided by the tunica albuginea of the penis. In this way outpouching does not occur, although postmicturition dribbling can still be a problem (Fig. 19.1).[21] Furthermore the re-stricture rate of ventrally placed grafts is three times higher than with dorsally placed grafts,[21] thus making dorsal stricturotomy and patch the treatment of choice.

A summary of the general principles of urethroplasty is provided in Table 19.4.

Strictures by site and type

Traditionally the urethra is subdivided into the posterior urethra surrounded by the sphincter mechanisms and the anterior urethra surrounded by the corpus spongiosum. These can be further subdivided as described below.

Posterior urethral strictures

These include strictures of the bladder neck, the prostatic urethra and the membranous urethra. Bladder neck strictures typically follow transurethral resection of the prostate when a bladder neck incision would have been more appropriate. These are best treated by a bladder neck incision which is usually curative. Strictures of the bladder neck following radical prostatectomy are usually far more complicated. They may be considered in three categories: those without associated urinary incontinence; those with associated urinary incontinence; and those with distraction. Those without incontinence may be treated by instrumentation, repeated if necessary.[25] Those with incontinence and those with distraction will almost certainly require further surgery. This may be endoscopic to deal with the stricture and then implantation of an artificial urinary sphincter to produce continence; or may involve a re-anastomosis of the urethra to the bladder neck, with or without implantation of an artificial sphincter, in those with distraction.

Prostatic urethral strictures occasionally follow retropubic prostatectomy or a transurethral resection for benign prostatic hyperplasia (BPH) when the postoperative course is complicated by infection. More commonly they follow 'new technology' treatment for BPH such as brachytherapy, cryotherapy and laser therapy.[26] Fortunately they are uncommon. Treatment generally involves either endoscopy or total prostatectomy and vesicourethral anastomosis if that fails.[27]

Membranous urethral strictures can be subdivided into sphincter strictures following prosta-

Table 19.4 Summary of the general principles of urethroplasty

1. Urethral dilation and visual internal urethrotomy are equally effective.
2. 50% of short bulbar strictures are cured by the very first dilation or urethrotomy.
3. Penile urethral strictures are rarely cured by dilation or urethrotomy.
4. If a patient develops a recurrent stricture after a previous urethrotomy and dilation however long the interval, further instrumentation is never curative.
5. The only curative alternative is urethroplasty.
6. Whenever a urethroplasty is indicated an anastomotic urethroplasty is preferable because it has a lower re-stricture rate, success is maintained long-term and the complication rate is lower.
7. Substitution urethroplasty is indicated for longer bulbar strictures and all strictures of the penile urethra.
8. For most urethral strictures requiring substitution urethroplasty a stricturotomy and patch is preferable to excision and a tube graft/flap.
9. Grafts and flaps are equally good in most circumstances.
10. In the bulbar urethra grafts are quicker and easier.
11. A dorsal stricturotomy and patch has a higher success rate and a lower complication rate than ventral stricturotomy and patch.
12. Buccal mucosal grafting has advantages for stricturotomy and patch in the bulbar urethra.
13. In the penile urethra a flap is quicker and easier.
14. When a circumferential repair is required a two-stage reconstruction is safer and more reliable than a one-stage technique.

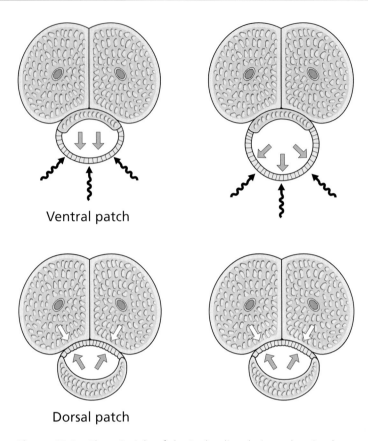

Ventral patch

Dorsal patch

Figure 19.1 The principle of the Barbagli technique showing how intraurethral pressure on voiding, coupled with the lack of external support, causes stretching and outpouching of a ventral patch. A dorsal patch, however, is well supported and outpouching does not occur. (Reproduced with permission from Andrich & Mundy 2000.[24])

tectomy for benign disease or pelvic fracture urethral distraction defects. Sphincter strictures usually respond to instrumentation and are best treated by urethral dilation as this is less likely than urethrotomy to cause further damage to the sphincter mechanism.[25]

Pelvic fracture urethral distraction defects (PFUDD) are typically described as membranous urethral strictures and are traditionally thought to be due to shearing through the membranous urethra as a consequence of the pelvic fracture injury.[28] In fact most evidence nowadays suggests that it is an avulsion injury rather than a shearing injury and one which causes avulsion of the membranous urethra from the bulbar urethra at the level of the perineal membrane rather than more proximally.[29]

Not everyone who suffers a pelvic fracture develops a distraction defect or even a stricture and in some instances occasional instrumentation may be all that is required to maintain normal voiding. For those patients with PFUDD a urethroplasty is the only option.

Principles of anastomotic urethroplasty for a PFUDD
In a PFUDD there has been no loss of urethral length; the problem is simply that the urethra has been disrupted and the two ends have become separated. What is then needed is a way of creating sufficient urethral length to connect the two ends. There are two general principles to achieve this:

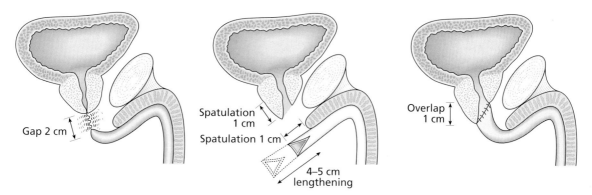

Figure 19.2 Mobilization of the bulbar urethra to overcome a short gap is dependent on the elasticity of the corpus spongiosum. As a consequence of this elasticity about 4–5 cm of urethral lengthening can be achieved. Given that spatulation on either side requires 1 cm overlap this means that a gap of 2 cm or thereabouts can be overcome in this way. (Reproduced with permission from Mundy 1997.[30])

1. mobilization of the bulbar urethra to capitalize on its intrinsic elasticity (Fig. 19.2)[14]
2. straightening out the natural curve of the bulbar urethra and converting it from a semicircle or five-eighths of a circle, which is its natural anatomical state, to the diameter of that same circle as shown in Figure 19.3.[30]

The natural perineal curve is caused by the urethra curving round firstly the fusion of the corpora cavernosa and secondly the underlying pubic symphysis more deeply. The first stage in straightening out the natural curve of the bulbar urethra is therefore to separate the crura as far forward as possible (Fig. 19.4) and lay the urethra in the groove between the two. If there is tension at the anastomosis then a wedge pubectomy of the inferior pubic arch is performed (Fig. 19.5). If tension remains then the urethra should be rerouted around the crus of the penis on one side. If it were possible to separate the crura further forwards than the usual 5 cm or so then rerouting would not be necessary. However if it is necessary to mobilize the urethra more distally than the crura can be separated, then it has to be higher and around the penis rather than higher and between the two crura of the penis (Figs 19.6 and 19.7).

Most PFUDDs are only 2–4 cm in length but using the four steps outlined above it is possible to overcome almost any length of gap and certainly up to 10 cm and occasionally longer. These four steps were described as a progression approach by Webster and Ramon,[31] bringing together concepts

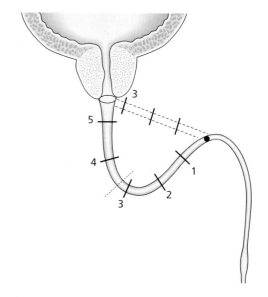

Figure 19.3 The normal course of the bulbar urethra is approximately five-eighths of a circle. This is caused by curving of the bulbar urethra around the fused corpora cavernosa and the underlying pubic symphysis. If this natural curve is eliminated by the maneuvers outlined, the distance between the apex of the prostate and the urethra in the region of the penoscrotal junction is approximately halved. (Reproduced with permission from Mundy 1997.[30])

described by Marion,[32] Turner-Warwick[14] and Waterhouse et al.[33] It is important to recognize that in using this approach the bulbar urethra is being mobilized as a flap which is therefore

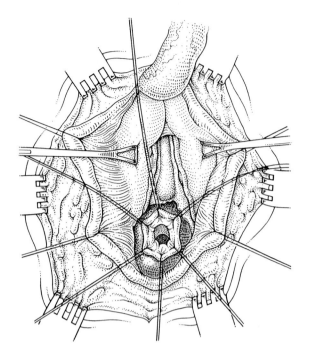

Figure 19.4 The intercrural plane has been incised. A Babcock forceps has been applied to each corpus to retract them away from the midline. On the deep aspect can be seen the dorsal vein of the penis in the midline and the dorsal neurovascular bundle on either side. (Reproduced with permission from Mundy 1997.[30])

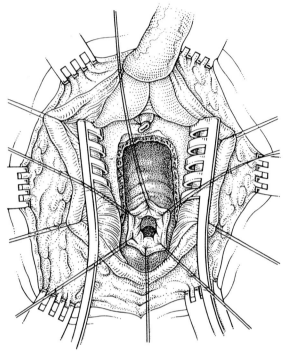

Figure 19.5 The corpora cavernosa are being held apart with a Travers retractor. The urethra is retracted upwards. The dorsal vein has been ligated and divided to allow a wedge resection of the underlying part of the inferior pubic arch. (Reproduced with permission from Mundy 1997.[30])

dependent on retrograde blood flow from the corpora cavernosa and from the glans backwards up the corpus spongiosum towards the bulb. Thus if the patient has a coexisting anterior urethral stricture or injury or was born with hypospadias such surgery may not be possible because of compromise to this retrograde blood flow.[14]

Anterior urethroplasty

In the anterior urethra strictures may be traumatic, iatrogenic due to instrumentation, idiopathic or infective/inflammatory in origin. In addition, congenital strictures and strictures complicated by an indwelling Urolume® stent are sometimes seen in the bulbar urethra. The penile urethra is additionally prone to strictures due to lichen sclerosus (BXO) or as a consequence of hypospadias surgery in the past.

In the bulbar urethra idiopathic and congenital strictures (there is considerable overlap), inflammatory strictures and iatrogenic/traumatic strictures are about equally common. Most short congenital/idiopathic strictures are amenable to excision and end-to-end anastomosis. The remainder usually require a stricturotomy and patch.

In the so-called developed world an increasing percentage (if not yet a majority) of penile strictures are due to hypospadias surgery or lichen sclerosus (BXO). Only a comparatively small number are idiopathic, traumatic or infective except in those areas of the world where gonococcal urethritis is still common. Thus the majority of penile urethral strictures will require excision and two-stage circumferential repair. Only a minority are amenable to an Orandi flap repair.

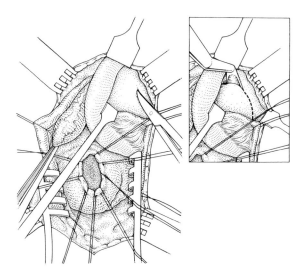

Figure 19.6 The urethra is retracted with a pair of forceps. The left crus of the penis has been retracted with a Langenbeck retractor to expose the pubic symphysis from above after division of the left side of the suspensory ligament of the penis. A trench has been cut through the pubis from above to connect with the inferior pubectomy, already cut from below. The Travers retractor exposes the apex of the prostate which is spatulated open with eight stay stitches. (Reproduced with permission from Mundy 1997.[30])

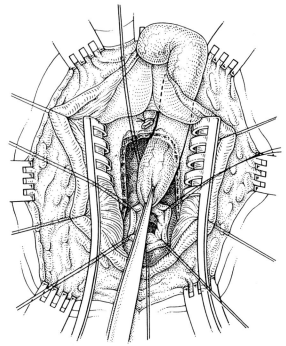

Figure 19.7 The mobilized urethra is now being rerouted around the left crus of the penis, through the trench cut in the pubis, to connect with the inferior pubectomy to allow a tension-free bulboprostatic anastomosis. (Reproduced with permission from Mundy 1997.[30])

Stricturotomy and patch procedure for a bulbar urethral stricture

The rationale for this, as described above, is that it is quick and easy and gives as good a result as anything else in most circumstances.[21] The stricturotomy should be placed dorsally and the patch therefore supported by the tunica albuginea.[34] This has the lowest re-stricture rate and the lowest complication rate. The bulbar urethra is mobilized for 2–3 cm on either side of the stricture which usually means throughout its length. It is then rotated and the stricturotomy performed in the dorsal midline (Fig. 19.8). Healthy urethra is opened for at least 1 cm on either side and further if there is any doubt. A suitable graft is then harvested, quilted in place onto the tunica albuginea (Fig. 19.9) and the urethra is then stitched round the margins of the graft, picking up the full thickness of the urethra together with the graft and a bite of the underlying tunica albuginea to help spatulate the stricturotomy open as well as to restore continuity. Nowadays, most surgeons use a buccal mucosal graft but a full thickness graft of penile shaft skin seems to give equally good results.[35]

The flap repair for complex bulbar strictures

Strictures that are due to ischemia, are actively infected, follow previous surgery or are full length or transsphincteric are best repaired with a flap. In all of these conditions it may not be possible to do a urethral mobilization and dorsal stricturotomy to place the flap; in such circumstances the stricturotomy and patch must be ventral. The flap is raised from penile shaft skin or failing that scrotal skin from a non-hair-bearing area, in all instances using

(a)

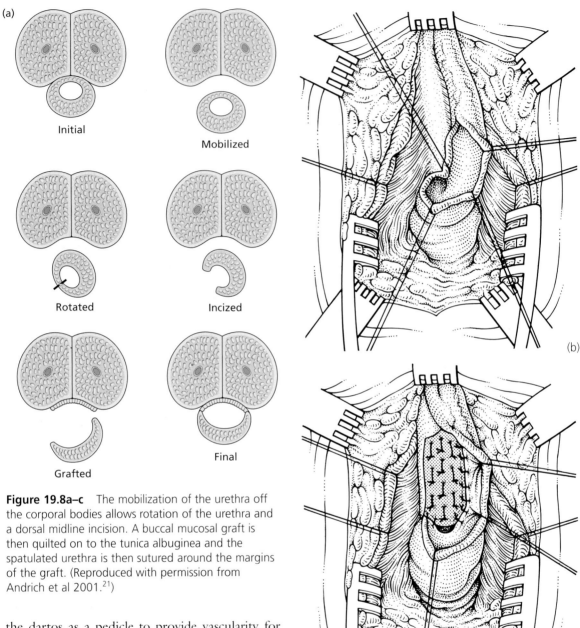

Initial

Mobilized

Rotated

Incised

Grafted

Final

(b)

(c)

Figure 19.8a–c The mobilization of the urethra off the corporal bodies allows rotation of the urethra and a dorsal midline incision. A buccal mucosal graft is then quilted on to the tunica albuginea and the spatulated urethra is then sutured around the margins of the graft. (Reproduced with permission from Andrich et al 2001.[21])

the dartos as a pedicle to provide vascularity for the skin paddle.[14,36] A wide dartos pedicle must be raised.

The Orandi flap repair of simple penile strictures

This flap is quick and easy to raise for a stricture of the penile urethra. The principle is the same as described above, i.e. a paddle of skin of adequate size is raised on the dartos as a pedicle.[22] This must be adequately but not excessively mobilized (Figs 19.10–19.13). The important point, as with all flaps/grafts, is to ensure adequate width. There is a tendency to make the flaps too narrow for fear of being unable to sew up the penile skin at the end of the procedure, thereby effectively recreating the stricture.

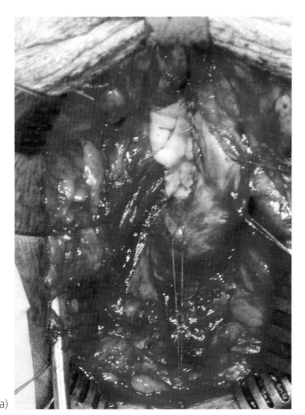
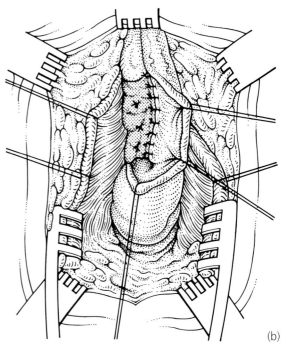

(a)

(b)

Figure 19.9 Operative photograph (a) and artist's diagram (b) of a Barbagli-type patch urethroplasty of the bulbar urethra. The bulbar urethra has been opened in the dorsal midline throughout its length and rotated with stay stitches to make the urethral lumen clearly visible. A patch of buccal mucosa has been quilted on to the tunica albuginea in the region of the stricturotomy. The left side of the spatulated urethra has been sutured to the left margin of the buccal mucosal graft. All that remains is to stitch the right margin of the urethra to the corresponding margin of the buccal mucosal graft.

Two-stage circumferential repair

In lichen sclerosus (BXO) and after hypospadias surgery the urethra will normally need to be excised.[17] As both conditions usually produce pronounced meatal stenosis and the meatus may be malpositioned then a glans cleft will need to be created via a graft laid into the glans cleft and quilted in place and onto the tunica albuginea up as far proximal as the point where healthy urethra is encountered (Fig. 19.14). The skin is then sewn to the margin of the graft (Fig. 19.15). In quilting the graft in place a slim layer of penile dartos should be interposed under the lateral margins of the graft so that it is easy to close the graft as a tube at the second stage (Fig. 19.16). The second stage is performed 3–6 months later when the graft is soft and pliable. This is then closed in three layers: the neourethra itself on the inside and the skin on the outside and, most importantly, a dartos layer between the two to waterproof the repair and reduce the risk of fistula formation which is the commonest complication of this procedure.

The future of urethral surgery

The results of anastomotic repair are so good and so well sustained that it seems unlikely that this will be superseded in due course by any technical development in urethroplasty surgery. The situation with substitution urethroplasty is different. Even with the flexible use of a variety of techniques there is still room for improvement and

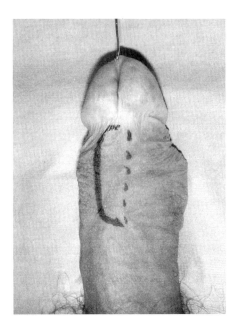

Figure 19.10   Orandi procedure – 1. The incision is outlined around a 2 cm wide patch of ventral penile skin. The skin and the full thickness of the subcutaneous tissue are incised along the bold line. The skin alone is incised along the dotted line, preserving the dartos layer which will become the vascular pedicle.

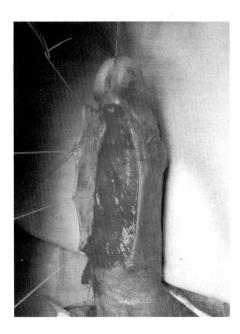

Figure 19.11   Orandi procedure – 2. The skin patch is now mobilized on the dartos pedicle.

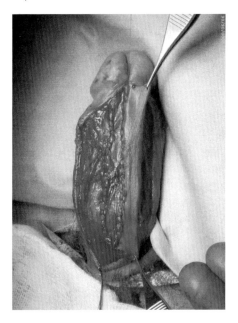

Figure 19.12   Orandi procedure – 3. The leading edge of the skin patch has been sutured to the adjacent margin of the urethra. The edges of the urethra have been oversewn for hemostasis.

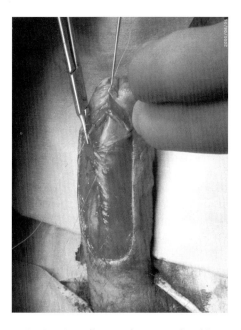

Figure 19.13   Orandi procedure – 4. The skin patch is flipped over with the dartos attached to be sutured to the other margin of the urethra – here nearing completion. The dartos layer is then tacked over the suture line to make it waterproof.

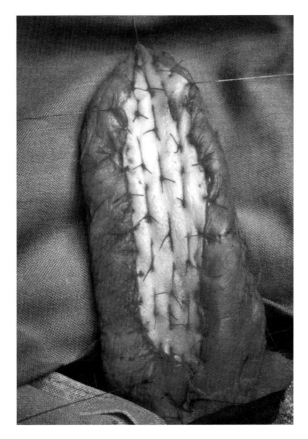

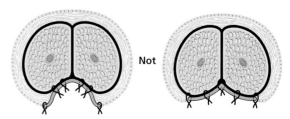

Figure 19.15 Diagram illustrating the interposition of a slip of dartos for each lateral margin of the graft to facilitate closure at the second stage.

Figure 19.14 In this patient the urethra has been excised following repeated failed operations for hypospadias. The glans cleft has been deepened and a 2.8 cm wide postauricular Wolfe graft has been quilted on to the tunica albuginea in the midline and on either side of it with quilting stitches at 0.5 cm intervals horizontally and longitudinally. On the lateral margins a thin slip of dartos has been incorporated.

current hopes are pinned on tissue engineering to provide an alternative to skin and buccal mucosa. On the other hand, the results of buccal mucosa grafts are so good that it is difficult to see that tissue engineering alone will make much difference. More interesting would be some way of prevent-ing the stricture process – perhaps by causing the urethral epithelium to revert to its normal pseudostratified columnar state – and thus prevent long-term re-stricturing, the problem with what is otherwise a very satisfactory procedure.

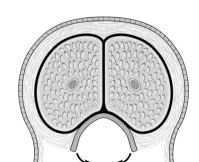

(b)

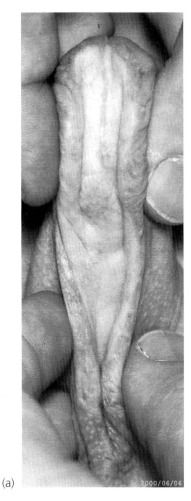

(a)

Figure 19.16 (a) The postauricular Wolfe graft has now matured and on clinical examination it can be seen that the graft is fixed in the midline but freely mobile on either side which allows the graft to be rolled inwards to allow easy closure at the second stage. (b) Diagrammatic illustration of clinical point.

References

1. Chambers R, Baitera B. The anatomy of urethral stricture. BJU 1977; 49:545–551.
2. Devereux M, Burfield G. Prolonged follow-up of urethral strictures treated by intermittent dilatation. BJU 1970; 42:231–239.
3. Romero Perez P, Mira Linares A. Complications of the lower urinary tract secondary to urethral stenosis. Actas Urol Esp 1996; 20(9):786–793.
4. Flocks H. The roentgen visualisation of the posterior urethra. J Urol 1933; 30:711–736.
5. Pansadoro V, Emiliozzi P. Internal urethrotomy in the management of anterior urethral strictures: long-term follow up. J Urol 1996; 156:73–75.
6. Steenkamp J, Heyns C, De Kock M. Internal urethrotomy versus dilatation as treatment for male urethral strictures: a prospective, randomized comparison. J Urol 1997; 157:98–101.
7. Heyns C, Steenkamp JW, De Kock ML, Whitaker P. Treatment of male urethral strictures: is repeated dilatation of internal urethrotomy useful? J Urol 1998; 160:356–358.
8. Harriss D, Beckingham IJ, Lemberger RJ, Lawrence WT. Long-term results of intermittent low-friction self-catheterization in patients with recurrent urethral strictures. BJU 1994; 74(6):790–792.
9. Milroy E, Chapple C, Wallsten H. A new stent for the treatment of urethral strictures: preliminary report. BJU 1989; 63:392–396.
10. Badlani G, Press SM, Defaclo A, et al. Urolume endourethral prosthesis for the treatment of urethral strictures disease: long-term results of the North American Multicenter Urolume trial. Urology 1995; 45(5):846–856.
11. Nissenkorn I, Shavel M. Polyurethane stent for treatment of urethral strictures. J Endourol 1997; 11(6):481–483.

12. Milroy E, Allen A. Long-term results of urolume urethral stent for recurrent urethral strictures. J Urol 1996; 155:904–908.

13. Mundy A. Results and complications of urethroplasty and its future. BJU 1993; 71:322–325.

14. Turner-Warwick R. Urethral stricture surgery. In: Munday A, ed. Current operative surgery – urology. London: Bailliére Tindall; 1988:160–218.

15. Koraitim M. The lessons of 145 posttraumatic posterior urethral strictures treated in 17 years. J Urol 1995; 153:63–66.

16. Greenwell T, Venn S, Mundy A. Changing practice in anterior urethroplasty. BJU Int 1998; 83:631–635.

17. Venn S, Mundy A. Urethroplasty for balanitis xerotica obliterans. BJU 1998; 81:735–737.

18. Jordan G, Devine P. Application of tissue transfer techniques to the management of urethral strictures. Semin Urol 1987; 5(4):228–235.

19. Jordan G. Principles of wound healing and tissue transfer techniques useful for genitourinary reconstructive surgery. Semin Urol 1987; 5(4):219–227.

20. Wessels H, McAninch J. Current controversies in anterior urethral stricture repair: free-graft versus pedicled skin-flap reconstruction. World J Urol 1998; 16(3):175–180.

21. Andrich D, Mundy A. The Barbagli procedure gives the best results for patch urethroplasty of the bulbar urethra. BJU Int 2001; 88:385–389.

22. Orandi A. One-stage urethroplasty. BJU 1968; 40(6):717–719.

23. Mundy A. The long-term results of skin inlay urethroplasty. J. Urol 1972; 107:977–980.

24. Andrich DE, Mundy AR. Urethral strictures and their surgical treatment. BJU Int 2000; 86:571–580.

25. Mark S, Perez L, Webster G. Synchronous management of anastomotic contracture and stress urinary incontinence following radical prostatectomy. J Urol 1994; 151(5):1202–1204.

26. Pansadoro V, Emiliozzi P. Iatrogenic prostatic urethral strictures classification and endoscopic treatment. Urology 1999; 53(4):784–789.

27. Theodorou Ch, Kastifotis Ch, Stournaras P, et al. Abdomino-perineal repair of recurrent and complex bladder neck prostatic urethra contractures. Eur Urol 2000; 38(6):734–741.

28. Pokorny M, Pontes J, Pierce J Jr. Urological injuries associated with pelvic trauma. J Urol 1979; 121:455–457.

29. Andrich D, Mundy A. The nature of urethral injury in cases of pelvic fracture urethral trauma. J Urol 2001; 165:1492–1495.

30. Mundy A. Reconstruction of posterior urethral distraction defects. Atlas Urol Clin North Am 1997; 5(1):139–174.

31. Webster G, Ramon J. Repair of pelvic fracture posterior urethral defects using an elaborated perineal approach: experience with 74 cases. J Urol 1991; 145(4):744–748.

32. Marion G. Traité d'urologie. Paris: Masson; 1928: Vol 1 & 2.

33. Waterhouse K, Abrahams JI, Caponegro P, et al. The transpubic repair of membranous urethral strictures. J Urol 1974; 111:188–190.

34. Barbagli G, Selli C, di Cello V, Mottola A. A one-stage dorsal free-graft urethroplasty for bulbar urethral strictures. BJU 1996; 78(6):929–932.

35. Iselin C, Webster G. Dorsal onlay urethroplasty for urethral stricture repair. World J Urol 1998; 16:181–185.

36. Quartey J. One-stage penile/preputial island flap urethroplasty for urethral stricture. J Urol 1985; 134:474–487.

20

Organ preserving therapies for penile carcinomas

Chryssanthos Kouriefs and Nicholas Watkin

Introduction

Penile carcinomas are rare. The incidence, in England and Wales, as reported by the National Office for Statistics, has remained relatively unchanged at 1.2–1.5 per 100 000 (male population) per year, between 1950 and 1999.[1] This compares to a similar incidence in other Western countries.[2] In some parts of the world (Mexico, China, Puerto Rico) however, penile cancer occurs with an incidence of 15–20/100 000/year.[3,4] Histologically, the majority (90%) are primary carcinomas, of which 95% are squamous cell carcinomas but sarcomas, melanomas and basal cell carcinomas have been reported.

The rarity of penile cancer makes it very difficult to conduct randomized control trials. In fact, there are no randomized trials to date leaving many question marks concerning the treatment of penile carcinomas. Available treatments include surgical amputation and penis preserving therapies. The latter may be surgical (circumcision, laser, glansectomy) or non-surgical (radiotherapy, immunotherapy, chemotherapy). Surgical amputation is the oldest of all modalities. In 1761 Morgani[5] mentioned the procedure of partial penectomy performed by Valsalva but it is Thiersch (quoted in Lewis[6]) who has been credited with the first detailed description of curative surgery for penile cancer, in 1931. Surgical amputation provides excellent local oncological control[7,8,9] but is associated with urinary and sexual dysfunction as well as enormous psychological morbidity.[10] Nowadays, the definitive management of penile carcinomas is stage dependent (Table 20.1) and with careful case selection, more and more patients can benefit from penile preserving therapies.

Data from retrospective studies suggest a statistically higher local recurrence rate following organ preserving therapies compared with penile amputation.[11] Most recurrences are surgically salvageable and the regional recurrence, metastasis and overall mortality are comparable to primary amputative surgical procedures.[11] Available retrospective series report good cosmetic and functional outcome with organ preserving therapies and an overall organ preservation of 60%.[11] This chapter will review the applicability of the available organ preserving therapies.

The management of penile carcinoma in situ

Penile carcinoma in situ (CIS) is a premalignant condition of the penis. It refers to two similar clinicopathological entities: 'erythroplasia of Queyrat' and 'Bowen's disease'. It is non-invasive

Table 20.1 TNM (1997) classification of penile carcinomas

A. Extent of primary tumor (T)
Tx: Primary tumor cannot be assessed
Tis: Carcinoma in situ
Ta: Non-invasive verrucous carcinoma
T1: Invades subepithelial connective tissues
T2: Invades corpus spongiosum/cavernosum
T3: Invades urethra or prostate
T4: Invades other adjacent structures

B. Extent of regional lymph nodes (N)
Nx: Regional lymph nodes cannot be assessed
N0: No regional lymph node metastasis
N1: Metastasis in single superficial inguinal lymph node
N2: Metastasis in multiple or bilateral superficial inguinal lymph nodes
N3: Metastasis in deep inguinal or pelvic lymph node(s), unilateral or bilateral

C. Extent of distant metastasis (M)
Mx: Distant metastasis cannot be assessed
M0: No distant metastasis
M1: Distant metastasis

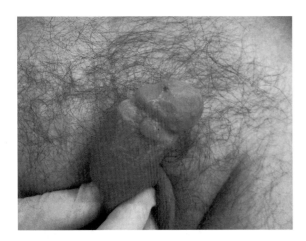

Figure 20.1 Superficially invasive (T1 stage) squamous cell carcinoma present at the coronal sulcus with coexisting carcinoma in situ of the glans penis.

and therefore highly amenable to curative penis preserving therapies. Invasive penile carcinomas and CIS commonly coexist in 25% of cases (Fig. 20.1) and generous deep biopsies are necessary to make that distinction before definitive treatment for CIS is initiated. Data on the management of CIS by topical chemotherapy, radiotherapy and laser surgery are derived from small reported series (Table 20.2).[12–21]

The first line treatment of penile CIS is topical chemotherapy with 5% 5-fluorouracil (5FU) cream (Efudix®). Goette and colleagues[12,13] reported a sustained 100% complete response rate at 5 years,

with 5% 5FU cream. Other series in the literature report the same high success.[14] Concerns were raised regarding the potential systemic toxicity from mucosal absorption of 5FU. Studies have however demonstrated that the absorption of 5FU from the genital mucosa is minimal and is therefore safe to use topically.[22] The superficial non-invasive nature of CIS makes it amenable to both CO_2 and Nd:YAG laser surgery. However, there are concerns that superficial invasion could be missed in the absence of histology.

Second line treatments for intractable or recurrent disease include radiotherapy, microscopically controlled surgical excision and excision combined with patch skin grafting. Surgical salvage can be performed by excising the epithelial and subepithelial tissues of the glans and replacing with either a full thickness skin graft from shaft skin, or partial thickness graft from a suitable donor site (Watkin and Bracka, personal communication). This can be particularly advantageous when coexisting balanitis xerotica obliterans (BXO) or unsightly scar tissue is present. Cosmetic results are excellent and long-term control rates are awaited.

Surgical penis preserving therapies for invasive tumors

Circumcision
Circumcision is by far the commonest intervention in the management of penile carcinomas. The majority of men who present with penile carci-

Table 20.2 Series reporting on the treatment of penile carcinoma in situ

Year	Authors	Treatment	Cases	Control (%)	F/u*
1975	Goette et al[12]	Topical 5FU	3	100	20–60
1976	Goette & Carson[13]	Topical 5FU	7	100	70
1971	Hueser & Pugh[14]	Topical 5FU	1	100	–
1988	Malloy et al[15]	Laser (Nd:YAG)	5	100	36
1995	Windahl & Hellsten[16]	Laser (CO₂/Nd:YAG)	4	100	31
1998	Tietjen & Malek[17]	Laser (KTP/Nd:YAG)	15	94	58
1998	Shirahama et al[18]	Laser (Nd:YAG)	10	100	72
1987	Bandieramonte et al[19]	Laser (CO₂)	4	100	6–36
1988	Bandieramonte et al[20]	Laser (CO₂)	3	100	7
1993	McLean et al[21]	EBRT	11	100	168

* Follow up in months. 5FU, 5-fluorouracil; EBRT, external beam radiotherapy.

noma are uncircumcised. Very few reports exist in the literature of penile carcinoma in uncircumcised men. It is indicated for symptomatic treatment of painful or bleeding preputial tumors as well as for acquired phimosis secondary to preputial or even large glandular tumors. It is always recommended before radiotherapy because it allows better targeting and definition of the tumor, it prevents preputial radiotherapy adverse reactions and above all, it facilitates surveillance for local recurrences. Most importantly, circumcision is a sufficient primary curative therapy for small low stage (Tis, Ta, T1) disease limited to the prepuce.[23]

The need for adequate resection margins cannot be sufficiently emphasized. In the presence of proximal preputial tumor, the circumcision margin will need to be extended to the shaft of the penis to ensure adequate resection.[9,24,25] High recurrence rates are reported in the literature and reinforce the need for close surveillance for early detection and salvage of local recurrence. Case selection is paramount to reduce local recurrence rates.

Glansectomy

Glansectomy is a new surgical technique used to treat penile carcinomas limited to the glans penis and prepuce. It refers to the isolation and excision of the glans. Frozen sections from the cavernosal bed and urethral stump are encouraged during the operation to ensure clear surgical margins. An end-shaft urethrostomy is fashioned and a urethral catheter is left in situ for about 5–7 days. It is combined with partial thickness skin grafting of the corporeal heads to create a neo-glans. Glansectomy is new and poorly reported in the literature. Davis et al[26] reported three cases of penile verrucous carcinoma (recurrent), angiosarcoma and melanoma limited to the glans. All three underwent glansectomy with clear surgical margins. There were no local recurrences at a follow up of 12–48 months. The patient with angiosarcoma, however, developed lung metastasis at 9 months, and died a year later. In all cases normal erection, sexual and urinating function resumed shortly after the operation. Hatzichristou et al[27] reported seven cases of verrucous carcinomas treated with glansectomy. They reported only one surgically salvaged recurrence at 3 months. All patients are alive and disease free at 18–65 months. Once again, all patients resumed normal erections with normal sexual and urinating

function following the procedure. Vaginal pain was reported by two of their partners which was attributed to the absence of the glans.

The two largest series are still to be published (Watkin and Bracka). Early reports suggest that the operation fulfils the requirements of very low recurrence rate (Watkin: 0%), good cosmetic result and preservation of sexual and urinary function (Figs 20.2–20.4). Unlike radiotherapy, it also allows detailed histological evaluation of the tumor. Case selection is important. Carcinomas should be low

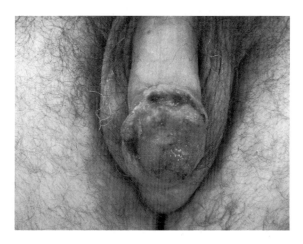

Figure 20.2 Invasive squamous cell carcinoma of the glans and distal shaft of the penis. This patient was suitable for glansectomy and skin graft reconstruction.

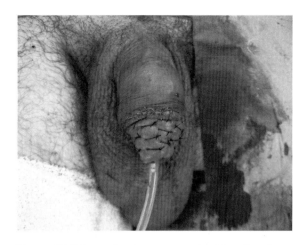

Figure 20.3 Immediately postoperative. The glans has been removed and the exposed corporeal heads have been covered with partial thickness skin, held in place by silk 'quilting' sutures.

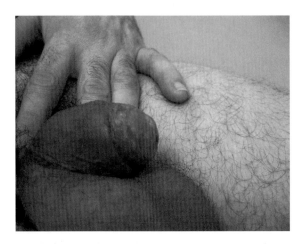

Figure 20.4 The same patient as Figure 20.3, 6 weeks later with maturing skin graft.

risk (low grade and stage T1/T2) and they should be at least macroscopically limited to the glans penis. Clear margins should be documented intra-operatively with frozen section biopsies from the cavernosal bed and urethral stump. Approximately 80% of all cases of invasive penile cancer are suitable for this procedure. Close follow up is mandatory as local recurrences are surgically salvageable when diagnosed early.

Laser surgery

There is considerable experience of the use of lasers to treat penile tumors.[15,16,17,19,28] The most widely used laser modes in penile carcinoma surgery are carbon dioxide (CO_2) and neodymium yttrium aluminum garnet (Nd:YAG) lasers since the pioneering work of Hofstetter and Frank in 1976.[29] CO_2 laser energy has a long wavelength (lambda = 10.6 μm) and a high frequency. It is readily absorbed by water, the primary constituent of human tissues. It has very low penetration power and is therefore unsuitable for deeply invading tumors. Nd:YAG has 10 times shorter wavelength (lambda = 1.06 μm) and therefore a higher penetration power of about 4–6 mm. It is important therefore to assess the depth of tumor prior to laser surgery. Depth of invasion can be assessed clinically as well as radiologically by ultrasound and MRI scans. A pretreatment deep incisional biopsy can give us similar but 'localized' information.

Both CO_2 and Nd:YAG lasers can be used to ablate (vaporize) or excise tumors. Excision laser surgery has the advantage of obtaining a tumor specimen for histological assessment. Laser surgery has excellent cosmetic and functional results. It has hemostatic properties and can be performed in the outpatient setting. However, it needs dedicated staff, training and expensive equipment. When compared to radiotherapy and chemotherapy, it provides histological specimens for examination and has fewer local acute reactions.

Laser surgery, as with most other organ pre-serving therapies, finds application in the palliative management of metastatic or even locoregionally advanced penile carcinomas as well as in the primary management of local disease with curative intentions. It has also been used as an adjuvant therapy to primary radiotherapy, chemotherapy or a combination of the two. Several studies in the literature report these applications of laser surgery. Malloy et al[15] reported on the primary treatment of 16 cases of penile carcinomas (five Tis, nine T1, two T2) with Nd:YAG laser between 1983 and 1986. They reported a local recurrence rate of 33% for stage T1 disease at a mean follow up of 27 months. The local control rate for carcinoma in situ at 26 months follow up was 100%. On the other hand, none of the stage T2 cases was tumor free by laser surgery alone. Windahl et al[16] treated 19 cases (four Tis, seven T1, eight T2), with CO_2 alone (eight cases) or in combination with Nd:YAG laser (11 cases), between 1980 and 1994. They reported two (11%) recurrences. They were both salvaged successfully with second laser surgery and were reported to be free of disease at 12 and 52 months. Tietjen et al,[17] from the Mayo Clinic, treated 30 cases of penile carcinomas with KTP or Nd:YAG lasers. These included 15 carci-nomas in situ (Tis), 14 stage T1 and one stage T2 carcinomas. In the Tis group, there was one (6%) recurrence at 5 months salvaged with second laser treatment. In the stage T1 group, they reported two (14.3%) recurrences at 3 and 7 months. Both cases were salvaged with second laser treatment. Finally, the only stage T2 case in the series recurred at 3 months and underwent amputation.

A study by Shirahama et al[18] demonstrates the importance of case selection. They selected patients with carcinomas less than 6 mm thick based on MRI and ultrasound scan assessments. This is the tissue penetration range for Nd:YAG laser beam. They treated 10 cases of carcinoma in situ and stage T1 penile carcinomas. Patients were all free of disease at 6 years. Two cases of stage T2 penile carcinoma were included in this series. These two patients were treated aggressively with a combination of chemoradiation and adjuvant laser surgery. Both patients were free of disease at 7 and 8 years of follow up. Few other studies demonstrate the potential advantage of aggressive combination therapies for advanced penile carcinomas.[30,31]

Surface glansectomy

Two reports describe a novel application of laser for organ preservation in superficial penile cancer limited to the glans penis. They refer to surface glansectomy. This technique, according to the authors, is useful in superficial lesions occupying more than 50% of the surface of the glans or when they are multifocal. They used CO_2 laser in both reports. In the first report in 1987,[19] they treated 47 patients with penile dermatoses. These included eight cases of invasive squamous cell carcinoma and four cases of Tis. They report one (12%) recurrence at 5 months, which was salvaged with a second laser treatment. Their follow up was 6–36 months. In their second report in 1988,[20] they treated 15 cases of penile dermatoses. These included three Tis, four stage T1 disease and three cases of residual disease postchemotherapy. They reported one (10%) recurrence/persistent disease, again salvaged with repeat laser surgery. All patients were reported to be free of disease at a short follow up of 2–48 months (median of 7 months).

Laser surgery versus surgical amputation

The available data to date demonstrates that laser surgery has significant anatomical and functional advantages over the traditional surgical amputation. However, as with any organ preserving therapy, in the context of penile carcinomas, the local recurrence is higher and a close follow up is mandatory to be able to diagnose these recurrences early and salvage them without compromising patient survival in an eager attempt to preserve phallic function. Patient selection is also very important. High stage disease tends to be resistant to laser monotherapy. In such cases, combination therapy may be considered. Finally, in laser surgery the depth of invasion of the tumor is important.

Tumors invading more than 6 mm into tissues might be unsuitable for laser surgery.

Mohs micrographic excision

Mohs micrographic surgery (MMS) – also known as microsurgery or even chemosurgery – refers to a surgical technique of excising accessible tumors under microscopic control.[32,33] The tumor is excised in horizontal slices and the undersurface of each slice is examined microscopically by systematic frozen sections. In the presence of disease on the frozen sections further slices of tissue are excised until the 'mapping' frozen section biopsies of the undersurface of the excised tissue are negative. At that point, another section of tissue is removed to ensure a clear resection margin. On excision, the tissue may be fresh (frozen-tissue MMS) or fixed by aluminum chloride (fixed-tissue MMS). The technique is most commonly used for skin cancers but the accessibility of penile carcinomas (most commonly on the glans) makes it suitable for such a technique. In case of large volume tumors, a debulking procedure is performed prior to the microscopically controlled stages.

Mohs et al[32] reported their 50 years' experience with this technique for treating penile malignancies. This is perhaps the only reported series of Mohs microsurgery for penile carcinomas in the literature. They treated 35 cases of penile carcinomas. In the analysis of their results, they concentrate on the 31 cases that they had followed up for at least 5 years. These comprised 21 cases of stage T1, eight cases of stage T2 and two cases of stage T3 disease (Jackson's clinical staging system). In eight out of these 31 cases, they were unable to render the patient disease free because of metastatic disease (six cases) or locally advanced disease (two cases). The success rate was stage dependent; 86% and 82% of stage T1 and T2 cases were tumor free compared to none of the two stage T3 cases. Out of the 23 successfully treated and tumor free cases, they report two (6%) local recurrences at a follow up of 5 years.

This technique is attractive because it allows reassurance of local complete excision and preservation of the phallic anatomy and function. Once again, the local failure rate is stage dependent and local recurrence is higher (32%) than amputation. Patient selection may allow a higher primary success rate and lower subsequent local recurrence rate. Further reports with this technique are necessary to allow comparison and reproducibility of results and outcome.

Non-surgical penis preserving therapies

Radiotherapy

Radiotherapy is a well-established primary therapy for penile carcinomas.[34] Its role in the management of regional lymphadenopathy and palliation for distant metastases is, however, beyond the scope of this chapter. The review will concentrate purely on the use of radiotherapy for local control and organ preservation.

Preradiotherapy circumcision is always recommended. It reduces the tumor volume, allows better definition and therefore targeting of the tumor and reduces the incidence of radiotherapy complications related to the foreskin. Above all, it allows better surveillance and detection of local recurrence by the patient and clinician. In an era of rapid technological advances and innovations, there are various effective techniques of radiotherapy. In Scandinavia and North America external beam radiotherapy is most popular, whereas in the UK and France brachytherapy (BRT) is favored. Brachytherapy is further divided into interstitial brachytherapy (IBRT) where the radiation source is implanted into the tumor itself and plesiotherapy where the radiation source surrounds the tumor. IBRT is more popular in France and plesiotherapy, also known as mold radioactive technique or contact brachytherapy, is more popular in the UK. There are no randomized controlled trials comparing one mode of therapy to another. Data derived from retrospective studies[8,11,21,35–38] suggest that the different radiotherapy techniques are equally effective (Table 20.3). The decision on the type of radiotherapy treatment mainly depends on local expertise.

Plesiotherapy

This technique involves the application of two cylindrical molds round the penis (Fig. 20.5). The inner piece is in direct contact with the penis and straightens it. The outer piece is loaded with radioactive wires, The most commonly used being radioactive iridium-192 wires. The patient's cooperation and dexterity are paramount for a

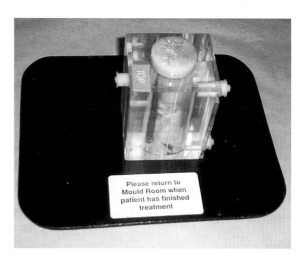

Figure 20.5 The plesiotherapy molds stabilize the irradiated penis in an upright position during treatment.

Table 20.3 Retrospective studies on the management of penile carcinomas by radiotherapy

Year	Authors	Cases	Mode of treatment	Local recurrence rate (%)	5-year survival rate (%)
2000	Cotsadze et al[11]	155	EBRT	15.3	86
1984	El-Demiry et al[35]	23	BRT	21.7	89
		10	EBRT	70	76
1981	Krieg & Luk[36]	41	EBRT	25	–
1996	Chaudhary et al[37]	23	IBRT	21.7	–
1993	McLean et al[21]	37	EBRT	39	62
1994	Ravi et al[38]	156	EBRT/BRT	33	87
1992	Horenblas et al[8]	–	EBRT	–	–

BRT, brachytherapy; EBRT, external beam radiotherapy; IBRT, interstitial brachytherapy.

successful treatment. The patient is shown how to apply the outer mold and how to take it off, for example when urinating. The loaded mold should be applied for about 12 hours a day for approximately 1 week. The patient is treated in an isolated room. A total dosage of 60 Gy is aimed for. The theoretical biophysical advantage of plesiotherapy, or brachytherapy in general (including IBRT) compared to external beam radiotherapy (EBRT), is the more targeted administration of radiation with higher biological effective tumor dose. In practical terms, the patient is in control of the timing of his treatment, the treatment is shorter and local complications usually occur after the completion of therapy and therefore do not interfere with the treatment. The main disadvantage is the need for isolation.

Interstitial brachytherapy

Interstitial brachytherapy (IBRT) shares some of the biophysical advantages of plesiotherapy. The radiation source is within the tumor mass and therefore provides a higher tumor biological radiation dosage. It involves the implantation of radioactive wires or needles through the tumor/penis. The most commonly used radioactive wires are iridium-192. The implantation necessitates general or regional anesthesia, which is obviously a practical disadvantage. The wires measure about 40 mm and are held in place by two external templates on either side of the penis. The templates have holes corresponding to each wire and the distribution of the holes ensures a uniform administration of radiation to the whole of the tumor.

The number and arrangement of the wires are determined by the size of the tumor. In general, penile tumors treated with primary radiotherapy tend to be small. In fact, most would agree to the safe treatment of tumors smaller than 4 cm. The wires therefore are usually arranged in two rows of four to six wires in each row. The total radiation dosage is aimed at 50–70 Gy, as with plesiotherapy and EBRT, at a rate of 0.5–1 Gy/hour. The total duration of treatment is 5–7 days. As with plesiotherapy, the treatment takes place in an isolated room.

External beam radiotherapy

Worldwide, external beam radiotherapy (EBRT) is the most popular and most commonly reported of the three radiotherapy techniques. It is usually a megavoltage fractionated technique during which the whole of the penis is irradiated. A wax mold is used to ensure uniform distribution of radiation. A total dose of 50–70 Gy is aimed for in 15–30 daily sessions for 3–8 weeks. The advantage of this mode of treatment is the outpatient setting. However, its lengthy character means that acute reactions occur during the course of the treatment and when severe, the treatment may have to be terminated.

Complications

Radiotherapy is not without its downside. The reported complication rate is very high and patients should be carefully counseled before treatment. Acute local reactions, mucositis, skin irritation and tissue edema occur early and virtually in everyone. As mentioned above, during EBRT, these reactions occur during the course of treatment and when severe can result in termination of the treatment. On the other hand, with BRT, which is shorter, they occur a few days after the end of treatment and subside within a few weeks with supportive management.

Late complications occur at a variable rate, often more than 40%.[39,40] Skin changes such as hypochromasia, telangiectasia and superficial necrosis are common (Fig. 20.6). The first two are of no clinical significance and superficial necrosis heals up spontaneously within a few weeks. In deeply invading tumors treated with high radiation doses, especially when postradiotherapy biopsies are performed, deep necroses can occur. This is perhaps the most serious complication. It is tumor volume and radiation dose dependent.[41] It is twice as common with BRT (15%) than EBRT (8%).[42] These necroses take a long time to heal and may get complicated or even not heal at all necessitating amputation. Large (> 4 cm) deeply invading tumors should therefore (when possible) not be treated with radiotherapy.

In the same way, small superficial tumors should be treated with low radiation doses to avoid unacceptable complications. If the foreskin is left in situ, sclerosis of the foreskin can result in phimosis that is best treated with circumcision. This is one of the reasons why circumcision is always encouraged before radiotherapy to the penis. Finally, urethral strictures occur in 5–40% of

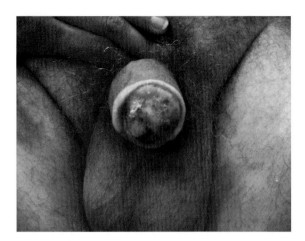

Figure 20.6 Long-term changes after radical radiotherapy for squamous cell carcinomas. Balanitis xerotica obliterans is also seen. There is atrophy of the glans with scarring, keratinization and recurrent meatal stenosis. The patient also admitted to partial erections.

cases.[35,38,39] These rates compare favorably to penile amputation. The great majority of these strictures occur at the meatus. They can be managed with instrumental dilation, meatotomy or even plastic reconstruction.

Effectiveness of radiotherapy

Data regarding the effectiveness of radiotherapy is derived from retrospective clinical studies (see Table 20.3).[8,11,21,35–38] The largest series, by Cotsadze et al,[11] reports on the treatment of 155 cases of invasive penile cancer (stage T2/T3 N0–N3) with external beam radiotherapy. They report a subjective response of 76.2% with complete disappearance of the tumor in 63.2%. The local recurrence in this study is 15.3% between 3 and 78 months of follow up. The overall 5- and 10-year survival rates were 86% and 82% respectively. They report an overall organ preservation of 64.5%. Response to radiotherapy was statistically different between staging groups (89.4% for T1 and 8.3% for T3, p < 0.05).

The figures reported by Cotsadze et al[11] are in agreement with other reported series. El-Demiry et al[35] reported on 33 cases treated with plesiotherapy (23 cases) and EBRT (10 cases). The recurrence rate for plesiotherapy was 21.7% and for EBRT 70% (selection bias). The overall 5-year survival for EBRT and brachytherapy were 76%

and 89% respectively, figures comparable to the 5-year survival following amputation of the penis in the same series. They concluded that what really determines the outcome of disease is not the mode of treatment but its inherent pathology, a concept with which most clinicians would agree.

Krieg et al[36] report a 25% local recurrence rate following EBRT. Their local control after radiotherapy and surgical salvage was 92% compared to a surgery-only local control rate of 88%. Chaudhary et al[37] reported on 23 cases treated with iridium-192 interstitial brachytherapy. They report a local recurrence rate of 21.7% (5 of 23), four of which were salvaged with surgical intervention. Of interest is the report by McLean et al[21] who included 11 cases of carcinoma in situ. They treated in total 37 cases of penile carcinomas with EBRT. In the invasive tumor group, they report a local recurrence of 39% all of which were surgically salvaged. The overall 5-year survival was 62%. In the carcinoma in situ group they report a 100% local control at 14 years of follow up.

Ravi et al[38] reported on 156 cases of invasive local penile carcinomas treated with brachytherapy (28 cases) or EBRT (128 cases). The local control rate was 65%, but 33% more were surgically salvaged. They report a 5-year disease free survival of 87%. They also observed that the recurrence rate was disease stage dependent. The same observation was made by Horenblas et al.[8] They reported a 100% recurrence rate in stage T3 disease. They also reported comparable local recurrence rates for laser and EBRT therapies.

Many other series[43,44,45] have produced figures comparable with the above studies. Although retrospective studies, their results are consistently reproducible. The local recurrence rate following primary radiotherapy is in the range of 15–40%, which is higher than the reported recurrence rate following penile amputation. The local recurrence rate seems to be unaffected by the mode of radiotherapy treatment used. However, with close follow up, the great majority of these recurrences are local and surgically salvageable. The combination of radiotherapy and salvage surgery when necessary raises the overall local control rate to levels comparable to amputation. The overall organ preserving rate is in the range of 60–80% with no compromise in the overall 5- and 10-year survival.

Most authors would agree that local recurrence rate correlates with inherent tumor factors such as stage and grade. Stage T1 tumors can be managed safely and effectively with primary radiotherapy. Most would agree that stage T3 and T4 tumors exhibit an unacceptably high recurrence rate, following primary radiotherapy, and should be managed with surgical amputation at the first instance. Opinions may be conflicting with stage T2 tumors. Patient selection is extremely important. Small, distal low-grade tumors could be safely managed with primary radiotherapy but close follow up is required to be able to surgically salvage any local recurrences without compromising overall survival. On the other hand, large, proximal and high grade tumors may be suitably managed with surgical amputation. Patients should be carefully counseled to be able to make an informed decision.

Chemotherapy

Penile squamous cell carcinomas are chemosensitive to some extent. Systemic chemotherapy has been used mainly as palliative treatment for disseminated or locoregionally advanced disease.[46–51] It has also been used as neoadjuvant therapy to downstage local tumors that would otherwise be unsuitable for organ preserving surgical intervention (cryodestruction, laser ablation, wedge resection).[42,52,53] It has gained little popularity as a primary curative therapy for local disease. Data on the use of systemic chemotherapy for penile carcinomas are derived from small series (Table 20.4).[11,51,53–55]

Bleomycin, methotrexate, cisplatin and vinblastine are perhaps the most commonly reported chemotherapeutic agents. They have a low indivi-

dual effectiveness of about 20% and their response is usually partial and short lasting.[51] They are commonly used in multidrug chemotherapy regimens or even in combination with other organ preserving therapies such as radiotherapy or immunotherapy.[11,53]

Sklaroff et al[54] reported methotrexate monotherapy in eight cases of invasive penile carcinomas with a 38.1% response rate. The response was short in all cases and a 100% local recurrence rate was reported at 2, 3 and 11 months. Ahmed et al[55] reported a 21% response rate with bleomycin monotherapy sustained for a median of 3 months. The same group treated 21 patients sequentially with bleomycin, cisplatin and methotrexate monotherapies and reported response rates of 21%, 25% and 61% respectively.[51] They observed that younger patients were statistically more likely to respond and responders lived significantly longer. Recently, Cotsadze et al[11] reported their experience in using systemic chemotherapy as a curative primary organ preserving therapy for local penile carcinomas. They treated 33 cases with four different chemotherapy regimens: bleomycin monotherapy (11 cases), vinblastine and bleomycin (11 cases), cisplatin and bleomycin (five cases) and cisplatin, vinblastine and bleomycin (six cases). They reported an overall 48.5% complete response rate after only one cycle of chemotherapy. Their organ preservation was increased to 60.6% by adjuvant cryodestruction in partial responders. None of the stage T3 cases exhibited complete response. The local recurrence rate was 18.7%, all of which were salvaged surgically. The 5- and 10-year survival rates were 78% and 73% respectively. There seemed to be no advantage in using multidrug chemotherapy compared to bleomycin monotherapy.

Table 20.4 Retrospective data on the management of penile carcinoma with systemic chemotherapy

Year	Authors	Cases	Mode of treatment	Response rate (%)	Local recurrence rate (%)
1980	Sklaroff & Yagoda[54]	8	MTX	38.1	100
1984	Ahmed et al[55]	14	B	21	–
1984	Ahmed et al[51]	21	B CP MTX	21 25 61	–
2000	Cotsadze et al[11]	33	B, VB+B, CP+B, CP+VB+B	48.5	18.7
1994	Mitropoulos et al[53]	12	CP+Interferon	75	50

B, bleomycin; CP, cisplatin; MTX, methotrexate; VB, vinblastine.

Mitropoulos et al[53] treated 12 cases (stage T2/T3) with immunochemotherapy (cisplatin and interferon-alpha). They reported a 75% response rate (33% complete and 42% partial) with a 50% local recurrence in the complete response group. All recurrences were surgically salvaged with amputation. Other studies report complete response rates between 14 and 37.5% with multidrug chemotherapies for the treatment of locoregionally advanced penile carcinomas.

Immunotherapy

The reported use of immunomonotherapy in the context of penile carcinomas is limited to verrucous carcinomas (VC).[56] Verrucous carcinomas are histologically non-invasive (stage Ta), well-differentiated squamous cell carcinomas. They do not metastasize and have a good prognosis. They are therefore ideal for organ preserving therapies. Radiotherapy induced anaplastic transformation of VC has been reported and radiotherapy is best avoided.[57]

There are only two reports of interferon-alpha monotherapy for VC; they are both from the same institution and overlap.[56] The authors reported the successful use of subcutaneous interferon-alpha for three cases of VC in young individuals. They used doses of $3–6 \times 10^6$ IU daily or three times weekly to cumulative doses of 165, 249, 426×10^6 IU. They reported no significant systemic adverse reactions. One case was a patient with recurrent tumor after multiple local surgical excisions. He refused amputation and was rendered tumor free after 5 months of interferon treatment. He remained tumor free at 10 years of follow up. In the second case, interferon was used as a primary therapy in a patient also refusing amputation. He was tumor free after 3 months and he was reported tumor free at 7 years' follow up. The final case was one of multiple penoscrotal VC. He was tumor free after 1 year of treatment and remained free at a short follow up of 4 months. These are the only reports of interferon-alpha monotherapy for treating penile carcinomas.

In contrast to these very good results, a group from France reporting on the treatment of VC in other parts of the body, including a penile VC (cumulative dose 522 IU), concluded that interferon monotherapy can slow down the growth of tumors and can be used as an adjuvant therapy

to surgical excision. It never prevents surgery or death.[58]

Interferon-alpha in combination with cisplatin-based chemotherapy has been used for the primary treatment of invasive penile carcinomas. Mitropoulos et al[53] reported on the management of 13 histologically proven localized invasive penile carcinomas with immunochemotherapy. They evaluated the response of 12 cases: four (33%) responded completely and five (42%) responded partially (defined as reduction in the size of tumor by more than 50%). Out of the complete responders, two (50%) recurred locally after a short period of time and were salvaged by local laser excision and partial penectomy. The partial responders all underwent partial penectomy.

Conclusions

Definitive management of penile carcinomas is stage dependent. Penile amputation with its associated psychosexual and urinary morbidity would be considered as perhaps inappropriate overtreatment of low stage disease (Tis–T1). Penis preserving therapies offer superior cosmetic and functional outcome in such cases. Topical chemotherapy (5% 5-fluorouracil cream) should be the first line treatment for carcinoma in situ. Non-surgical therapies (radiotherapy, chemotherapy and immunotherapy) are associated with a high local recurrence rate and close follow up is necessary. Glansectomy can treat up to stage T2 disease and it appears to have a higher local control rate. Glans resurfacing with split skin grafting offers excellent cosmetic results. Long-term outcome results of glansectomy are however awaited.

References

1. Cancer trends in England and Wales, 1950–1999. http://www.statistics.gov.uk.
2. Cancer 1971–1997 [CD-ROM]. London: Office for National Statistics, 1999.
3. Burgess JK, Badalament RA, Drago JR. Penile carcinoma. Clinical presentation, diagnosis and staging. Urol Clin North Am 1992; 19:247–255.
4. Persky L. Epidemiology of carcinoma of penis. Recent Results Cancer Res 1977; 60:97.
5. Morgani GB. The seats and causes of disease. 1761:Book IV, letter L, article 50.
6. Lewis L. Young's radical operation for the cure of cancer of the penis: a report of 34 cases. J Urol 1931; 26:295.

7. Ekstron T, Edsmyr F. Cancer of the penis: 229 cases. Acta Chir Scand 1958; 115:25–45.

8. Horenblas S, Van Tinteren H, Delemarre JFM, et al. Squamous cell carcinomas of the penis. II. Treatment of the primary tumour. J Urol 1992; 147:1533–1538.

9. McDougal WS, Kirchner FK, Edward RH, Killian LT. Treatment of carcinoma of the penis: the case of primary lymphadenectomy. J Urol 1986; 136:38–41.

10. Opjordsmoen S, Fossa SD. Quality of life in patients treated for penile cancer. A follow-up study. Br J Urol 1994; 74(5):652–657.

11. Cotsadze D, Matveev B, Zak B, Mamaladze V. Is conservative organ-sparing treatment of penile carcinoma justified? Eur Urol 2000; 38:306–312.

12. Goette DK, Elgart M, DeVillez RL. Erythroplasia of Queyrat. Treatment with topically applied fluorouracil. JAMA 1975; 232(9):934–937.

13. Goette DK, Carson TE. Erythroplasia of Queyrat. Treatment with topical 5-fluorouracil. Cancer 1976; 38(4):1498–1502.

14. Hueser JN, Pugh RO. Erythroplasia of Queyrat: report of a patient successfully treated with topical 5-fluorouracil. Can Med Assoc J 1971; 104:148.

15. Malloy TR, Wein AJ, Carpiniello VL. Carcinoma of penis treated with Neodymium YAG laser. Urology 1988; 31(1):26–29.

16. Windahl T, Hellsten S. Laser treatment of localised squamous cell carcinoma of the penis. J Urol 1995; 154:1020–1023.

17. Tietjen DN, Malek RS. Laser therapy of squamous cell dysplasia and carcinoma of the penis. Urology 1998; 52:559–565.

18. Shirahama T, Takemoto M, Nishiyama K, et al. A new treatment for penile conservation in penile carcinoma: a preliminary study of combined laser hyperthermia, radiation and chemotherapy. Br J Urol 1998; 82:687–693.

19. Bandieramonte G, Lepera P, Marchesini R, et al. Laser microsurgery for superficial lesions of the penis. J Urol 1987; 138:315–319.

20. Bandieramonte G, Santoro O, Boracchi P, et al. Total resection of glans penis surface by CO_2 laser microsurgery. Acta Oncol 1988; 27(5):575–578.

21. McLean M, Ahmed M, Warde P, et al. The results of primary radiation therapy in the management of squamous cell carcinoma of the penis. Int J Radiat Oncol Biol Phys 1993; 25(4):623–628.

22. Dillaha CJ, Jansen GT, Honeycutt WM, Holt GA. Further studies with topical 5-fluorouracil. Arch Dermatol 1965; 92:410.

23. Bissada NK. Conservative extirpative treatment of cancer of the penis. Urol Clin North Am 1992; 19(2):283–290.

24. Das S. Penile amputations for the management of primary carcinoma of the penis. Urol Clin North Am 1992; 19(2):277–282.

25. Skinner DG, Leadbetter WF, Kelley SR. The surgical management of squamous cell carcinoma of the penis. J Urol 1972; 107:273.

26. Davis JW, Schellhammer PF, Schlossberg SM. Conservative surgical therapy for penile and urethral carcinoma. Urology 1999; 53:386–392.

27. Hatzichristou DG, Apostolidis A, Tzortzis V, et al. Glansectomy: an alternative surgical treatment for

28. Rothenberger KH, Hofstetter A. Laser therapy of penile carcinoma. Urologe A 1994; 33(4):291–294.

29. Hofstetter A, Frank F. The Nd:YAG laser in urology. Basel: Hoffman-LaRoche; 1980.

30. Kuroda M, Tsushima T, Nasu Y. Hyperthermotherapy added to the multidisciplinary therapy for penile cancer. Acta Med Okayama 1993; 47:169–174.

31. Obama T, Mitsuhata N, Yoshimoto J, et al. Combination therapy with continuous infusion of peplomycin, radiation and hyperthermia in advanced penile cancer: a case report. Nishinihon J Urol 1981; 43:769–774.

32. Mohs FE, Snow SN, Larson PO. Mohs micrographic surgery for penile tumours. Urol Clin North Am 1992; 19(2):291–304.

33. Vidaurre MI, Manrique HI, Jaka SJP, et al. Verrucous carcinoma of the penis: local excision with Mohs micrographic technique. Arch Esp Urol 1996; 49(9):959–964.

34. Harden SV, Tan LT. Treatment of localised carcinoma of the penis: A survey of current practice in the UK. Clin Oncol 2001; 13:284–288.

35. El-Demiry MIM, Oliver RTD, Hope-Stone HF, Blandy JP. Reappraisal of the role of radiotherapy and surgery in the management of carcinoma of the penis. Br J Urol 1984; 56:724–728.

36. Krieg RM, Luk KH. Carcinoma of the penis. Review of cases treated by surgery and radiation therapy 1960–1977. Urology 1981; 18(2):149–154.

37. Chaudhary AJ, Ghosh S, Bhalavat RL, et al. Interstitial brachytherapy in carcinoma of the penis. Strahlenther Onkol 1999; 175(1):17–20.

38. Ravi R, Chaturvedi HK, Sastry DVLN. Role of radiation therapy in the treatment of carcinoma of the penis. Br J Urol 1994; 74:646–651.

39. Koch MO, Smith JA Jr. Local recurrence of squamous cell carcinoma of the penis. Urol Clin North Am 1994; 21(4):739–743.

40. Gerbaulet A, Lambin P. Radiation therapy of cancer of the penis. Indications, advantages and pitfalls. Urol Clin North Am 1992; 19(2):325–332.

41. Delannes M, Malavaud B, Doucher J, et al. Iridium-192 interstitial therapy for squamous cell carcinoma of the penis. Int J Radiat Oncol Biol Phys 1992; 24:479–483.

42. Pizzocaro G, Piva L, Bandieramonte G, Tana S. Up-to-date management of carcinoma of the penis. Eur Urol 1997; 32:5–15.

43. Mazeron JJ, Langlois D, Lobo PA, et al. Interstitial radiation treatment for carcinoma of the penis using Iridium-192 wires: the Henri Mondor experience (1970–1979). Int J Radiat Oncol Biol Phys 1984; 10:1891–1895.

44. Neave F, Neal AJ, Hoskin PJ, et al. Carcinoma of the penis: a retrospective review of treatment with iridium mould and external beam irradiation. Clin Oncol 1993; 5:207–210.

45. Suchaud JP, Kantor G, Richaud P, et al. Curiethérapie des cancers de la verge: analyse d'une serie de 53 cas. J Urol (Paris) 1989; 95:27–31.

46. Shammas FV, Ous S, Fossa SD. Cisplatin and 5-fluorouracil in advanced cancer of the penis. J Urol 1992; 147(3):630–632.

Buschke–Lowenstein tumours of the penis. Urology 2001; 57:966–969.

47. Corral DA, Sella A, Pettaway CA, et al. Combination chemotherapy for metastatic or locally advanced genitourinary squamous cell carcinoma: a phase II study of methotrexate, cisplatin and bleomycin. J Urol 1998; 160(5):1770–1774.

48. Haas GP, Blumenstein BA, Gangliano RG, et al. Cisplatin, methotrexate and bleomycin for the treatment of carcinoma of the penis: a Southwest Oncology Group study. J Urol 1999; 161(6):1823–1825.

49. Roth AD, Berney CR, Rohner AS, et al. Intra-arterial chemotherapy in locally advanced or recurrent carcinomas of the penis and anal canal: an active treatment modality with curative potential. Br J Cancer 2000; 83(12):1637–1642.

50. Kattan J, Culine S, Droz JP, et al. Penile cancer chemotherapy: twelve years' experience at Institut Gustave-Roussy. Urology 1993; 42(5):559–562.

51. Ahmed T, Sklaroff R, Yagoda A. Sequential trials of methotrexate, cisplatin and bleomycin for penile cancer. J Urol 1984; 132(3):465–468.

52. Bandieramonte G, Lepera P, Mogha D, et al. Neoadjuvant chemotherapy and conservative surgery for exophytic T1N0 carcinoma of the penis. Fourth International Congress on Anticancer Chemotherapy, Paris. 1993:Abstract 178.

53. Mitropoulos D, Dimopoulos MA, Kiroudi-Voulgari A, et al. Neoadjuvant cisplatin and interferon-alpha 2B in the treatment and organ preservation of penile carcinomas. J Urol 1994; 152(4):1124–1126.

54. Sklaroff RB, Yagoda A. Methotrexate in the treatment of penile carcinoma. Cancer 1980; 45(2):214–216.

55. Ahmed T, Sklaroff R, Yagoda A. An appraisal of the efficacy of bleomycin in epidermoid carcinoma of the penis. Anticancer Res 1984; 4(4–5):289–292.

56. Maiche AG, Pyrhonen S. Verrucous carcinoma of the penis: three cases treated with interferon-alpha. Br J Urol 1997; 79:481–483.

57. Fukunaga M, Yokoi K, Miyazawa Y, et al. Penile verrucous carcinoma with anaplastic transformation following radiotherapy. A case report with human papilloma virus typing and flow cytometric DNA studies. Am J Surg Pathol 1994; 18(5):501–505.

58. Risse L, Negrier P, Dang PM, et al. Treatment of verrucous carcinoma with recombinant alpha-interferon. Dermatology 1995; 190(2):142–144.

21

Reducing medical errors in urology

*Jonathan P Coxon, Sophie H Pattison
and Peter K Stevenson*

Introduction

There can be little doubt that urologists, like all health care professionals, are facing increased pressure from various groups to respond to the issue of medical error. Politicians, the media, patients and fellow health care workers are amongst those who are providing this increased scrutiny. Recent work highlighting the prevalence of adverse events in health care, along with increasing coverage of high profile cases, has provided the ethical and financial impetus for action to be taken to address this sizeable problem. In this chapter we give a brief summary of some of this background before introducing some novel practical approaches that can we can all use to combat the danger of introducing error into our work.

Background

That it is possible to suffer undesirable outcomes from medical management has of course long been recognized, and been described with phrases such as 'iatrogenic injury'. However, there has previously been a greater tendency to leave the description of such events at that, and not to explore their root causes and examine to what extent they may be thought of as *preventable*. There is of course a natural reluctance to admit to our potential human errors or failures in our systems, which must partly account for previous inadequate appreciation of this problem. As discussions of our medical management and patient interaction continue to become more open, so discussions of our mismanagement should continue to do likewise. The hope of course is that lessons can be learnt and, exemplifying the clinical governance concept, changes implemented.

The growing interest in patient safety issues has been developing for several years. A major early contribution came from the Harvard Medical Practice Study, published in 1991.[1,2] The authors appreciated that despite escalating malpractice claims, little accurate information was available regarding the incidence of adverse events. To address this, they looked retrospectively at over 30 000 medical records, from 1984. Their definition of an adverse event was quite strict, namely an injury that was due to medical management and which led to prolonged hospitalization, disability at discharge, or death. They reported an adverse event rate of 3.7% of hospitalizations, with 0.5% of patients dying at least partly as a result. These findings were shocking to many at the time, and considerable debate ensued. They did not, however, attract as much media attention as might have been expected.

Other studies were published in the following years, a notable one being the Quality in Australian Health Care Study.[3] This included more minor events, and also those where other variables had meant an error in management had not progressed to an adverse consequence (a so-called *near miss*). This study reported an adverse event rate of 16.6%, half being considered preventable. A higher death rate, 1 in 123 cases, was also found. No large scale studies have been performed in the UK, but Vincent et al[4] carried out a pilot study which reported an adverse incident rate of 10.8%, at a cost of an average of 8.5 additional bed days per event.

These and other studies give an idea of the serious magnitude of this problem. Together with the increased media attention that inevitably transpired, fuelled further still by other high profile medical error cases such as the wrong-sided nephrectomy in Wales in 2000,[5] they served to demand a response.

In July 2000, the UK Department of Health published a document *The NHS – An Organisa-*

tion With a Memory.[6] It was so named as it took note of numerous examples where the NHS had not learnt lessons from previous mistakes, and took steps to address how this could be resolved. To provide an illustration, the Chief Medical Officer quoted the fatal errors of intrathecal vincristine injections which had occurred twelve times over the previous 15 years. Unfortunately, Wayne Jowett was to suffer this same fatal outcome just 6 months later. This naturally increased pressure further still.

It had become clear that it was necessary to examine errors thoroughly and work out why they were happening. It was appreciated that errors rarely have much intention behind them, but are still made, a key message of the patient safety ethos. This is a problem that various other high risk industries have been facing up to for considerably longer than the NHS, in an attempt to reduce errors in realms where they can have obvious disastrous consequences. Considerable work has been focused on 'human factors' (HF) training, namely psychologically based examination of how workers interact with each other and the systems in which they work. It was appreciated that much of the thinking behind causation of accidents, and actions taken to remedy these, could be transferred over from work in these industries to the high risk environment of health care.[7] We can draw particular experience from HF training in aviation. In this industry, there is an obvious huge incentive not to make the costliest of errors. Aviation is renowned as a good model for safety following investment of considerable time and money in understanding and reducing errors.[8]

It was thus with the help of a commercial pilot and Chief Instructor in Human Factors Training, working with a consultant urologist, that a Patient Safety Training course was devised. This course looks to adapt the concepts successfully put to use in aviation safety training, applying them to the field of health care. The course aims to predict, recognize, manage, follow up and prevent errors. Some of the key points are described here.

Risk-conscious culture

Of vital importance is to instill a risk-conscious culture into our working practice. As suggested above, little progress can be made without bringing appreciation and discussion of medical error much more to the fore. We must encourage ourselves to accept that errors are commonplace, and are unlikely ever to be eliminated – that 'to err is human'. Our realistic goal cannot be to entirely eradicate all adverse incidents in urology, but rather to introduce ourselves to alternative methods of examining and responding to them.

Within this culture, a central concept is to move away from an environment where it is felt the priority is to find the culpable individual, to 'point the finger'. Rather, once the universality of error is accepted, we should focus instead on the learning potential that analyzing it can bring, and how this is likely to provide an emotionally positive result, rather than the negative one which might otherwise be feared. The aim is to move away from the 'blame culture', seeking out these alternative goals instead.

Error chains and root cause analysis

It is crucial then to shift beliefs away from the view that accidents are attributable to a single error by a single person, and that when there are especially disastrous consequences this must be due to a particularly terrible blunder. The aim is to abandon this 'person approach' in favor of a more holistic 'systems approach'. The key concept is that accidents almost always represent the end result of a series of faults and errors involving several workers. These make up the 'error chain'. It is appreciated in HF science that there are many common themes running through varying error chains, which explains the benefits to be enjoyed by employing this concept in different industries. Of all the aspects outlined in this chapter, this has probably been discussed most widely in the medical literature[7,9–11] and is briefly summarized here.

A simple diagrammatic representation of an error chain is illustrated in Figure 21.1. The term 'error chain' is really a misnomer, which has stuck. Firstly, it can be seen that not all the contributing factors should be thought of as distinct 'errors' made by those working in a system. Secondly, 'chain' might imply a linear progression of events, but it is much more common for a number of interacting strands, separate in time and space, to come together towards a final outcome. Alternatives such as 'accident fault tree' have thus been suggested.

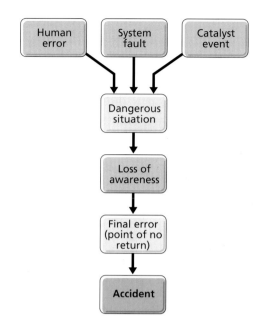

Figure 21.1 A schematic representation of the anatomy of an error chain, based partly on work by Reason.[7,9]

Table 21.1 Examples of human errors (active failures)

Miscommunication
Picking up wrong item
Failing to carry out a check
Not seeking clarification of instruction
Forgetting to carry out a procedure
Consciously deciding to depart from protocol

Table 21.2 Examples of system faults (latent failures)

Staff/bed shortages
Unreliable equipment
Poor protocols
Similar drug names/packaging
Inadequate communication systems
Overworked staff

In any case, a vital concept to convey is that the accident process tends to begin with *latent* system failures – faults which pre-exist in the system, waiting to interact with ongoing events and potentially cause sufficient disruption to allow events to progress with adverse consequences. Operators within this system provide the active human errors made nearer the time of the accident, and there often also tends to be a contribution from so-called *catalyst events*, which are essentially outside the control of the system or its operators.

The dangerous situation is thus created. If operators are not aware of this, then it may be allowed to progress towards an irreversible accident.

Human errors

While human errors will almost always play some part in an error chain, it is emphasized that these errors, or active failures, made at the 'sharp end' of the system, are often not of a catastrophic nature as is commonly misconceived. They are actually often rather mundane, as illustrated in Table 21.1. It is the close-knit combination with other interacting factors that creates the adverse consequences. Dyer[12] (and personal communication) outlines as an example the error chain leading to

the wrong kidney being removed in the case mentioned earlier which began simply with a senior house officer (SHO) writing 'left' instead of 'right' on an admission card.

System failures

These are the pathogens lurking in the system, or 'accidents waiting to happen'. They can effectively lead the unwary into the trap of contributing to a major accident (Table 21.2). These error-inducing conditions usually find their origins in decisions or oversights from higher levels of management. Such failures may lie dormant in an ongoing system for many years, waiting to interact with a particular combination of accompanying events to help trigger an error chain. Tragically, in the analysis of many disasters, it is discovered that workers in the field knew of these system faults but insufficient action had been taken to rectify them. The onus is clearly on us to actively seek out and eliminate these faults in our working environments before they have chance to slot into an evolving error chain.

Catalyst events

These events, beyond workers' control, may involve such phenomena as coincidences or enforced changes of plan. They are unfortunate occurrences that would have been difficult to predict and take account for in advance. Similarly, one can think of an unlikely convergence of a number of variably related problems at the same time as a catalyst event, as they happen to come together powerfully to help create an unsafe situation.

Such events may provide the impetus required to energize an error chain to which operator errors and system failures have already contributed. Examples are listed in Table 21.3.

If the creation of an unsafe situation is accompanied by 'loss of awareness' of the situation on the part of the workers involved, the danger is that this false mindset takes control and makes us blind to ensuing error. At this stage, there is often a more rapid progression of a small number of errors towards a point of no return and the resultant accident.

Analyzing error chains in this way, digging out the causes at the roots of an incident, is termed *root cause analysis*. The emphasis here is always on finding contributing causes behind any human failures, to try to understand how a worker was presented with the opportunity to make whichever error was made. Judgmental descriptions (e.g. 'poorly', 'unwisely', etc.) are avoided in the analysis, concentrating instead on a purely factual presentation of events, focusing on establishing clear cause and effect relationships.

With this approach, it is hoped that changes can be made to a system (including training of those behind human errors) that would reduce the opportunity for error in the future.

Red flags

These represent a concept largely new to most health care workers, taken directly from the aviation industry. They are essentially warning signs,

metaphorical flags to wave when there is increased *potential* that workers may be in an evolving error chain. There is an important distinction between these and the actual components of an error chain, as outlined above. Red flags are often subtle symptoms and signs, picked up in the way workers are behaving, thinking or interacting as a team.

Their origins can be traced back to analysis of cockpit voice recordings, or 'black boxes'. This revealed a number of recurrent and similar examples of certain patterns of dialogue or evidence of altered teamwork. It was realized, with the luxury of retrospect, that these could have been interpreted as clues that things were amiss, but they had not been acknowledged as such. It is often difficult for us to appreciate we are in an insidious error chain, instead only noticing a variety of seemingly unrelated trivial distractions or irritations. It is hoped that raising awareness of the potential importance of such nuances and discussing how best to respond to them may allow some error chains to be halted before they reach undesirable outcomes.

It is accepted that not all error chains will present any red flags to pick up on, and that sometimes they may appear after it is too late for any successful preventative intervention. However, with these exceptions borne in mind, red flags are presented as potentially invaluable in certain scenarios.

Table 21.4 outlines twelve examples of red flags. It can be seen from this list that some of these 'flags' may well relate to the same underlying

Table 21.3 Examples of catalyst events

| Coincidental similar appearance/name |
| Unusual anatomy |
| Interrupted sentence |
| Very rare medical condition |
| Convergence of numerous events at same time |
| Enforced change of plan |

Table 21.4 Twelve red flags

1.	Deviation/sudden changes of plan
2.	Missing steps/information
3.	Unusual responses/ambiguities
4.	Fixation
5.	Confusion
6.	Unease/fear
7.	Denial/inaction
8.	Fatigue
9.	Broken communications
10.	Juniors cut short
11.	Hardware alarms
12.	Time distortion/event runaway

phenomenon, but which can present itself or be sensed in different ways. Rather than go through all the suggested red flags in detail, we shall expand on three of them to exemplify their potential use:

Red flag: 'Broken communications'

These may take the form of unfinished sentences, such as: *'I think we should…'; 'Perhaps if we gave him some…'.*

It is important to register such instances, and at least contemplate and then confront the potential reasons that they were not completed. These include:

- Unforeseen or ambiguous events may have arisen which interrupt or distract the speaker. These may need addressing, but attention should also be directed to the speaker's concerns.
- The speaker may not wish to 'cause a scene'.
- The speaker may simply not be able to formulate a statement that makes sense. They may have a genuine concern that they cannot communicate, or simply are unsure of the details.
- They may not wish to dwell on the subject to which they are alluding and any resultant potentially unpleasant repercussions.

In all, efforts should be made to encourage the completion of the unfinished communication, which may or may not reveal danger of error.

Red flag: 'Unease/fear'

This may present in an especially subtle way, but may underlie a crucial warning that workers could be entering a dangerous situation. We make the comparison between how our response to a patient with an obvious clinical sign such as cyanosis has become engrained in us through our training, while little attention is usually paid to teaching us how to spot unease in our coworkers and how we should respond to this. It is vital that the cause for this unease is explored and either resolved as non-consequential, or acted upon if appropriate. We must become more prepared to accept that our colleagues may be interpreting a situation in a different way from ourselves, and must deal with this before we can progress effectively as a team. Responses under this heading may be characterized by thoughts such as: *'The staff nurse sounds nervous'; 'My SHO is sweating and seems to want to interrupt'.*

Red flag: 'Denial/inaction'

It is remarkably common to find evidence of denial when analyzing an error chain retrospectively. It can be attributed to one of two major causes:

1. It can be thought of as expression of the 'flight' component of the natural autonomic response. While we do not usually physically flee a stressful situation, which may be leading towards a possible accident, we may have a tendency to do this mentally by denying any problem.
2. Certain individuals may find themselves in denial as an expression of reluctance to accept implied criticism of their management of a situation, with obvious resultant potential cause for error.

Responding to red flags

First, it is important to appreciate that we should be watchful for red flags both in ourselves and in those working with us. It can be especially difficult to fully acknowledge these various sensations and behaviors within oneself. It can take considerable conscious effort to register them and take active measures to explore them.

Ideally we should be constantly vigilant for error, but this is probably not practical. The value of red flags is that each one that is observed can serve as a cue to step up our vigilance for possible error, thus leading to safer practice.

One can debate how many red flags one should observe before making some active response to address them. It can probably be appreciated that some of those we have suggested may present not uncommonly, perhaps in isolation. Therefore, commenting on every appearance of a red flag may sometimes occur so frequently as to be counterproductive. But as more are noted, so the risk of danger is heightened. From the aviation experience, analysis of various accidents has revealed an average of between four and six red flags having presented themselves at some stage. Importantly though, various workers will often notice some but not all. By speaking up and communicating these observations effectively, information is efficiently distributed amongst the team, who collectively may then become aware of several warning signs. This is an illustration of *synergy*, whereby the total knowledge acquired by a team is greater than each member's individual contribution. A priority in responding to red flags then is voicing concerns effectively, and this is discussed below.

When focusing on how to tackle these warnings, one should try as much as possible to calmly stand back from a situation and reassess it as completely as possible. We describe a parallel from aviation, involving a pilot pulling up to a safe altitude, before recommencing a landing procedure which had produced some red flags. There is often ample opportunity early on in an error chain to halt events in good time and avoid an accident, by effectively taking stock of a situation and carrying out appropriate corrective actions.

As soon as red flags have been highlighted, whether or not an error then ensues, action should be initiated as soon as possible to lessen the likelihood of such a situation recurring. Measures to be taken would include early communication with as many health care workers as may be appropriate as well as with patients and relatives. This should include an accurate handover of all relevant events and meticulous note-keeping.

The value of a good *debriefing* following any accident or near miss cannot be overemphasized. Debriefing is best done as early as possible, while a good deal of the relevant personnel can be brought together and events are still fresh in the mind. One of its primary aims should be to divert thoughts from any focus on blame and concentrate rather on lessening any distress incurred as a result of the incident, as well as highlighting the lessons that can be learnt and any changes to practice that might be recommended as a result.

Debriefing tends to be much appreciated by those undergoing it, and we suggest it should be done a good deal more than it is at present. We propose that it need not just be done when things have gone wrong, but can also be used to give purely positive feedback, thus reinforcing good practice.

A good debriefing along with accurate event reporting and subsequent root cause analysis will be hugely beneficial in achieving effective follow up for any incident.

Speaking up (effectively)

Through a working knowledge of error chains and red flags, it is hoped that we will become more alert to errors. This will only be useful if we are able to express these concerns effectively, or be open to concerns expressed by others. There are many examples of major disasters where 'subordinates' were aware of evolving error chains and gave a precise warning but received an inadequate response from a team leader. In the case of the wrong-sided nephrectomy in Wales in 2000, the investigators heard how a medical student expressed her concern that the wrong kidney was being removed, but it seems that this warning was not heeded.[12]

We stress that drawing attention to unsafe or inappropriate patient care is not an optional extra for all of us working in health care, but that we are duty bound to bring such circumstances to the attention of those in a position to act upon them. For example, this is outlined in clauses 11–13 of the Code of Conduct of the UKCC[13] (now the Nursing and Midwifery Council).

To help juniors during a potentially stressful occasion where they feel there is a need to speak up, we argue that being aware of a framework may be very useful.

Again we draw directly on experience from aviation, where just such a framework exists and is well known by all those working in the field. This is the PACE approach, incorporating four levels of intervention strategies: *P*robe, *A*lert, *C*hallenge, *E*mergency. These are arranged so as to minimize potential areas of conflict through a diplomatic strategy, creating potential for educational opportunity along the way, but allowing for step-wise persistence that concerns are effectively communicated.

Level 1: Probing

Initially of course we must be aware that, especially if more junior, our interpretation of a situation as potentially dangerous may well be faulty. However, we cannot work effectively as a team while this thought lingers, so it must still be addressed. By probing for answers to a query, we may satisfy ourselves that the situation is in fact safe, and may well have enjoyed a valuable educational experience without creating a potentially awkward scene. Open questions are often very useful, forcing the responder to actively process a more considered reply. Useful phrases may include: '*Can I just check...*'; '*Could you tell me why...*'; '*Could you confirm for me that...*'. In the majority of cases, this will be sufficient to trigger appropriate responses from the team, and ensure any required actions are employed. Should we feel that there are issues that remain to be resolved, we would consider stepping up to the next level.

Level 2: Alerting

Now the aim is to directly alert our colleagues to the fact that we still have a particular concern, and that we are not satisfied it has been dealt with adequately. In this and the next two levels, airline staff are even trained to use and recognize specific phrases that serve as markers for having reached a particular level of this hierarchy. Here, for example, one would state: '*I am not happy...*'. One would then go on to specifically outline the concern that prompted this statement.

Level 3: Challenging

If there was still an inadequate response, and it is suggested that this would be unusual, our priority is now to leave the team leader with little doubt that we believe we are in an unsafe situation, and to challenge him or her to make a change of plan. As we ascend each level, it is of course useful to try to adopt an increasingly assertive tone. The chosen recognized phrase in aviation here is simply: '*You must listen...*'. Such a statement can have a powerful effect, and should help make progression to the final level very rare indeed.

Level 4: Emergency

At this stage, the team member is effectively declaring an emergency, and that further progression along a likely error chain must be halted at all costs: '*We must stop...*'.

The aviation industry has found these tactics extremely useful in approaching this naturally difficult scenario, and we suggest that they are easily transferable to our own practice.

Situational awareness

The principal aim here is to demonstrate how perception of ongoing events may often not be as accurate as we would wish, leaving obvious opportunity for error. This concept is crucial to considerations of human error. It is common for those caught up in an evolving error chain to be totally convinced that what they are doing is right, and they will be aware of no reason to suspect they may have incorrectly interpreted the details of a particular situation. It is this loss of awareness that allows an error chain to be perpetuated.

In the dynamic working environment, an operator has to make numerous decisions; to make these safely the operator should acquire and maintain high situational awareness. This relies on three essential components:

1. Having access to all relevant data, through the senses.
2. Processing this data into an accurate mental model.
3. Updating the model as the situation changes.

Thus faults in any of these stages can cause the operator to lose awareness.

A 'mental model' refers to the framework within which an individual makes sense of a situation – the broad interpretation of what is perceived. There are more obvious variables which can mean that someone is not able to gain access to all the required data. For example, problems such as visibility, noise, personal sensory deficits and distraction would all serve to impede accurate delivery of relevant details. Similarly, we must appreciate that the system we work in may not be designed in such a way as to present data to us in an optimal fashion. It follows that we may suffer difficulties in extracting required information. Time constraints in stressful scenarios may compound these problems.

More subtle forces account for faults in processing of data. To provide an early illustration, we ask people to count the number of times the letter 'F' appears in the following text (for those who have not seen this before, try to cover up the answer below!):

FINISHED FILES ARE THE RESULTS OF YEARS OF SCIENTIFIC STUDY COMBINED WITH THE EXPERIENCE OF YEARS

In general, about two-thirds of people fail to get the correct answer, when allowed to look at this for about 1 minute. Some will see the true number (six) straightaway. From this, we raise the following points:

- Even an apparently simple task can be poorly executed as the brain scans quickly for an answer.

- We might be quite confident that we are enjoying high situational awareness and be blissfully unaware that we are wrong.
- It is difficult to check our own work. Those who see less than six (often seeing only three) can look back at this for a considerable amount of time without being able to find the others.
- Efficient communication raises the team's awareness to greater than some individuals'. Those who could see all six could help raise others' awareness by sharing this information. This is another example of *synergy*.

Patterns of loss of situational awareness

It is interesting to consider three broad ways that situational awareness may be lost, allowing an error chain to be perpetuated:

1. *Convincing* error chain: Here workers believe they are in control of a situation and have interpreted all its components accurately, but in fact are unaware of danger that is developing. A simple medical example would be making an incorrect diagnosis.
2. *Confusing* error chain: In this case, workers may be faced with a series of apparently contradictory indications, and are thereby unable to form a working mental model within which to operate. They may thus become incapacitated to work safely, as they are absorbed by efforts to make sense out of non-sense. Medically, we could equate this to being unable to make a diagnosis.
3. *Fixating* error chain: This issue was alluded to in discussion on red flags. Here, one aspect of a situation assumes inappropriately high importance in the mind of an individual, who exposes himself to being unaware of potentially dangerous events occurring around him. In our profession, we could think of a scenario where we make a correct initial diagnosis but fail to notice another condition that has arisen.

One of the strongest influences on our formation of mental models is our *expectation*. What we are expecting to perceive has a natural tendency to potentially alter how we process information. Partly relying on expectation is usually an extremely efficient and sensible way for the brain to operate, having to make sense as it does from the torrent of data to which it is exposed and by which it could otherwise be overwhelmed.

To effectively take 'short cuts', the brain fills in a large amount of detail in our perception, based partly on what we are expecting, from memory. This memory may be very new, or old. So we form our mental model and this framework influences how we interpret further data. We need then only handle the much smaller amount of data needed to update this overall impression. We are always scanning our surroundings, rapidly seeking out details which, based on our knowledge and experience, we may expect to have changed. The price paid for this efficient approach is introducing the possibility of bias or distortion in our perception.

Change blindness

A number of serious accidents in high risk areas can be attributed to perception errors. With retrospect, investigators may wonder how workers seemed, for example, to have missed large changes apparently occurring right before their eyes. The important difference is that such occurrences would be much more obvious to those *expecting* them to happen. Without this expectation, we are naturally more prone to miss vital changes and thus be 'blind' to a dangerous situation. This tendency is termed *change blindness*.

There are a number of other dangers with the inherent mechanism of forming mental models which create the potential for arriving at false models which may be difficult to dislodge. These include 'primacy effect', 'confirmation bias', 'assumed connection' and 'environmental capture'.

- *Primacy effect*: This describes a tendency we have to favor our first hypothesis, and stand by it, potentially being resistant to other possible interpretations of a situation. This would seem to be mainly a consequence of mental modeling. Once we have formed the model, we will initially assimilate further data with respect to this framework of ideas, and so it is easier to process those data which neatly fit within it.
- *Confirmation bias*: This related phenomenon more directly describes how we seek indications that uphold our theory (often the initial one). We are biased towards evidence confirming our impression, interpret essentially neutral evidence as supporting it, and even subconsciously

reject that which contradicts it. In a medical setting, primacy effect and confirmation bias are probably most simply illustrated by the tendency we may have to stick with our initial diagnosis of a patient's condition, and confirm this with evidence that does not necessarily completely prove it.

- *Assumed connection*: Again this relates to how we like to form one mental model, making it easier to manage a great deal of information at once. By trying to fit details into one mental model, we may assume certain details are connected in some way, when they may be quite independent. We re-emphasize that this discussion only relates to tendencies, which will be stronger in some situations than in others. Assumed connection could be illustrated by a presumption that a patient's rapid deterioration after administering certain medication is related to that drug's effects, when these events may be coincidental.

- *Environmental capture*: This refers to the potential for losing awareness by being carried along by familiar cues in our immediate environment, which can prompt rather automatic, sub-conscious responses. Most of us can relate to setting off to drive a familiar route with the intention of stopping off somewhere, and then finding ourselves at the final destination, not completely recalling how we got there and quite forgetting to make any stops along the way! It is not difficult to see how this type of phenomenon can lead to the potential for error in the workplace, when rather more may be at stake. This could involve an operation with which we have become extremely familiar, and so perhaps unwittingly complacent.

Engendering an appreciation of these in-built difficulties in maintaining high situational awareness is half the battle won; it follows that we should be seeking out ways of actively counteracting them. We suggest some mechanisms which may be employed to meet this aim, as outlined below:

1. Expect errors. Give at least some consideration to the 'worse case scenario'.
2. Use a form of *briefing* to ensure that as many people have access to as many facts as possible from the outset. This is the earliest opportunity to raise situational awareness.
3. Regularly encourage measures to break our concentration on particular aspects and take account of the wider picture.
4. Look for and *respond to* red flags.
5. Employ 'focused vigilance' in areas where we believe consequential errors are most likely.
6. Communicate our thoughts, distributing them amongst the team. This collective process will raise overall awareness and allow discussion of any inconsistencies which should be addressed.
7. It may be appropriate to delegate more tasks to others in time of crisis. This prevents us becoming overloaded with thoughts and procedures, which would hinder accurate mental modeling.
8. Reiterating familiar advice, we must discipline ourselves in getting *back to the basics*, which can be forgotten as we are carried along with the intricacies of a developing error chain.

Communication issues

It is appreciated that many of us will have been given advice on various communication issues in the past, but our aim here is to emphasize specific aspects that we can focus on in the context of patient safety.

Communication is one of the very core concepts of any realistic approach to this field. We suggest it is not far from a universal truth to state that *every* human error accident will involve some form of communication failure.

Some of the time the breakdown may stem from someone withholding some information. This is partly addressed in the section on 'Speaking up' above. On other occasions it may be that communication is attempted but not completed successfully. It is of course far more common that errors of omission are implicated than there having been an excess of information communicated. Alternatively, sufficient information may have been contained in a message, but this was not processed efficiently.

We encourage an understanding that the communication process represents more than just the sending and receiving of a message. We maintain instead that it is a multistage process, with each stage representing a potential source of error. It is important to emphasize that these stages are to be found not just in the way the message is sent, but also in how it is received.

Problems in sending

1. The person sending the message should be looking to address the correct *need* in the first instance. Failing to do so may result from a situational awareness problem.

2. We need to carefully choose the *format* of a message, namely how it is to be sent. We may for example, choose an inappropriate medium for conveying the message or, in verbal communication, send it with misleading body language or tone of voice.

3. We *encode* the message, choosing the exact words to use. There are a host of potential errors here, important ones being the use of ambiguous pronouns (he, she, it, them, etc. which of course can be interpreted as applying to the wrong subject) or unnecessary jargon.

4. Errors can appear in actual *transmission* of the message. For example a simple 'slip of the tongue', missing out a word or even a letter, can ascribe a whole new meaning to a communication. In addition, problems with accents should not be ignored.

Problems in receiving

The first stage here is *detecting* the message. This can be affected by 'noise' of any kind, which corrupts the message after it has been transmitted. As a result, for example, missing information may never be acquired, and indeed a receiver may 'fill in' any resultant gaps, according to anticipation.

Subsequent stages include *decoding* (assigning meaning to detected words) and *comprehending* (understanding the entire concepts and implications of the message). Expectation of a message's content may still adversely influence communication in these stages. If attention wanders, we may begin to anticipate what is being communicated to us, as our brains 'race ahead', with obvious possible error-inducing implications.

Solutions to communication problems

One of the concepts on the course that we believe is most vital is that of '*readback*'. Readback represents virtually the last line of defense in the communication process. Quite simply, it involves reading back a summary of that message which has been given, highlighting the crucial components within it, thus quickly demonstrating that the message has been conveyed safely. This may often seem more difficult to do when time is short, but it is precisely then that readback can be most valuable. It is easy to see in so many accidents how an accurate readback, which would have clearly revealed a miscommunication, could have instantly prevented progression. For those who think it could be unusual introducing this to standard practice, we remind them how universally it is used with more mundane tasks such as telephone banking and even ordering a pizza!

Other suggested solutions to communication problems are largely direct and logical responses to the problems outlined above. For example the danger of a receiver predicting or not expecting a certain part of a message can partly be addressed by emphasizing more important information first, while the receiver's attention is high, and by making efforts to focus attention with well-chosen phrases. These might include: 'This isn't what you might expect, but…', 'This is a change of plan…'.

Thus by making small changes both in the way messages are sent and received, extra safety barriers are employed which can help to avert communication failures.

Other aspects of patient safety

Other important issues to consider would include adverse incident reporting and litigation. While these are vital to any consideration of patient safety, our approach to these is perhaps not as novel as other parts of this discussion, and so is expanded little here. Essentially, every effort should be made to encourage more incident reporting, ensuring we all know its process, and are aware of the considerable benefits. Good reporting provides the information which can be used to analyze incidents in the way we have discussed. A move towards collecting incident reports on a national basis, exemplified by the National Patient Safety Agency in the UK, reflects this emphasis.[14]

With regard to litigation, most urologists are well briefed in this matter, and we prefer to emphasize an approach that focuses primarily on patient safety, which should have the direct consequence of lessening litigation risk.

To make our patients safer, and our work less likely to attract lawyers and adverse publicity, we must appreciate the value of arming ourselves with defenses such as error awareness, effective teamwork and efficient communication. These are goals we must seek to focus on, perhaps through specific courses such as Patient Safety Training, to complement our ongoing specialized training.

References

1. Brennan TA, Leape LL, Laird NM, et al. Incidence of adverse events and negligence in hospitalized patients. Results of the Harvard Medical Practice Study I. NEJM 1991; 324:370–376.

2. Leape LL, Brennan TA, Laird N, et al. The nature of adverse events in hospitalized patients. Results of the Harvard Medical Practice Study I. NEJM 1991; 324:377–384.

3. Wilson RM, Runciman WB, Gibberd RW, et al. The quality in Australian health care study. Med J Aust 1995; 163:458–471.

4. Vincent C, Neale G, Woloshynowych M. Adverse events in British hospitals: preliminary retrospective record review. BMJ 2001; 322:517–519.

5. Dyer C. Surgeons cleared of manslaughter after removing wrong kidney. BMJ 2002; 325:9.

6. Department of Health. The NHS – an organisation with a memory: report of an expert group on learning from adverse events in the NHS. London: DoH, 2000.

7. Reason J. Understanding adverse events: human factors. Qual Health Care 1995; 4:80–89.

8. Helmreich RL. On error management: lessons from aviation. BMJ 2000; 320:781–785.

9. Reason J. Human error. New York: Cambridge University Press, 1990.

10. Vincent CA, Taylor-Adams S, Stanhope N. Framework for analysing risk and safety in clinical medicine. BMJ 1998; 316:1154–1157.

11. Stanhope N, Vincent CA, Adams S, et al. Applying human factors methods to clinical risk management in obstetrics. Br J Obstet Gynaecol 1997; 104:1225–1232.

12. Dyer C. Doctors go on trial for manslaughter after removing wrong kidney. BMJ 2002; 324:1476.

13. Knape J. Just do it. Nursing Times 2001; 97(45):24.

14. Mayor S. NHS introduces new patient safety agency. BMJ 2001; 322:1013.

Index

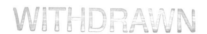